W9-AGI-102

C'EST À TOI!

Level One

Authors

Karla Winther Fawbush

Toni Theisen

Dianne B. Hopen

Linda Klohs

Contributing Writers

Sarah Vaillancourt

Christine Gensmer

EMC/Paradigm Publishing, Saint Paul, Minnesota

Credits

Editor
Sarah Vaillancourt

Associate Editor
Christine Gensmer

Assistant Editors
Tim Fulford
Diana Moen

Language Specialist
Sandrine Noyelle

Desktop Production Specialist
Bradley J. Olsen

Design
The Nancekivell Group

Illustrator
Hetty Mitchell

Cartoon Illustrator
Steve Mark

Consultants

Augusta DeSimone Clark
St. Mary's Hall
San Antonio, Texas

Michael Nettleton
Smoky Hill High School
Aurora, Colorado

Mirta Pagnucci
Oak Park River Forest High School
Oak Park, Illinois

Ann J. Sorrell
South Burlington High School
South Burlington, Vermont

Nathalie Gaillot
Language Specialist
Lyon, France

ISBN 0-8219-1422-7

Published by EMC/Paradigm Publishing
875 Montreal Way
St. Paul, Minnesota 55102

Printed in the United States of America
2 3 4 5 6 7 8 9 10 XXX 03 02 01 00 99 98

To the Student

C'EST À TOI! (*It's Your Turn!*), as your book's title suggests, invites *you* to express yourself in French by interacting with your classmates. Either in pairs or in small groups, you'll be talking right away about subjects that interest both you and French-speaking teens: music, sports, leisure activities, food, etc. Don't hesitate to practice your French every chance you get both during and outside of class. You will make mistakes, but your ability to speak French and your confidence will improve with continued practice.

Bienvenue au monde francophone! (*Welcome to the French-speaking world!*) You are beginning an exciting journey of discovery. You will not only visit many of the countries where people speak French every day, but you will also learn how to communicate and interact with them. In addition, as you are exposed to new ways of thinking and living in other cultures, your horizons will widen to include different ways of seeing and evaluating the world around you. Learning how to speak French will not only open the door to the French-speaking world, it will give you a knowledge, insight and appreciation of French culture. Language and culture go hand in hand, and together they reflect the spirit of the francophone world. An appreciation of French culture helps you understand what we have in common with French speakers and how we differ. And learning about an important world culture and its language will help you appreciate your own culture and language even more.

People speak French well beyond the borders of France itself. Nearly 200 million people worldwide use French in their daily lives. On our continent, French speakers live in places like Louisiana, New England and Quebec. Besides in Europe, people also speak French in Africa and Asia, as well as in the Caribbean. Obviously, these diverse French speakers come from a wide variety of cultural backgrounds. Communicating with them will help you understand their way of life and give you a more global perspective. During your lifetime, you will hopefully be able to use your French as you visit at least one of these lands. But even if your travels abroad are limited to "living the language" in your classroom, you will be exposed to a new way of viewing the world.

Internationally, French is one of the primary languages, and people who speak and understand it are an asset in the world of work. Knowing French can expand your career options in areas such as international trade or law, investment, government service, technology and manufacturing. Multinational companies hire hundreds of thousands of Americans who have proficiency in at least one world language. Just knowing French will not assure you of the job you want, but, combined with another specialization, it will increase your employment opportunities. French may be the key that gives you the competitive edge in the global marketplace. Whatever your reasons for learning French, **bon voyage** as you begin to discover the culture and language of the French-speaking world, and **bonne chance** (*good luck*)!

Table of Contents

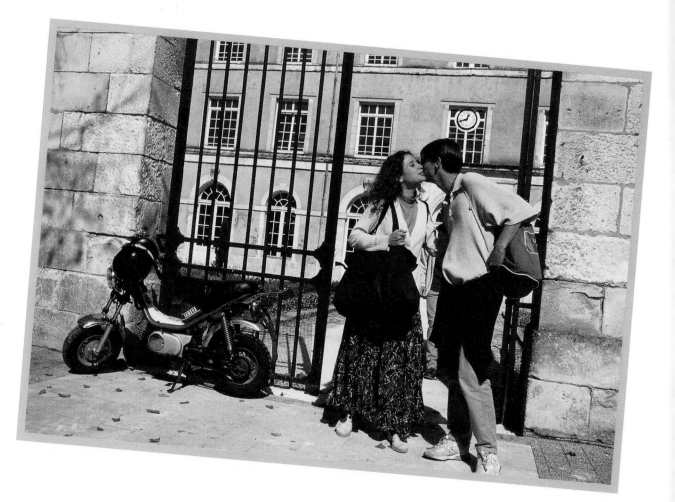

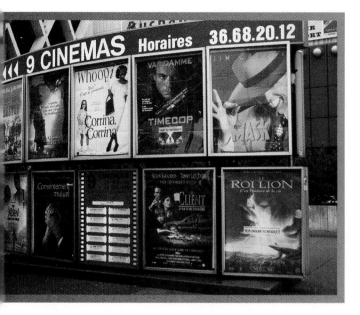

Unité 2 Qu'est-ce que tu aimes faire? 17

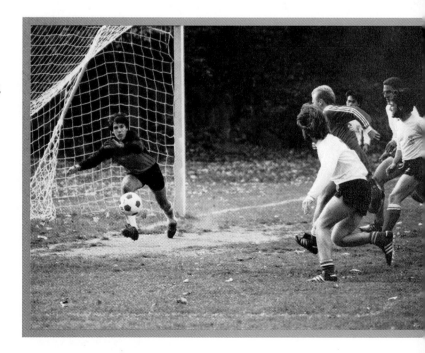

Unité 3 Au café 53

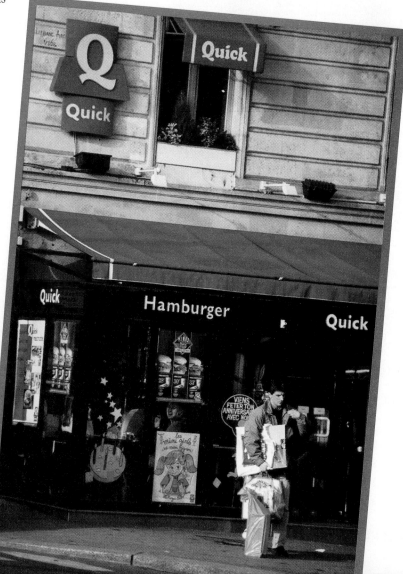

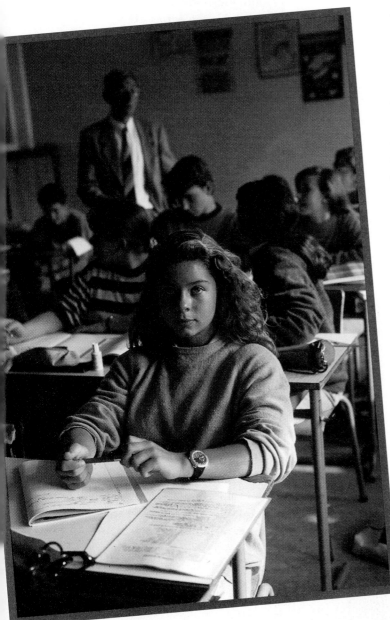

Unité 5 En famille   123

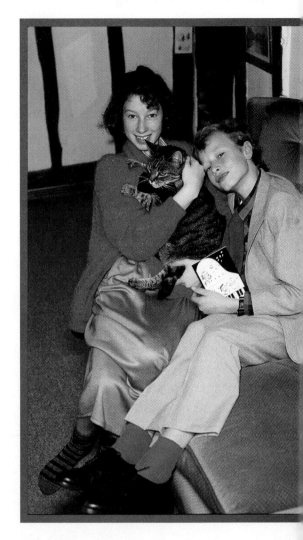

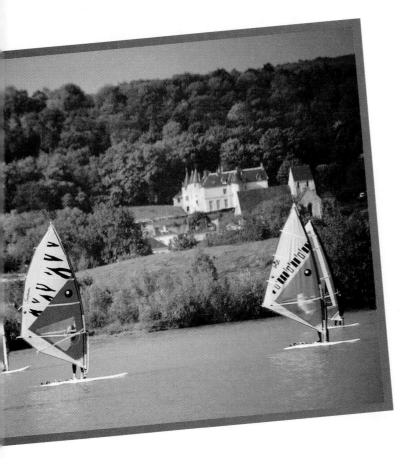

Unité 7 On fait les magasins. 203

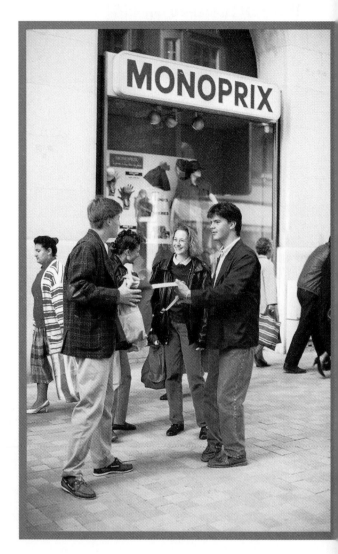

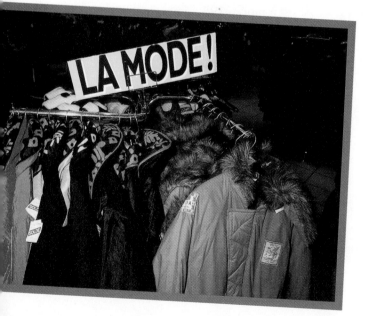

Unité 8 On fait les courses. 241

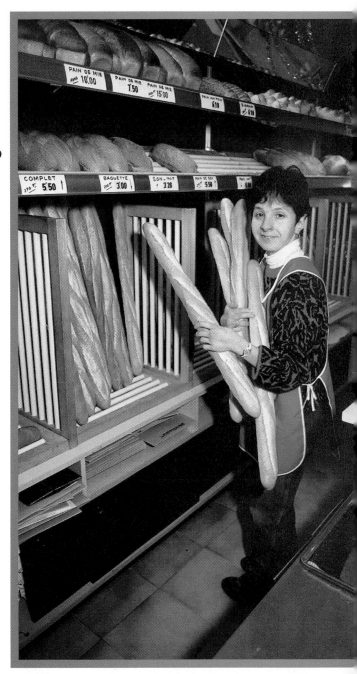

Unité 9 À la maison 279

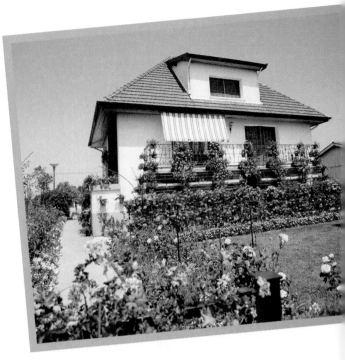

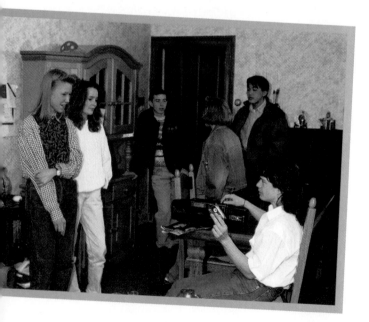

Unité 10 La santé 315

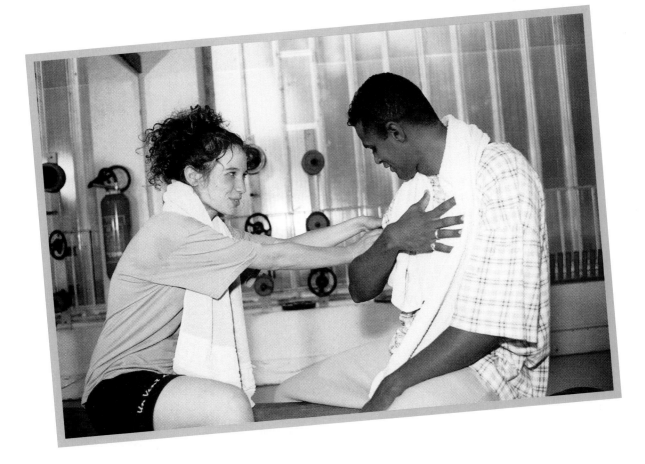

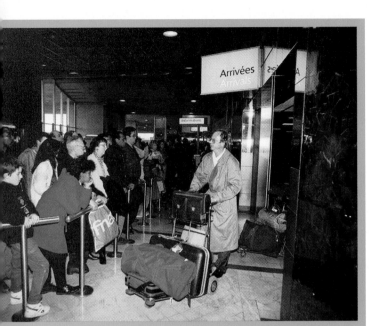

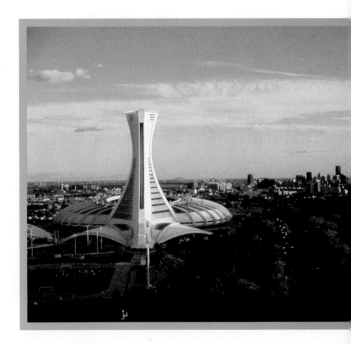

Unité 12 À Paris   383

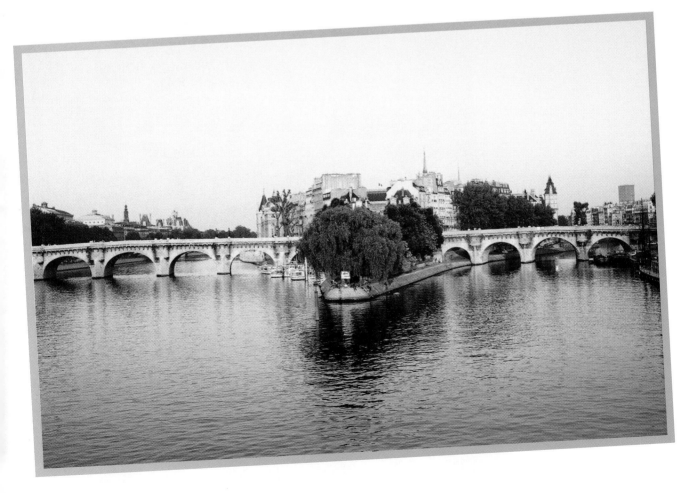

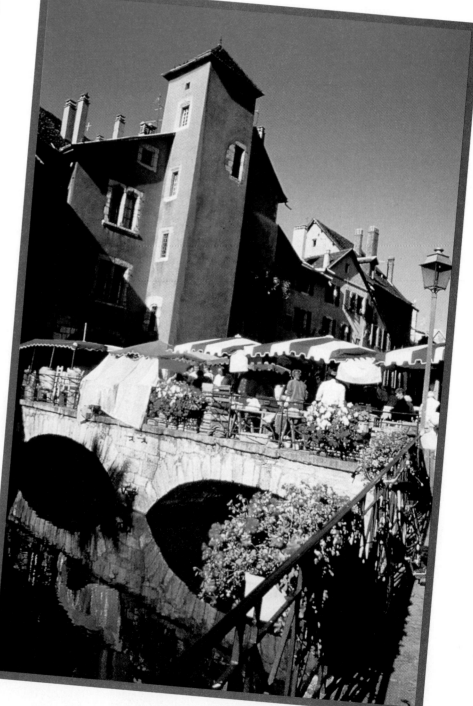

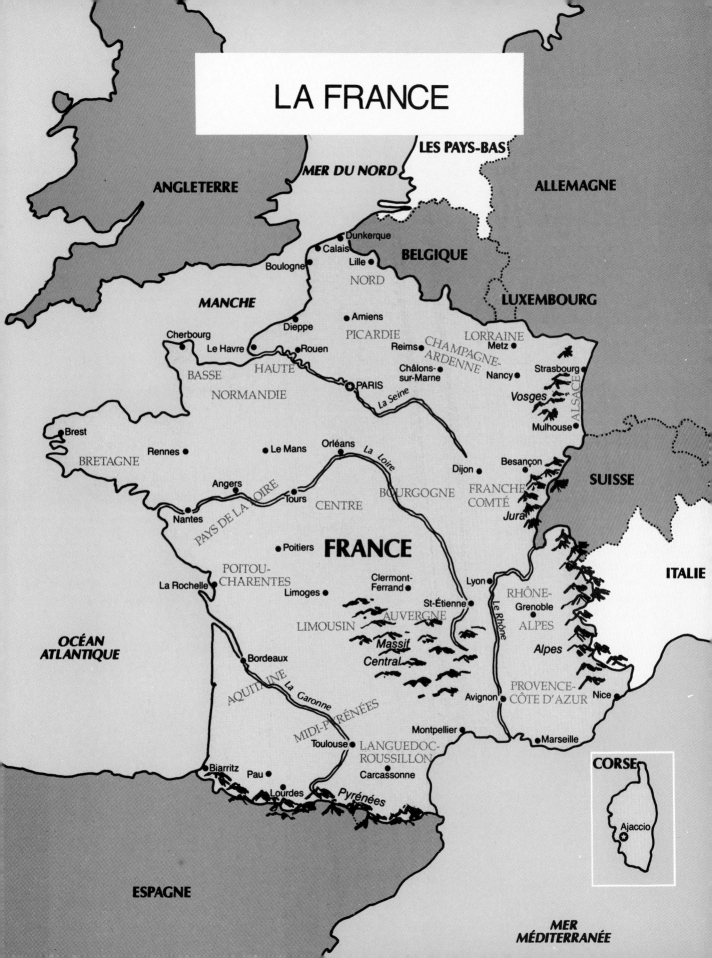

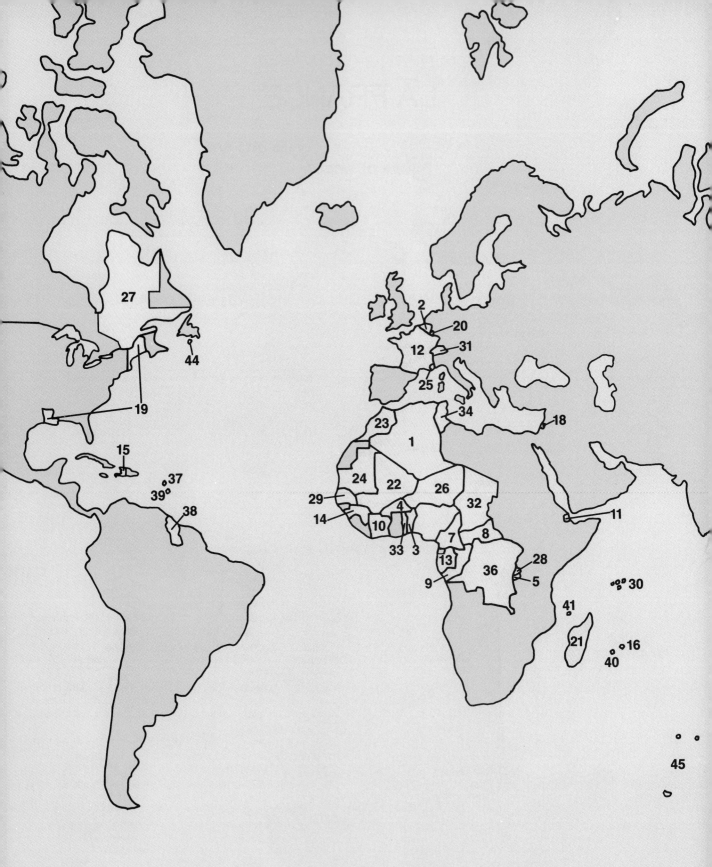

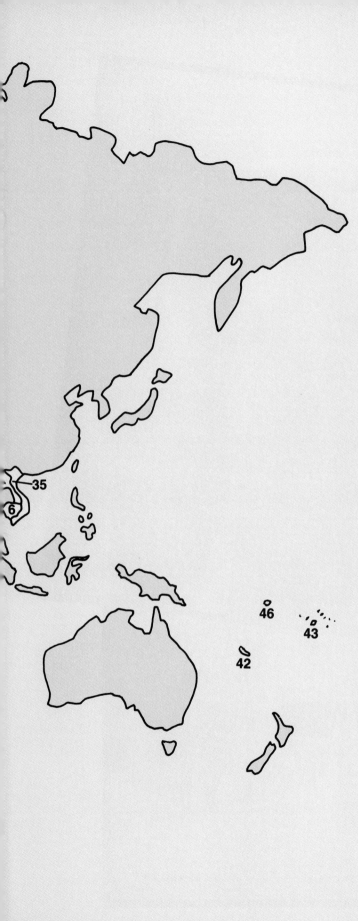

Les pays francophones

It's not only in France that people speak French. In more than 30 countries of the world, there are about 200 million people who speak French either as their mother tongue or as an unofficial second language. These countries are called *les pays francophones* (French-speaking countries). They are very different. There are European countries, of course, like France and Switzerland, and there is Canada, but there are also African countries and tropical islands.

1. **l'Algérie**
2. **la Belgique**
3. **le Bénin**
4. **le Burkina-Faso**
   (la république du...)
5. **le Burundi**
   (la république du...)
6. **le Cambodge**
7. **le Cameroun**
   (la république du...)
8. **Centrafricaine**
   (la république...)
9. **le Congo**
   (la république du...)
10. **la Côte-d'Ivoire**
11. **Djibouti**
    (la république de...)
12. **la France**
13. **le Gabon**
    (la république du...)
14. **la Guinée**
15. **Haïti**
    (la république d'...)
16. **l'île Maurice**
17. **le Laos**
18. **le Liban**
19. **la Louisiane, la Nouvelle-Angleterre**
20. **le Luxembourg**
21. **Madagascar**
    (la république de...)
22. **le Mali**
    (la république du...)
23. **le Maroc**
24. **la Mauritanie**
    (la république de...)
25. **Monaco**
26. **le Niger**
27. **le Québec**
28. **le Ruanda**
29. **le Sénégal**
    (la république du...)
30. **les Seychelles**
31. **la Suisse**
32. **le Tchad**
33. **le Togo**
34. **la Tunisie**
35. **le Viêt-nam**
36. **le Zaïre**
    (la république du...)

La France d'outre-mer

Did you know that the islands of *Martinique* and *Guadeloupe* (more than 6,000 kilometers from Paris) are, in fact, French? They are overseas departments or *départements d'outre-mer (les DOM)*. There are four in all. The others are *la Guyane française* and *la Réunion*.

The inhabitants of these islands have the same rights as the mainland French. They have the same government with the same president and the same system of education, and they often take trips to France.

There are also overseas territories or *territoires d'outre-mer (les TOM),* which are more independent and have their own system of government.

les départements
37. **la Guadeloupe**
38. **la Guyane française**
39. **la Martinique**
40. **la Réunion**

les territoires
41. **l'île Mayotte**
42. **la Nouvelle-Calédonie**
43. **la Polynésie française**
44. **Saint-Pierre-et-Miquelon**
45. **les Terres australes et antartiques françaises**
46. **Wallis-et-Futuna**

The Francophone World

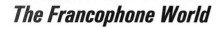

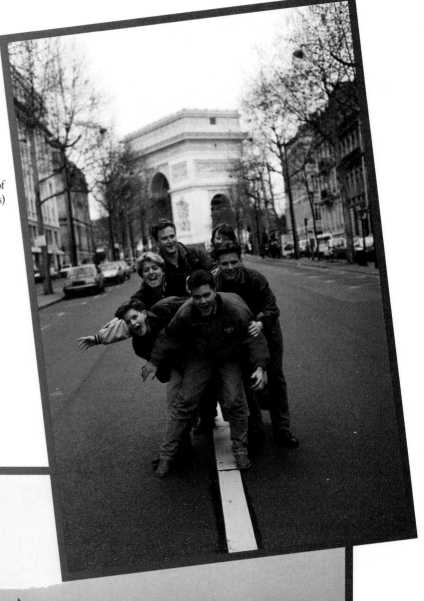

near the Arch of
Triumph (Paris)

windsurfing in the Mediterranean
(Saint-Tropez)

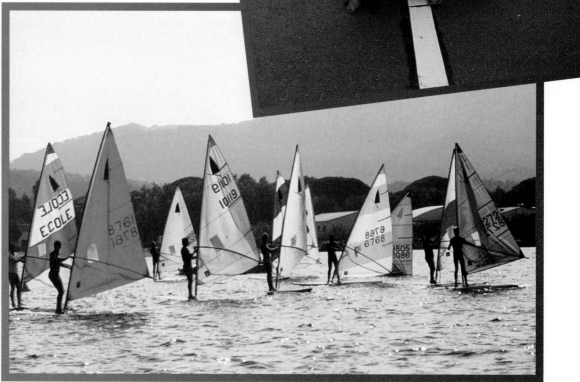

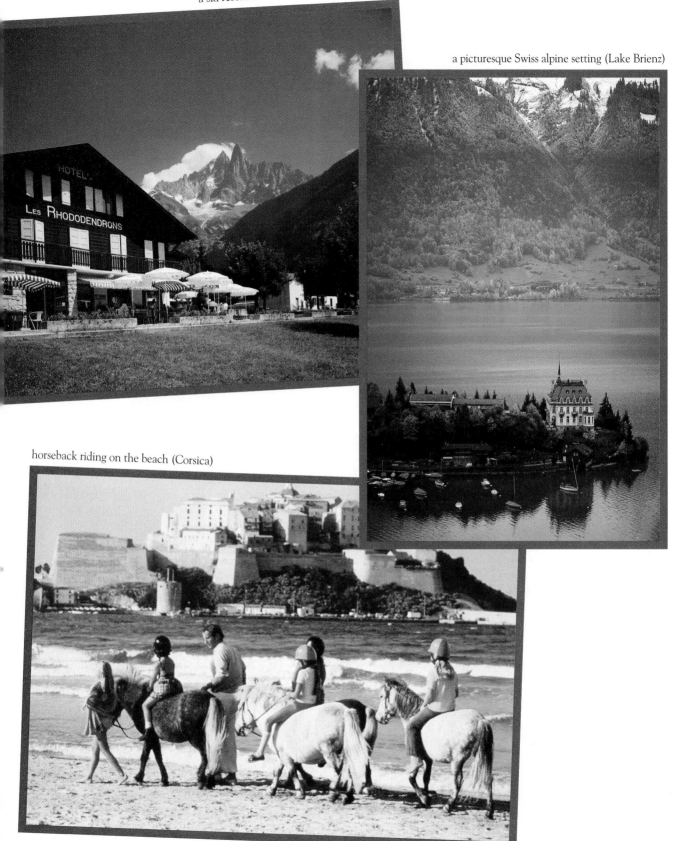

a ski resort in the French Alps (Chamonix)

a picturesque Swiss alpine setting (Lake Brienz)

horseback riding on the beach (Corsica)

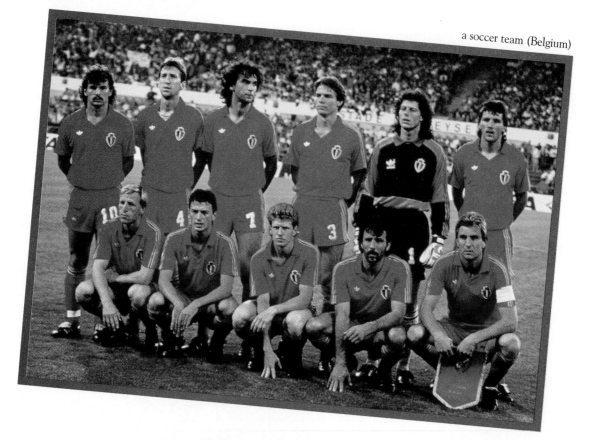

a soccer team (Belgium)

the Casino in Monte Carlo (Monaco)

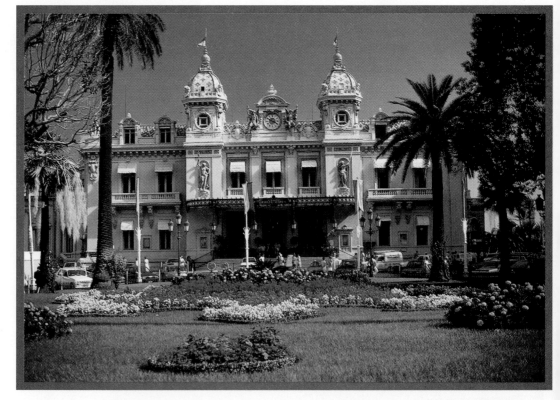

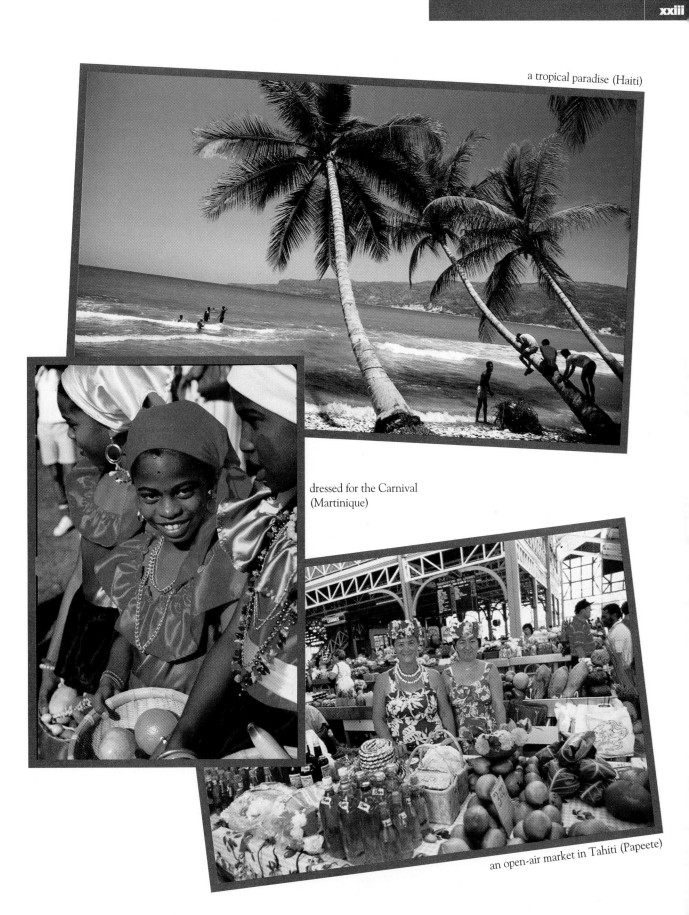

a tropical paradise (Haiti)

dressed for the Carnival
(Martinique)

an open-air market in Tahiti (Papeete)

traveling by camel in Morocco (Agadir)

the village market day
(Senegal)

shopping in the old quarter of a Tunisian city (Mahdia)

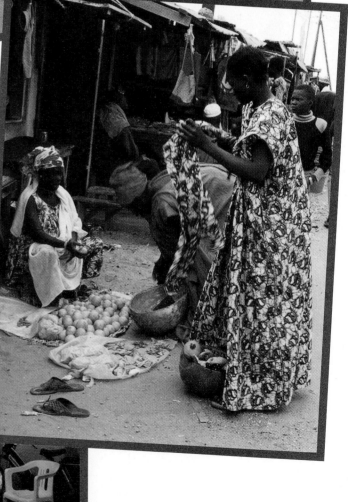

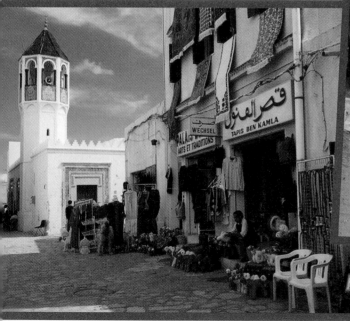

the Ice Palace at the Winter Carnival (Quebec City)

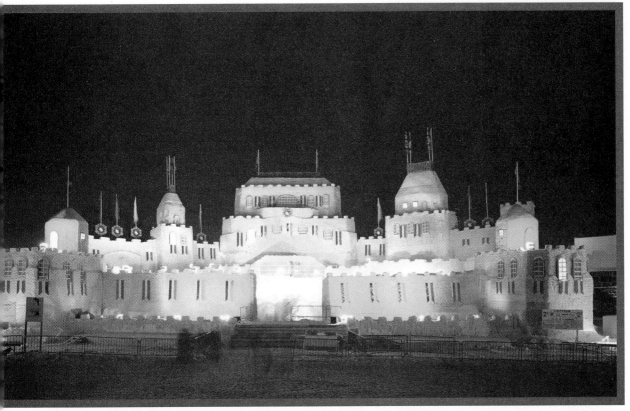

Mardi Gras (New Orleans)

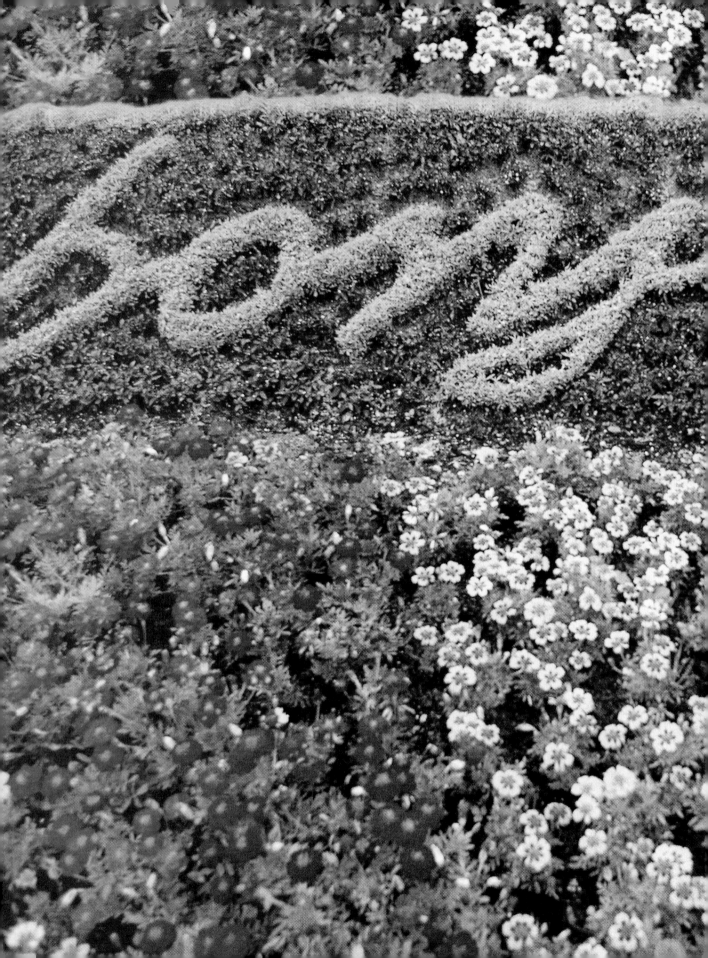

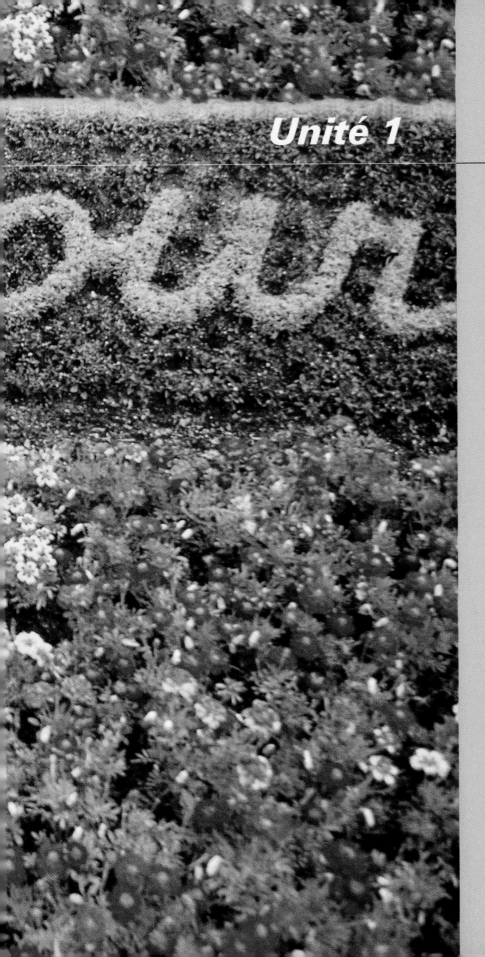

Unité 1

Salut! Ça va?

In this unit you will be able to:

➤ greet someone

➤ leave someone

➤ thank someone

➤ introduce yourself

➤ introduce someone else

➤ ask someone's name

➤ tell someone's name

➤ give telephone numbers

➤ restate information

Leçon A

In this lesson you will be able to:

➤ greet someone
➤ introduce yourself
➤ introduce someone else
➤ ask someone's name
➤ tell someone's name

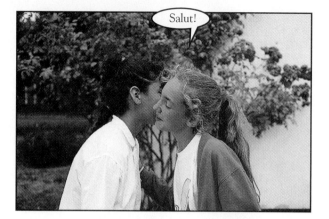

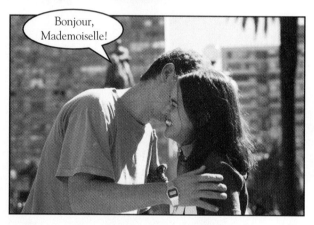

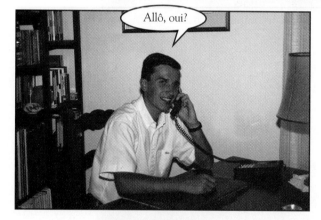

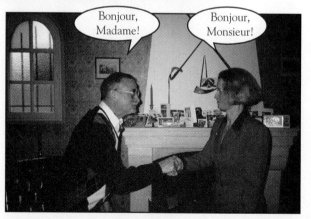

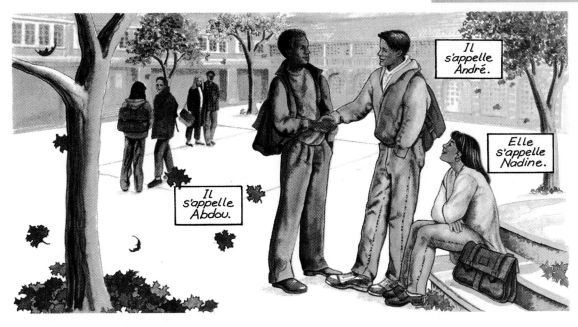

André is talking with Nadine in the school courtyard between classes.
André's friend Abdou joins them.

Abdou: **Eh, salut, André!**
André: **Tiens, bonjour, Abdou! Je te présente Nadine.**
Abdou: **Pardon, tu t'appelles comment?**
Nadine: **Je m'appelle Nadine.**
Abdou: **Bonjour, Nadine.**

Enquête culturelle

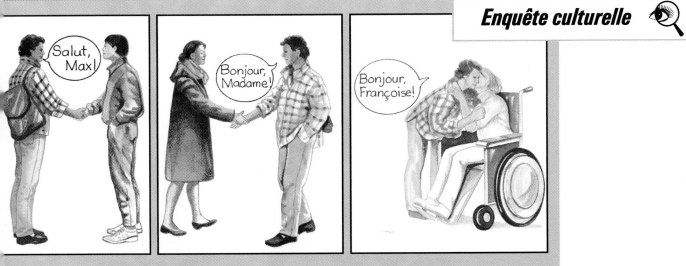

French people often shake hands when they greet and say good-bye to each other.
Their handshake consists of just one up-and-down motion, unlike the American
handshake which involves several movements. Friends and family members say
hello and good-bye to each other with two to four kisses (**bises**) on alternating
cheeks. Girls and women kiss each other and male friends as well. The number of
kisses varies according to the region of the country. Boys and men usually shake
hands with each other instead of kissing.

bonjour

French speakers change the way they talk depending on the situation. They will often use slang and casual speech when talking to friends and family. Teenagers will use more formal words with adults as a sign of respect. For example, a student would say hi to a friend with either **Salut** or **Bonjour**, but would generally say **Bonjour, Monsieur** (*Mr.*), **Bonjour, Madame** (*Mrs.*) or **Bonjour, Mademoiselle** (*Miss*) to a teacher. In writing, these titles are abbreviated as follows:

Monsieur = **M.**   Madame = **Mme**   Mademoiselle = **Mlle**

The school courtyard, **la cour**, is a very popular meeting place for French students between classes and before and after school. Teenagers talk with their friends and play games there.

1 Answer the following questions.

1. What are three words for saying hello in French? Which one can you say only when talking on the phone?

2. What do boys do when they say hello to each other?

3. What do girls do when they say hello to friends?

4. Where can students meet between classes? Does your school have one?

French teens get together in *la cour* during lunch hour. (Verneuil-sur-Seine)

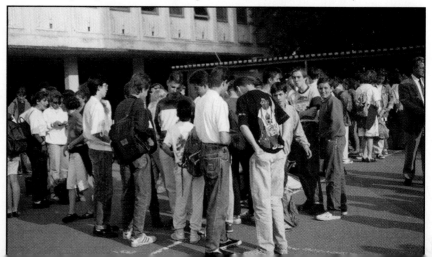

2 *Choisissez la bonne réponse.* (Choose the correct answer.)

1. How does Abdou say hello to André?
   a. Pardon.
   b. Tiens.
   c. Salut.

2. How does André introduce Nadine to his friend?
   a. Je te présente Nadine.
   b. Je m'appelle Nadine.
   c. Bonjour, Nadine.

3. What does Abdou say when he doesn't hear Nadine's name?
   a. Eh....
   b. Tiens....
   c. Pardon....

4. What does Abdou say to Nadine to find out her name?
   a. Tu t'appelles comment?
   b. Je te présente Nadine.
   c. Je m'appelle Nadine.

5. How does Nadine give her name?
   a. Tu t'appelles comment?
   b. Je m'appelle Nadine.
   c. Je te présente Nadine.

6. What does Abdou say after meeting Nadine?
   a. Tiens, Nadine.
   b. Bonjour, Nadine.
   c. Eh, Nadine.

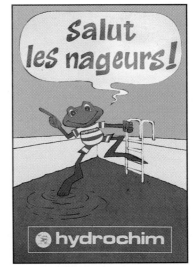

3 What do you say in French when . . .

1. you greet a friend in the hall at school?
2. you introduce your friend to another classmate?
3. you ask a new student his or her name?
4. you tell your teacher the new student's name?
5. you tell someone your name?
6. someone tells you his or her name?

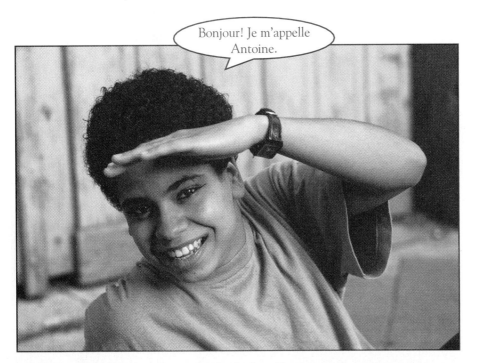

Tu t'appelles comment?

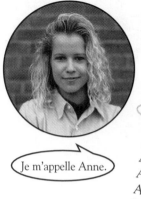

Je m'appelle Anne.

prénoms de filles

Adja
Aïcha
Amina
Anne
Anne-Marie
Antonine
Arabéa
Ariane
Assia
Béatrice
Caroline
Catherine
Cécile
Chloé
Christine
Claudette
Clémence
Delphine
Denise
Diane
Élisabeth
Fatima
Florence
Françoise
Gilberte
Isabelle
Jamila
Jeanne
Karima
Karine

Laïla
Lamine
Latifa
Magali
Malika
Margarette
Marie
Marie-Alix
Martine
Michèle
Myriam
Nadia
Nadine
Nathalie
Nicole
Nora
Patricia
Renée
Sabrina
Saleh
Sandrine
Sonia
Sophie
Stéphanie
Sylvie
Valérie
Véronique (Véro)
Yasmine
Zakia
Zohra

Je m'appelle Malick.

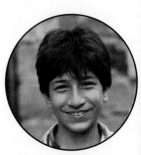

Je m'appelle Zakia.

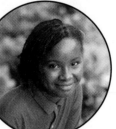

prénoms de garçons

Abdel-Cader
Abdou
Abdoul
Ahmed
Alain
Alexandre
Amine
André
Assane
Benjamin
Bruno
Charles
Christophe
Clément
Damien
Daniel
David
Dikembe
Djamel
Édouard
Emmanuel (Manu)
Éric
Étienne
Fabrice
Fayçal
Frédéric (Fred)
Guillaume
Hervé
Jean
Jean-Christophe

Jean-François
Jean-Philippe
Jérémy
Karim
Khaled
Khadim
Laurent
Louis
Luc
Mahmoud
Malick
Mamadou
Marc
Max
Michel
Mohamed
Nicolas
Normand
Olivier
Ousmane
Patrick
Paul
Pierre
Raphaël
Robert
Salim
Théo
Thibault
Thierry
Vincent

Je m'appelle Salim.

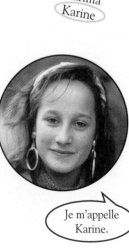

Je m'appelle Karine.

Je m'appelle Frédéric.

What's in a name?

First names can reflect a person's religious or cultural background. For example, children called Paul and Anne may have been named after saints, while the names Charles and Catherine may refer to former French royalty.

Last names, or surnames, often explain where a family was from originally or the family's occupation. The name Dubois ("from the woods") means that the family lived near a forest; the name Meunier ("miller") indicates that the family milled flour.

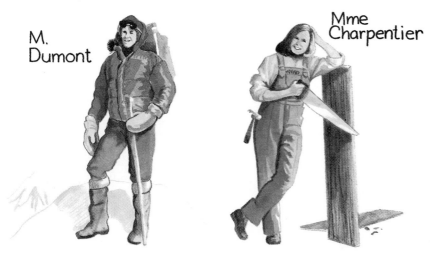

M. Dumont

Mme Charpentier

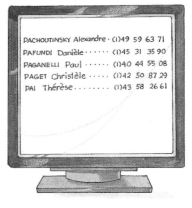

Today, names reflect the multicultural makeup of French society. When looking up a last name in the phone book or on the Minitel (a tele-communication system), you will find family names from a variety of French-speaking countries and other areas of the world.

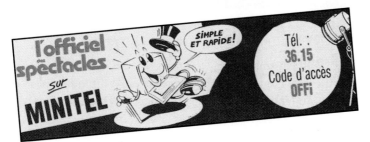

French-Canadian families pass along first names, such as Serge, Robert, Muguette and Céline, from generation to generation. Paquette, Charbonneau, Levesque and Poitras are examples of surnames from Quebec.

In French-speaking Africa, first names may indicate on what day a child was born, his or her birth order or the name of a nearby lake or town. For example, a boy called Fez or Fes would be named after a city in Morocco. African surnames vary from country to country: Kourouma (the Ivory Coast), Moutawakel (Morocco), Senghor (Senegal).

Il s'appelle Serge Desrosiers.

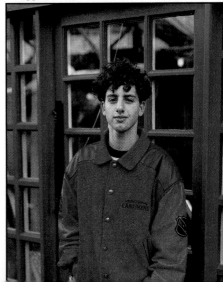

Communication

Modèle:

Nicolas (shaking hands with
Sandrine):   Bonjour.

Sandrine (shaking hands with
Nicolas):   Salut.

Nicolas: Tu t'appelles comment?

Sandrine: Je m'appelle Sandrine.
           Tu t'appelles comment?

Nicolas: Je m'appelle Nicolas.

4   It's the first day of school and you're in French class. You have already chosen a French name and now you want to practice asking and giving names with a classmate before you meet the new French exchange student. With your partner:

1. Shake hands (the way French people do).
2. Greet each other.
3. Ask each other's new French name.
4. Answer.

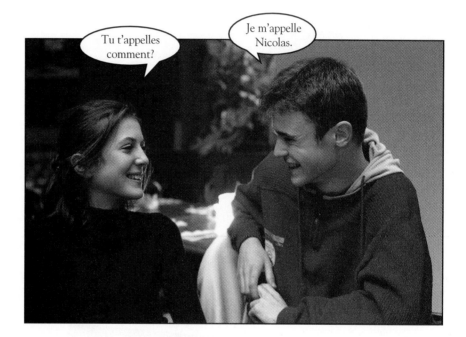

5   With two of your classmates, play the roles of a student, the student's friend and the new French exchange student who's attending your school this year. The student must introduce this new exchange student to his or her friend in French class.

1. The student and exchange student greet each other.
2. The student introduces the exchange student to the friend.
3. The exchange student greets the friend by name.
4. The friend greets the exchange student. Then the friend asks for the exchange student's name again.
5. The exchange student gives his or her name.
6. The friend greets the exchange student by name.

Modèle:

Janine: Tiens, salut!

Zakia: Bonjour, Janine.

Janine: Je te présente Pierre.

Zakia: Bonjour, Pierre.

Pierre: Salut. Tu t'appelles
        comment?

Zakia: Je m'appelle Zakia.

Pierre: Bonjour, Zakia.

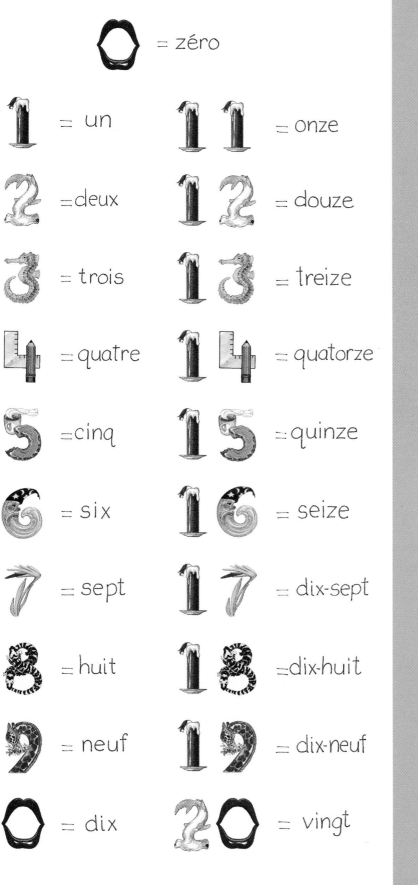

Leçon B

In this lesson you will be able to:

➤ **introduce yourself**
➤ **greet someone**
➤ **leave someone**
➤ **thank someone**
➤ **give telephone numbers**
➤ **restate information**

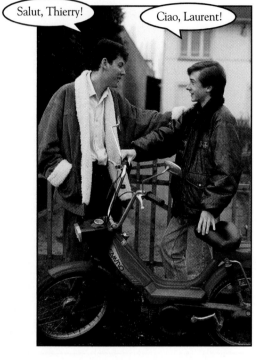

Salut, Thierry!

Ciao, Laurent!

a = a	**b** = bé	**c** = cé
d = dé	**e** = e	**f** = effe
g = gé	**h** = hache	**i** = i
j = ji	**k** = ka	**l** = elle
m = emme	**n** = enne	**o** = o
p = pé	**q** = ku	**r** = erre
s = esse	**t** = té	**u** = u
v = vé	**w** = double vé	**x** = iks
y = i grec	**z** = zède	

é = e accent aigu

à = a accent grave

ï = i tréma

ô = o accent circonflexe

ç = c cédille

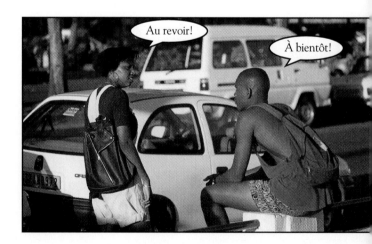

Au revoir!

À bientôt!

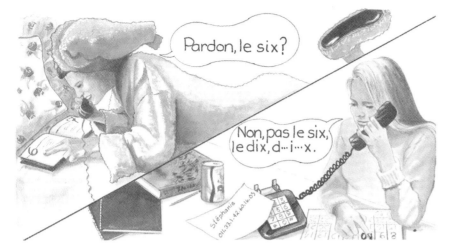

Jessica Miller, an American high school student, is planning to visit her French pen pal, Stéphanie Dufresne. Jessica calls Stéphanie to tell her when she will be arriving.

Jessica: **... seize, zéro trois.**
Stéphanie: **Allô, oui?**
Jessica: **Stéphanie? Bonjour! C'est Jessica Miller.**
Stéphanie: **Ah, salut, Jessica! Ça va?**
Jessica: **Ça va bien, merci. Écoute, j'arrive le dix.**
Stéphanie: **Pardon, le six?**
Jessica: **Non, pas le six, le dix, d... i... x.**
Stéphanie: **Ah, d'accord.**
Jessica: **À bientôt, Stéphanie.**
Stéphanie: **Au revoir.**

Enquête culturelle

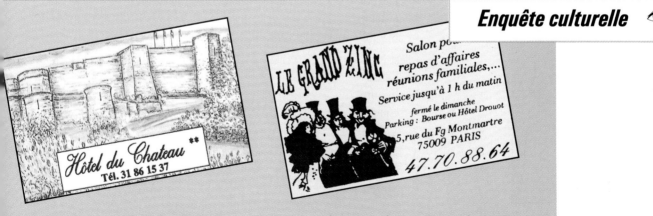

Stéphanie Dufresne's phone number is 42.60.16.03. Phone numbers in France have eight digits and are divided into four groups of two numbers, which are often separated by periods. If the first group of numbers is in the 40s, the phone number is for Paris or its suburbs. When calling Paris from the United States, Jessica begins by dialing "011" (international long distance), "33" (the country code for France) and then "1" (the city code for Paris).

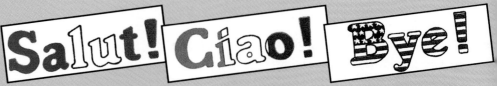

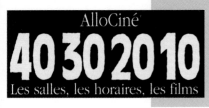

AlloCiné
40 30 20 10
Les salles, les horaires, les films

Although **Au revoir** may be used at any time to say good-bye in French, teenagers often say **Salut**. Two other words you may hear are **Ciao**, borrowed from Italian, and even "Bye." **Allô** is used only when answering the phone. **À bientôt** (*See you soon*) may also be said to end a conversation in French.

1   *Choisissez la bonne réponse.*

1. What word for hello is used when you answer the phone?
2. What do French speakers say when they want someone to repeat something?
3. How many digits are there in a French phone number?
4. What is the first digit in a Parisian phone number?
5. What word means both hello and good-bye in French?
6. What is the Italian word for good-bye that French people use?

    a. Allô.
    b. four
    c. Pardon?
    d. Salut.
    e. eight
    f. Ciao.

2   *Choisissez la bonne réponse.*

1. Allô, oui?
   a. J'arrive le dix.
   b. À bientôt.
   c. Bonjour! C'est Philippe.

2. C'est Myriam.
   a. Salut.
   b. Écoute.
   c. Ciao.

3. Ça va?
   a. Ah, d'accord.
   b. Ça va bien.
   c. Merci.

4. J'arrive le sept.
   a. Pardon, le dix-sept?
   b. Tu t'appelles comment?
   c. Pas le sept?

5. À bientôt.
   a. Tiens, bonjour.
   b. Au revoir.
   c. N... e... u... f.

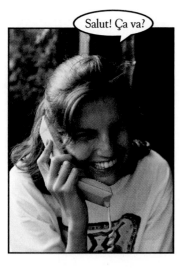

Salut! Ça va?

3   What would you say in French in the following situations?

1. You answer the phone.
2. Someone asks you how it's going.
3. Someone asks you when you're arriving.
4. You're not sure you've heard someone correctly.
5. Someone asks you to spell your first and last names.
6. Someone tells you good-bye.

Communication

4 You are going to make a name tag for the new French exchange student, but you aren't sure how to spell his or her name. With a partner, play the roles of the student and the exchange student. In the course of your conversation:

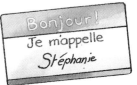

1. The student greets the exchange student.
2. The exchange student greets the student and asks how things are going.
3. The student says things are going well and then asks if the exchange student's name is spelled a certain way (incorrectly).
4. The exchange student says no and spells his or her name correctly.
5. The student repeats the correct spelling.
6. The exchange student agrees.
7. The student says OK, thank you, and says he or she will see the exchange student soon.
8. The exchange student says he or she will see the student again soon.

Modèle:

Laura:	Bonjour, Stéphanie.
Stéphanie:	Salut, Laura. Ça va?
Laura:	Ça va bien, merci. Ah... Stéphanie, c'est S... t... e... f... a... n... e... e?
Stéphanie:	Non, c'est S... t... e accent aigu... p... h... a... n... i... e.
Laura:	S... t... e accent aigu... p... h... a... n... i... e.
Stéphanie:	Oui!
Laura:	D'accord, merci. À bientôt.
Stéphanie:	À bientôt.

5 You need to call certain people but you don't have their telephone numbers. Fortunately, your partner does. As your partner reads you each person's telephone number in French, use the accompanying telephone to dial these eight-digit numbers, touching each set of numbers in order. For example, you say **Stéphanie?** Your partner replies **Ah... Stéphanie... zéro cinq, vingt, zéro neuf, quinze**. Then you dial 05.20.09.15 on the phone. Your partner will watch to see that you dial correctly.

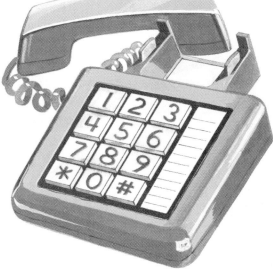

1. M. Paquette:
   dix-neuf, zéro deux, zéro trois, douze
2. Marie-Alix:
   vingt, quinze, seize, zéro un
3. Théo:
   treize, dix, quatorze, dix-sept
4. Mme Bérenger:
   zéro six, zéro quatre, onze, dix-huit

Nathalie et Raoul

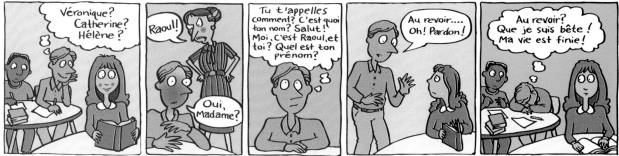

C'est à moi!

Now that you have completed this unit, take a look at what you should be able to do in French. Can you do all of these tasks?

➤ I can say hello, hi, thanks and good-bye, and can greet my friends and adults appropriately.

➤ I can introduce myself.

➤ I can introduce my friends to each other and tell their names.

➤ I can count from 0 to 20.

➤ I can spell names and other important information.

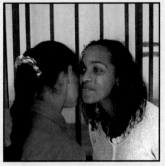

Friends greet each other with kisses (*bises*) on the cheek. (French West Indies)

Here is a brief checkup to see how much you understand about French culture. Decide if each statement is true or false.

1. When French teenagers talk to each other, they say **Monsieur**, **Madame** or **Mademoiselle.**
2. In French-speaking Africa, a child's first name may be the name of the weekday on which he or she was born.
3. You say **Allô** when answering the phone in French.
4. The French shake hands the same way Americans do.
5. French last names, such as Meunier and Dubois, indicate what work the family did or where they came from.
6. As soon as you meet someone in France, you should greet that person with two to four kisses on his or her cheeks.
7. French teenagers talk to their friends only in class or on the telephone.
8. French-Canadian first names are passed along from grandparents to parents to children.

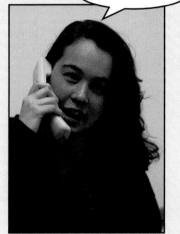

D'accord. Au revoir.

Communication orale

Imagine that a family in your town or city has a French teenager staying with them. The teenager speaks very little English. With a classmate, play the role of an American student who is a friend of this family and the role of the visiting teenager. The family has asked the American student to phone this French teenager so that he or she will have someone to talk to who can speak French. The American student agrees to do this because he or she is eager to practice speaking French.

Before beginning, the French person writes his or her American phone number on a small sheet of paper and gives it to the American student without saying anything. As the student pretends to dial the phone number, he or she says the numbers out loud in French one at a time. During the course of the phone call, turn away from each other to talk as though you are on the phone.

1. The French student answers the phone.
2. The American student greets the French student and introduces himself or herself.

3. The French student greets the American student.
4. Tell each other your name and spell it so that the other person is sure to understand.
5. Ask each other how things are going.
6. Tell each other that things are going well.
7. Tell each other good-bye and that you will see each other soon.

Communication écrite

After you and your partner finish talking on the phone in the preceding activity, your teacher wants to know exactly what each of you said. Begin by writing out the French words for the phone number of the French student, digit by digit. Then write out in dialogue form the entire conversation you had with your partner to give to your teacher. As you write out the conversation, remember to write the name of the person speaking before each line of dialogue.

Communication active

To greet someone, use:

Salut!	*Hi!*
Bonjour!	*Hello!*
Allô?	*Hello? (on telephone)*
Ça va?	*How are things going?*

To say good-bye to someone, use:

Au revoir.	*Good-bye.*
Ciao.	*Bye.*
Salut.	*Good-bye.*
À bientôt.	*See you soon.*

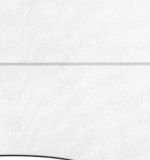

Bonjour! Je m'appelle Jérémy.

To introduce yourself, use:

Je m'appelle Valérie.	*My name is Valérie.*
C'est Patrick.	*This is Patrick.*

To introduce someone else, use:

Je te présente Malika.	*Let me introduce you to Malika.*
C'est Luc.	*This is Luc.*

To ask someone's name, use:

Tu t'appelles comment?	*What's your name?*

To tell someone's name, use:

Il s'appelle Mahmoud.	*His name is Mahmoud.*
Elle s'appelle Yasmine.	*Her name is Yasmine.*

To thank someone, use:

Merci.	*Thanks.*

To give a telephone number, use:

Dix-neuf, zéro cinq, dix, douze.	*Nineteen, zero five, ten, twelve.*

To restate information, use:

Raoul, R... a... o... u... l.	*Raoul, R . . . a . . . o . . . u . . . l.*

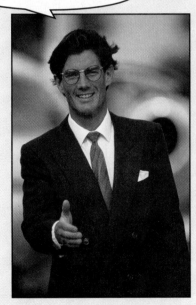

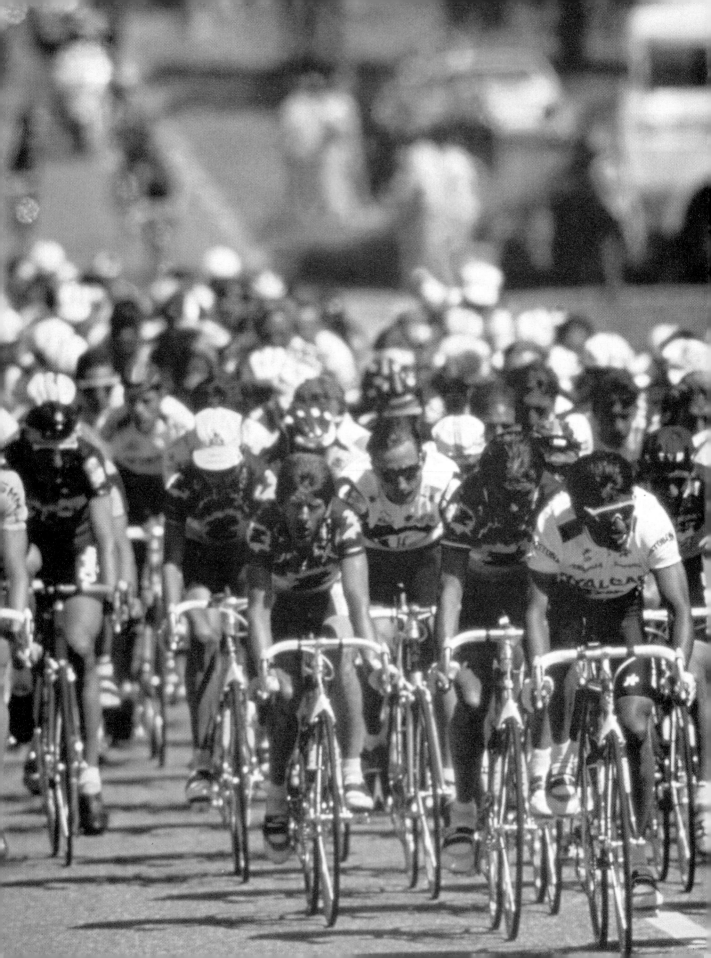

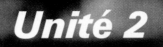

Unité 2

Qu'est-ce que tu aimes faire?

In this unit you will be able to:

➤ **express likes and dislikes**

➤ **agree and disagree**

➤ **give opinions**

➤ **ask for information**

➤ **invite**

➤ **refuse an invitation**

Leçon A

In this lesson you will be able to:

➤ **express likes and dislikes**

➤ **ask for information**

➤ **invite**

➤ **refuse an invitation**

➤ **agree and disagree**

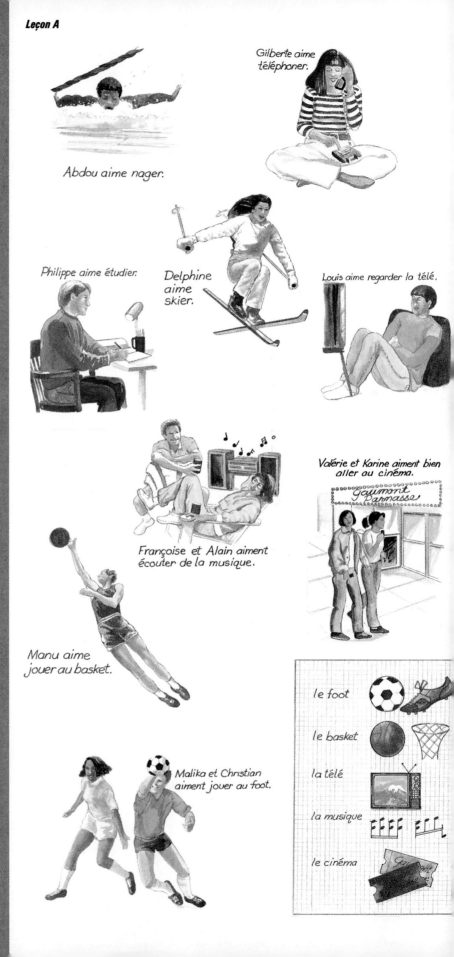

Abdou aime nager.

Gilberte aime téléphoner.

Philippe aime étudier.

Delphine aime skier.

Louis aime regarder la télé.

Françoise et Alain aiment écouter de la musique.

Valérie et Karine aiment bien aller au cinéma.

Manu aime jouer au basket.

Malika et Christian aiment jouer au foot.

le foot

le basket

la télé

la musique

le cinéma

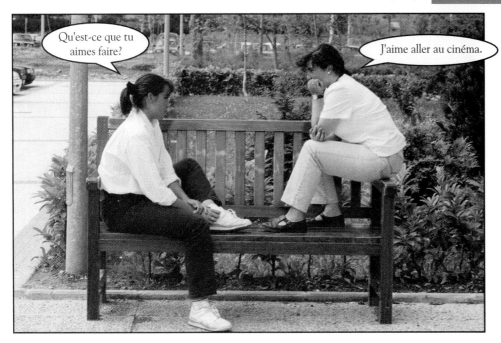

> Qu'est-ce que tu aimes faire?

> J'aime aller au cinéma.

It's Wednesday afternoon. Since Valérie and Karine don't have classes, they talk about what they're going to do this afternoon.

Valérie: **Dis, qu'est-ce que tu aimes faire?**
Karine: **J'aime aller au cinéma. Pourquoi?**
Valérie: **On passe un bon film au Gaumont. On y va?**
Karine: **Pas possible. J'étudie pour l'interro, demain.**
Valérie: **D'accord. Alors, à demain.**

Enquête culturelle

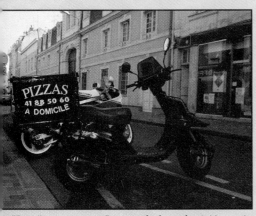

"Pizza" is a cognate. Can you find another? (Angers)

It's not hard to figure out what the French word **musique** means. **Musique** is a cognate, a word that has a similar spelling and meaning in both French and English. Originally, many of these words may have been borrowed from one language to another. Words like **basketball, télévision, skier** and **téléphoner** are examples of cognates. Learning to recognize cognates is an easy way to increase your French vocabulary.

French teenagers usually don't have school on Wednesday afternoon, but they may attend classes on Saturday morning. Students use Wednesday afternoon to see their friends, practice sports, shop and study. Few French teens have part-time jobs. They need to study quite a bit each evening because teachers often assign a lot of homework.

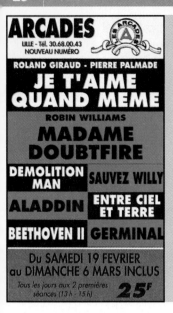

ARCADES
LILLE - Tél. 30.68.00.43
NOUVEAU NUMÉRO

ROLAND GIRAUD · PIERRE PALMADE
JE T'AIME QUAND MÊME

ROBIN WILLIAMS
MADAME DOUBTFIRE

DEMOLITION MAN | **SAUVEZ WILLY**

ALADDIN | **ENTRE CIEL ET TERRE**

BEETHOVEN II | **GERMINAL**

Du SAMEDI 19 FEVRIER
au DIMANCHE 6 MARS INCLUS

Tous les jours aux 2 premières
séances (13 h - 15 h) **25ᶠ**

How many American movies can you see at this theater? (Paris)

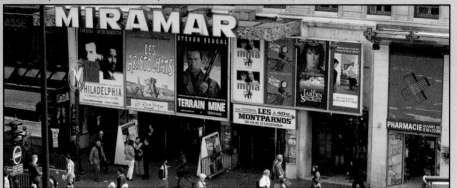

Going to movies is a popular leisure activity for French speakers of all ages. Paris has the largest number of movie theaters of any city in the world. Many films from countries other than France are shown as well. On certain days of the week movie theaters offer reduced prices for students.

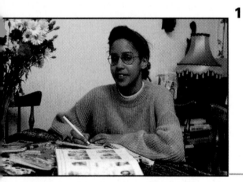

French teenagers have many hours of homework each night.

1 Answer the following questions.

1. How is the daily school schedule of Valérie and Karine different from yours?
2. What can you say in French to refuse an invitation?
3. How does a French speaker say good-bye when he or she will see the person the next day?
4. Why is it difficult for students in France to have part-time jobs?
5. Are only French movies shown in France?

2 *Choisissez la bonne réponse.*

1. What word does Valérie use to get Karine's attention?
   a. Dis.
   b. D'accord.
   c. Alors.

2. How does Valérie ask Karine what she likes to do?
   a. Pourquoi?
   b. Qu'est-ce que tu aimes faire?
   c. On y va?

3. How does Valérie say that there's a good movie?
   a. On passe un bon film.
   b. J'étudie pour l'interro.
   c. J'aime aller au cinéma.

4. What does Karine say to refuse Valérie's invitation?
   a. D'accord.
   b. Pas possible.
   c. Alors.

5. When does Karine have a test?
   a. À demain.
   b. Le six.
   c. Demain.

6. How does Valérie respond when Karine says she has to study?
   a. D'accord.
   b. Ciao.
   c. Pas possible.

7. How does Valérie tell Karine when they'll see each other again?
   a. Au revoir.
   b. Salut.
   c. À demain.

3 | *C'est à toi!* (It's your turn!) *Questions personnelles.*

1. Qu'est-ce que tu aimes faire?
2. Tu aimes aller au cinéma?
3. Tu aimes jouer au foot?
4. Tu aimes jouer au basket?
5. Tu aimes écouter de la musique?
6. Tu aimes regarder la télé?

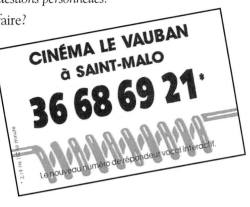

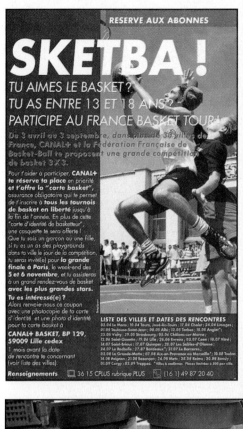

Structure

Subject pronouns

To talk to or about people, use subject pronouns to replace their names. Subject pronouns are either singular (referring to one person) or plural (referring to more than one person). In French the singular subject pronouns are **je**, **tu**, **vous**, **il**, **elle** and **on**. The plural ones are **nous**, **vous**, **ils** and **elles**.

Singular		Plural	
je	*I*	**nous**	*we*
tu		**vous**	*you*
vous	*you*		
il	*he*	**ils**	
elle	*she*	**elles**	*they*
on	*one/they/we*		

Tu aimes aller au cinéma?   *Do you like to go to the movies?*

Oui, **j'**aime aller au cinéma.   *Yes, I like to go to the movies.*

Note that **je** becomes **j'** when the next word begins with a vowel sound.

The pronoun **on** is singular even though it often refers to more than one person.

On passe un bon film au Rex.   *They're showing a good movie at the Rex.*

Il replaces a masculine name; **elle** replaces a feminine name.

Valérie? **Elle** va au cinéma.   *Valérie? She is going to the movies.*

Elles refers to two or more women. **Ils** refers to two or more men or to a combination of men and women.

Nicolas et Renée? **Ils** aiment skier.   *Nicolas and Renée? They like to ski.*

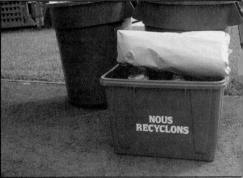

Nous recyclons. Et vous? (Canada)

Pratique

4 While paging through a French magazine, you come across the following headlines and advertisements. Tell what subject pronoun is found in each one.

Il jouait du piano assis...
1.

Nouvelle Peugeot 405 MI 16.
Elle met tout son talent à vos pieds.
5.

—Vous avez gagné 100f—
2.

On aime...
on déteste
fleurs
CD
tomates
6.

JE DESIRE M'ABONNER A PARIS MATCH
3.

Ils ont dit « oui »,
comme au cinéma !
7.

TU AS JOUÉ ?
4.

Nous allons à la plage!
8.

5 You are describing various people at your new school to a family member. Unfortunately, you can't remember any of their names. Select the appropriate subject pronoun you could use to describe each person or group of people from the following list:

| il | elle | ils | elles |

1.

3.

5.

2.

4.

6.

tu vs. *vous*

In French **tu** and **vous** both mean "you," but they are used in different ways. When you talk to one person,

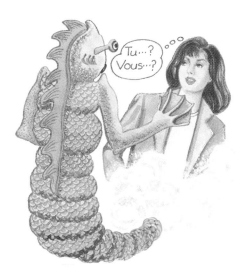

use **tu** with:	use **vous** with:
1. a friend	1. an adult you don't know
2. a close relative	2. a distant relative
3. a person your own age	3. a person older than you
4. a child	4. an acquaintance
5. a pet	5. a person of authority, such as a teacher

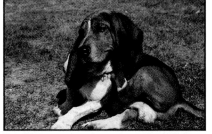

Dis, Toutounne, qu'est-ce que tu aimes faire?

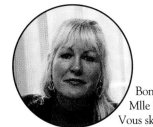

Bonjour, Mlle Dufresne! Vous skiez?

When you talk to more than one person, always use **vous**.

Qu'est-ce que **tu** aimes faire, Nadine?	*What do you like to do, Nadine?*
Vous skiez, Mlle Dufresne?	*Do you ski, Miss Dufresne?*
Karine et Luc, **vous** étudiez?	*Karine and Luc, are you studying?*

Pratique

6   Since Karine can't go to the movies, Valérie has asked you to go with her. On the way to the theater, you meet and speak French with many different people. Indicate whether you should use **tu** or **vous** with each person or group of people.

1. Karine's mother
2. a lost five-year-old
3. your math teacher
4. your friend Bruno
5. Bruno's dog, Milou
6. two secretaries from the office at school
7. your 15-year-old cousin Thierry
8. your grandfather's brother
9. your classmates Sophie and Béatrice
10. a police officer

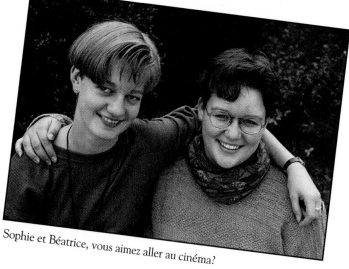

Sophie et Béatrice, vous aimez aller au cinéma?

Infinitives

A verb expresses action or a state of being. The basic form of a verb is the infinitive, the verb form found in the end vocabulary of this textbook and in French dictionaries. Many French infinitives end in **-er**. Some of the verbs you have already seen that end in **-er** are **présenter, arriver, étudier, nager, jouer, skier, regarder, écouter, téléphoner, aimer** and **passer**.

Pratique

7 | List the infinitives ending in **-er** that are found on the following page taken from a beginning French dictionary.

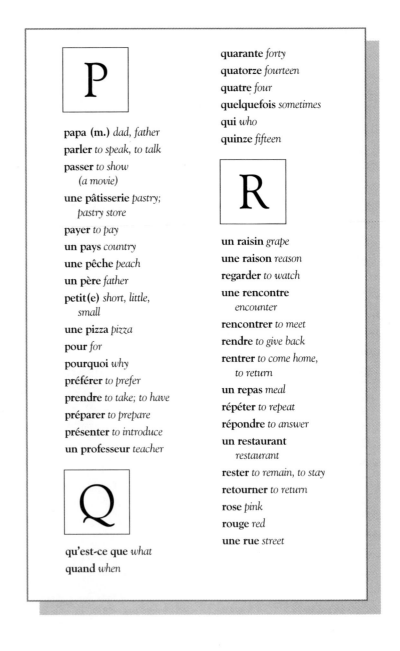

P

papa (m.) *dad, father*
parler *to speak, to talk*
passer *to show (a movie)*
une pâtisserie *pastry; pastry store*
payer *to pay*
un pays *country*
une pêche *peach*
un père *father*
petit(e) *short, little, small*
une pizza *pizza*
pour *for*
pourquoi *why*
préférer *to prefer*
prendre *to take; to have*
préparer *to prepare*
présenter *to introduce*
un professeur *teacher*

Q

qu'est-ce que *what*
quand *when*

quarante *forty*
quatorze *fourteen*
quatre *four*
quelquefois *sometimes*
qui *who*
quinze *fifteen*

R

un raisin *grape*
une raison *reason*
regarder *to watch*
une rencontre *encounter*
rencontrer *to meet*
rendre *to give back*
rentrer *to come home, to return*
un repas *meal*
répéter *to repeat*
répondre *to answer*
un restaurant *restaurant*
rester *to remain, to stay*
retourner *to return*
rose *pink*
rouge *red*
une rue *street*

8 | Tell what some of your friends like to do, according to the illustrations.

Modèle:

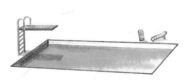

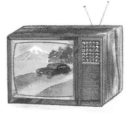

1. Marc aime....

4. Vincent aime....

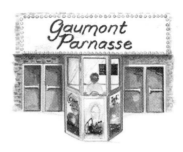

Karima aime **aller au cinéma**

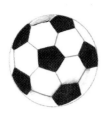

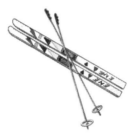

2. Fatima aime....

5. Caroline aime....

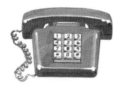

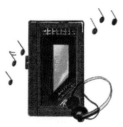

3. Louis aime....

6. Anne aime....

Present tense of regular verbs ending in *-er*

Many verbs whose infinitives end in **-er** are called regular verbs because their forms follow a predictable pattern. Regular **-er** verbs, such as **jouer**, have six forms in the present tense. To form the present tense of a regular **-er** verb, first find the stem of the verb by removing the **-er** ending from its infinitive.

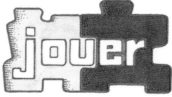

Now add the endings (**-e, -es, -e, -ons, -ez, -ent**) to the stem of the verb depending on the corresponding subject pronouns.

jouer

Subject Pronoun + Stem + Ending

je	**jou**	e	Je **joue** au foot.	*I play soccer.*
tu	**jou**	es	Tu **joues** bien.	*You play well.*
il/elle/on	**jou**	e	Elle **joue** le six.	*She plays on the sixth.*
nous	**jou**	ons	Nous **jouons** au basket.	*We play basketball.*
vous	**jou**	ez	Vous **jouez** demain?	*Are you playing tomorrow?*
ils/elles	**jou**	ent	Ils **jouent** au tennis.	*They are playing tennis.*

Remember that **je** becomes **j'** when the next word begins with a vowel sound: **J'étudie pour l'interro.**

Each present tense verb form in French consists of only one word but has more than one meaning.

André **nage** bien.   { *André swims well.* / *André is swimming well.*

André **nage** bien?   *Does André swim well?*

If an infinitive ends in **-ger**, its **nous** form ends in **-eons**.

Nous **nageons**.   *We are swimming.*

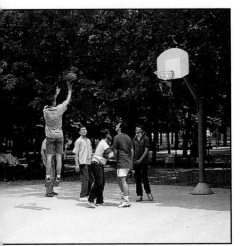

Ils jouent au basket.
(Paris)

Pratique

9 | Tell whether the following people play soccer or basketball.

Modèles:

nous
Nous jouons au foot.

Sandrine
Sandrine joue au basket.

1. Karim

2. vous

3. je

4. Florence et Alexandre

5. tu

6. Mlle Larue

7. David et Jean-François

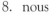

8. nous

0 Complete each short dialogue with the correct form of the appropriate verbs from the following list. Try to use each verb at least once.

| regarder | étudier | aimer | passer | écouter | jouer | arriver |

1. Qu'est-ce que vous... faire?
   Nous... nager.

2. Tu... la télé?
   Non, j'... de la musique.

3. Tu... au basket?
   Non, je... au foot.

4. Vous... le sept?
   Non, nous... le neuf.

5. On... un bon film au Gaumont. On y va?
   Pas possible. J'... pour l'interro.

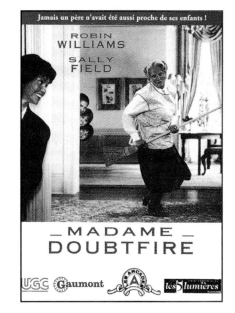

Jamais un père n'avait été aussi proche de ses enfants !

ROBIN WILLIAMS
SALLY FIELD

_ MADAME _
DOUBTFIRE

UGC   Gaumont   les 5 lumières

---

1 The Bouchards have invited the Robidoux family to spend the day at their cabin. Describe what everyone is doing.

Modèle:
Édouard joue au basket.

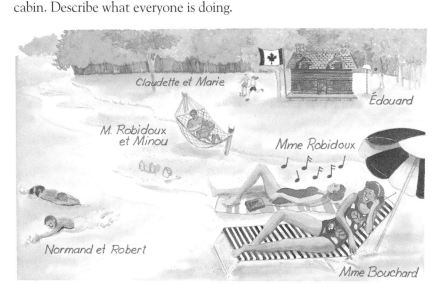

Claudette et Marie

Édouard

M. Robidoux et Minou

Mme Robidoux

Normand et Robert

Mme Bouchard

---

2 With a partner, talk about what various people are doing right now. Student A asks questions and Student B answers them. Follow the model.

1. Mme Gagner (regarder la télé/téléphoner)
2. Karine et Manu (étudier/jouer au basket)
3. tu (jouer au foot/écouter de la musique)
4. Diane et Nadia (arriver le dix/arriver le neuf)
5. tu (aimer aller au cinéma/aimer regarder la télé)

Modèle:
Éric (nager/skier)
Student A: Éric nage?
Student B: Non, il skie.

Communication

13 You would like to know what some of your classmates' favorite activities are. Draw a grid like the one that follows. In the grid write the question you will ask and add any three activities you can express in French. Then poll ten of your classmates to determine which of these three activities is the most popular. In your survey:

1. Ask each classmate what he or she likes to do, giving him or her your three choices.
2. As each classmate answers your question, make a check by the appropriate activity to indicate that he or she likes to do it. (You may check as many activities as your classmate names.)
3. After you have finished asking questions, count how many people like each activity and be ready to share your findings with the rest of the class.

Modèle:

Cécile: Qu'est-ce que tu aimes faire? Nager? Jouer au basket? Regarder la télé?

Daniel: J'aime nager.

Qu'est-ce que tu aimes faire?	1	2	3	4	5	6	7	8	9	10
nager	✔									
jouer au basket										
regarder la télé										

14 Working in pairs, take turns asking each other what you like to do. Make a grid like the one that follows and mark your partner's responses with a check in the appropriate column.

Modèle:

Frédéric: Tu aimes aller au cinéma?

Laurent: Oui.

Tu aimes...	oui	non
aller au cinéma?	✔	
étudier?		
nager?		
jouer au foot?		
jouer au basket?		
skier?		
regarder la télé?		
écouter de la musique?		
téléphoner?		

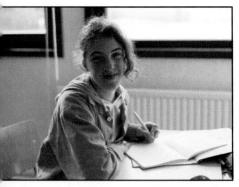

Tu aimes étudier?

5 Which of the nine activities whose names you have learned in this lesson are your favorites? Classify these activities by making a list of them beginning with the one you like the most and ending with the one you like the least. (You may need to refer back to Activity 14 to remember all nine of these activities.) When you have finished, read your list to a partner and compare your preferences.

6 It's the last class of the day. You and a friend pass notes back and forth to find out about your plans for after school. In these notes:

1. Student A tells Student B what two other friends are doing and asks Student B if he or she would like to do it also.
2. Student B either accepts Student A's invitation or refuses it and gives a reason for his or her refusal.
3. Student A says OK and that he or she will see Student B either soon or tomorrow.

For example:

> Abdou et Marie-France jouent au foot. On y va?
>
> Pas possible. J'étudie pour l'interro.
>
> D'accord. À demain.

Unpronounced consonants

Prononciation

A consonant in French generally is not pronounced when it is the last letter of a word. Say each of these words:

salut   alors   comment   pas   pardon   d'accord

The consonant **h** is never pronounced in French. Say each of these words:

Catherine   Hervé   Nathalie   Thierry

Leçon B

In this lesson you will be able to:

➤ express likes and dislikes
➤ agree and disagree
➤ ask for information

Ils aiment faire du sport.

Malick et Nicole aiment faire du roller.

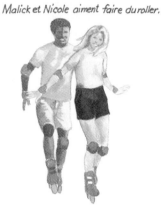

Marc et Renée aiment faire du footing.

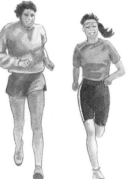

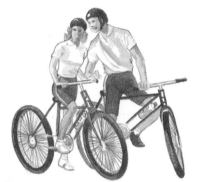

Fabrice et Karine aiment faire du vélo.

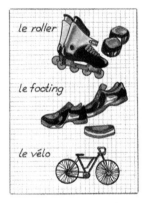

le roller

le footing

le vélo

M. Vinay aime
un peu le
camping.

Yasmine et Anne-Marie
aiment bien
les sports.

Patrick aime
beaucoup les
films.

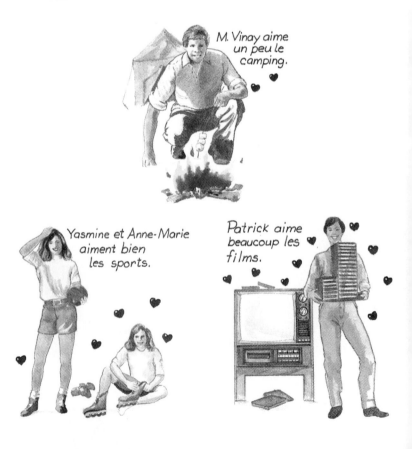

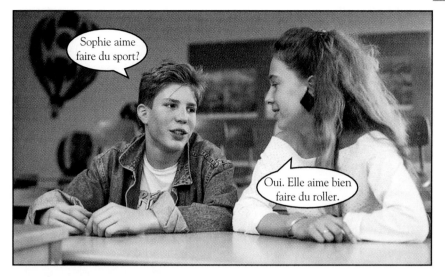

Jérémy wants to ask Sophie out. To find out what Sophie likes to do, he asks her friend Martine some questions.

Jérémy:	**J'aime bien Sophie. Elle aime faire du sport?**
Martine:	**Oui. Elle aime bien faire du roller, du footing, du vélo.**
Jérémy:	**Elle écoute de la musique?**
Martine:	**Oui. Elle aime beaucoup le rock et le reggae. Elle aime un peu le jazz.**
Jérémy:	**Super! Moi aussi, j'aime beaucoup le rock. Bon, je téléphone à Sophie.**

Enquête culturelle

After school many French teenagers play sports, listen to music or watch TV. When they have free time in the evening, they often get together with their friends at sidewalk cafés or at home. Many high school students like to dance at weekend parties, called **soirées.** Younger teens usually call their parties **boums.** Older teens and adults often go out to dance and listen to music at **les boîtes** and **les clubs** (*dance clubs*).

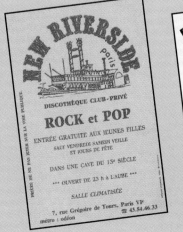

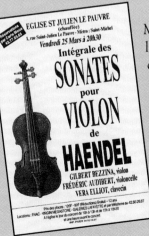

Many French speakers listen to music from other countries, including England and the United States. Teens may like **le rock, le rap, le reggae, la techno, le jazz, le hard, le funk, la dance** or **la musique classique,** for example.

In France teenagers can't get a driver's license until they are 18 years old. They often walk, bike, ride mopeds, use inexpensive public transportation or even hitchhike to get to school or to recreational activities.

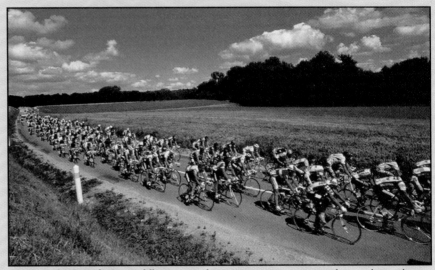

Racers in the *Tour de France* fall into one of two categories: *grimpeurs*, who excel in scaling mountains, and *sprinters*, who do best in speeding over short distances.

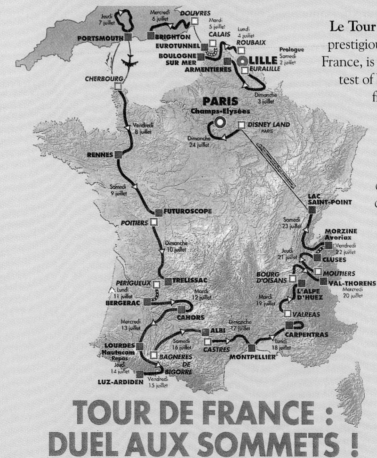

Le Tour de France, the most prestigious sporting event in France, is an annual endurance test of bicycling skill that was first organized in 1903. For 24 days in July, racers cover over 2,000 miles. The distance covered each day depends on the difficulty of the terrain. The most challenging laps wind through the mountain passes of the Alps and the Pyrenees. The **Tour de France féminin** also takes place in July.

TOUR DE FRANCE : DUEL AUX SOMMETS !

1   *Choisissez la bonne réponse.*

1. What is the French word for "running"?
2. Where do French teenagers often get together after school or in the evening?
3. What is the word 11- to 13-year-old students use for a "party"?
4. What do older students call a "party"?
5. Where would you go to dance in a French-speaking country?
6. Name a kind of music that is popular in France.
7. At what age can the French get a driver's license?
8. What is the name of the most famous sporting event in France?

    a. boîte
    b. 18
    c. techno
    d. Le Tour de France
    e. café
    f. boum
    g. soirée
    h. footing

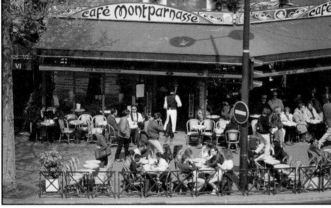

Where do the French often meet with their friends? (Paris)

2   *Répondez en français.* (Answer in French.)

1. Jérémy aime bien Sophie?
2. Qu'est-ce que Sophie aime faire?
3. Sophie écoute de la musique?
4. Sophie aime un peu le rock?
5. Jérémy aime aussi la musique?
6. Jérémy téléphone à Martine?

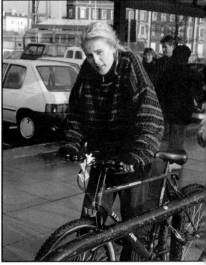

Sophie aime bien faire du vélo.

3   *C'est à toi!*

1. Tu aimes faire du sport?
2. Tu aimes le roller?
3. Tu aimes le footing?
4. Tu écoutes de la musique?
5. Tu aimes le reggae?
6. Tu aimes regarder la télé?
7. Tu aimes le camping?
8. Tu nages bien?

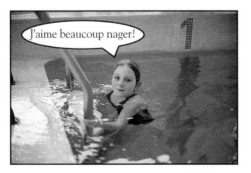

Structure

Position of adverbs

Adverbs describe verbs, adjectives and other adverbs. Adverbs tell how, how much, where, why or when. Note that French adverbs usually come right after the verbs they describe.

beaucoup	J'aime **beaucoup** le rock.	*I like rock a lot.*
bien	J'aime **bien** la musique.	*I (really) like music.*
un peu {	J'aime **un peu** le jazz.	*I like jazz a little.*
	J'aime **un peu** écouter le reggae.	*I like to listen to reggae a little.*

Pratique

4 | Tell how much you like what is indicated by using **beaucoup, bien** or **un peu**.

1. faire du roller
2. regarder la télé
3. le jazz
4. faire du vélo
5. le camping
6. faire du footing
7. le reggae
8. téléphoner

Modèle:

le rock
J'aime beaucoup le rock.

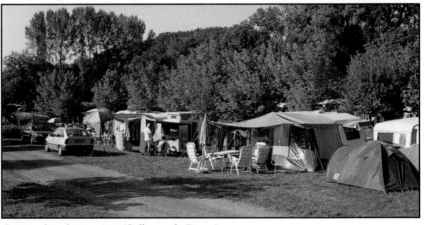

On aime bien le camping. (Collonges-la-Rouge)

5 | You just finished conducting a survey on how much your friends like running, in-line skating, soccer and basketball. Tell how much they like each individual sport and how much they like sports in general.

Modèle:

Max aime beaucoup le footing. Il aime un peu le roller, le foot et le basket. Il aime un peu les sports.

	le footing	*le roller*	*le foot*	*le basket*
Max	beaucoup	un peu	un peu	un peu
Sylvie	un peu	un peu	un peu	un peu
Nadia	beaucoup	un peu	beaucoup	beaucoup
Salim	beaucoup	beaucoup	beaucoup	beaucoup
Pierre	un peu	un peu	beaucoup	un peu
Chloé	un peu	beaucoup	un peu	un peu

6 People like to do the things that they do well. Tell what you and your friends like to do and then say that you do it well.

1. Bruno/jouer au foot
2. je/skier
3. Marc et Benjamin/ jouer au basket
4. Latifa/nager
5. Anne-Marie et Alain/skier
6. nous/étudier

Modèle:

Martine/jouer au basket

Martine aime jouer au basket. Elle joue bien.

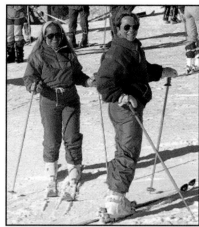

Anne-Marie et Alain skient bien.

Communication

7 Try to guess how much your partner likes certain activities. On a sheet of paper number from 1 to 8 and predict whether your partner will say he or she likes each activity in the following list a lot or a little. Beside the number on your paper that refers to each activity, write **beaucoup** or **un peu.** When you have finished, get together with your partner to check the accuracy of your guesses. Ask each other questions based on your predictions. If your partner's answer matches your prediction, circle it. See who has the most correct guesses.

Modèle:

Emmanuel: Tu aimes beaucoup le camping?
Diane: Oui, j'aime beaucoup le camping.
Emmanuel: (Circles beaucoup on his sheet of paper.)

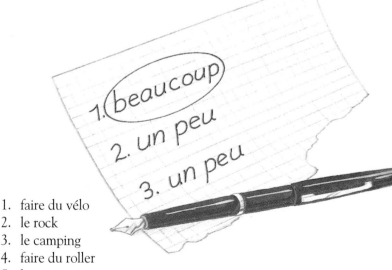

1. faire du vélo
2. le rock
3. le camping
4. faire du roller
5. le reggae
6. faire du footing
7. le jazz
8. les films

8 You have just put some photos of your friends in your album. Now you need to write captions for these photos. On a piece of paper, write a sentence for each one, giving the name of the person and telling what he or she likes to do. You may want to tell how much the person likes doing the activity by using **beaucoup, bien** or **un peu** in your caption. The first one has been written for you.

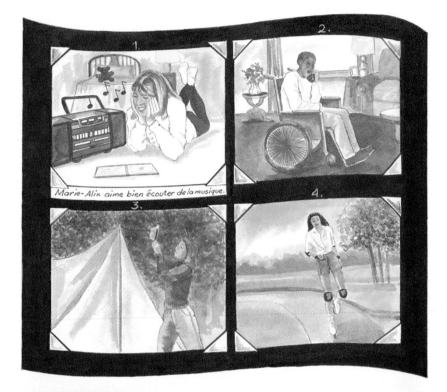

Marie-Alix aime bien écouter de la musique.

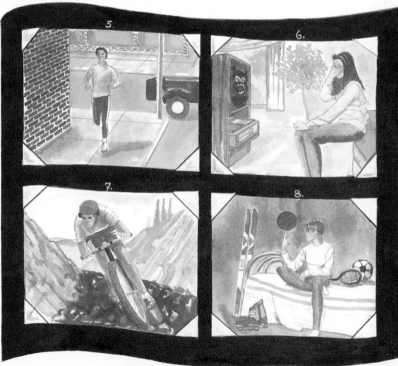

Music is an international language. **Le rock, le jazz** and **le reggae** sound familiar to teenagers all over the globe because of an increasing trend toward world music.

What kinds of music do you listen to? Chances are that French speakers listen to the same sounds that you do. Music is an important part of a teenager's life in French-speaking countries, just as it is for English-speaking teens. Of course, tastes in music vary from person to person.

Shopping for CDs or cassettes is a favorite activity of many adolescents in France. In fact, music lovers of all ages shop at a large music store in Paris that occupies four stories!

Performers from all over the world appear at the Zénith and at Bercy, two popular concert halls in Paris. When students' favorite artists perform at these halls, concerts sell out in no time.

Traditional French songs are usually poetic and melodious. The lyrics often have a message or a feeling to convey to the listener. The messages change, but the songs typically deal with love, peace, family, daily life and politics.

Mise au point sur... la musique

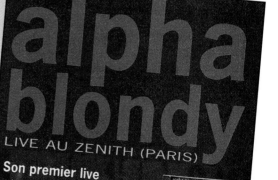

The Virgin Megastore on the Champ-Élysées sells music recordings of all kinds. (Paris)

L'ÉVÉNEMENT MUSICAL DE LA RENTRÉE

NRJ PARIS 00.3

LE MÉGA MUSIC DANCE À BERCY

MD

solidarité sida

SAMEDI 24 SEPTEMBRE À BERCY à 20h30 Plus de 30 artistes pour chanter et danser avec vous

alpha blondy

LIVE AU ZENITH (PARIS)

Son premier live
inclus :
"Jerusalem",
"Cocody Rock",
"Masada"
...
+ 1 inédit

alpha blondy LIVE AU ZENITH (PARIS)

LIVE

EMI

RAP, HOUSE, FUNK, TECHNO LA DANCE, C'EST

3 6 1 5 DE LA DANCE

LES RAVES, LES BONS PLANS, DES CD'S ET DES VOYAGES A GAGNER, ETC.

CHAQUE SEMAINE, LES CHARTS DE REFERENCE :

**TOP DANCE
MAXI DANCE
FREQUENCE DANCE**

POSEZ VOS QUESTIONS A **SPEEDY J**

The words of contemporary songs are more daring than those of the past. Topics include women's issues, antiracism, the environment and the difficulty of city life. The music and the lyrics are fairly aggressive, especially those of **le rock** and **l'alternative**. Their strong rhythm encourages dancing. **Le rap**, still popular in France, was influenced by the same movement in the United States. In fact, many French-speaking teenagers listen to songs in English and know the words, even though they may not know what these words mean.

At dance clubs and on the radio, teenagers listen to a variety of music formats, such as **le disco, le funk, la new wave, le rock, le hard** and **l'alternative. La cold** is a type of music that originated in England and now has a certain following in France. **La techno**, another popular type of music, is based on an industrial, synthetic sound. **La dance** also has a synthetic sound and a rhythm that makes it popular for dancing. Even though **le jazz** originated in the United States, many teens in France listen to it as well. Clubs, such as Le Petit Journal Montparnasse, New Morning and the Jazz Club Lionel Hampton, have helped establish Paris as one of the jazz capitals of the world.

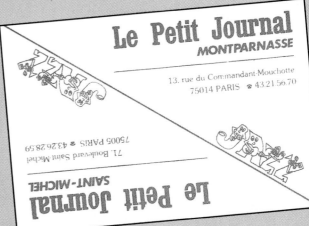

Teenagers all over the world listen to a wide variety of sounds. A wave of multiculturalism has swept across the music scene, influencing and expanding tastes. For example, singers from Quebec, such as Céline Dion, have become international stars. Other examples of the trend toward international music are **la musique créole**, exported from Martinique, and **l'african beat** or **le world beat**, from French West Africa. A style of reggae, sometimes called **le raggamuffin**, has also attracted many listeners. But no matter where a song originates, its music and lyrics reflect the lifestyles of its writers and performers.

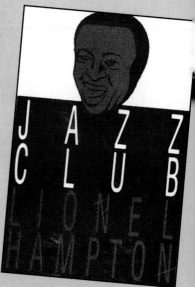

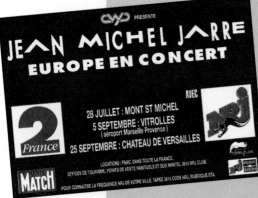

9 | Answer the following questions.

1. What is the major music trend in France?
2. What are the names of two concert halls in Paris?
3. What are two words that describe traditional French songs?
4. What are three topics that may be included in contemporary songs?
5. What are two styles of music that are based on a synthetic sound?
6. What kind of music is played at Le Petit Journal Montparnasse?
7. What is a type of music that has been exported from Martinique?
8. What is another name for **l'african beat**?

Eddy Mitchell
en concert

juin
22 Clermont-Ferrand
23 Toulouse
24 Pau
25 Istres

juillet
1ER Sully / Loire
2 Maubeuge
3 Braine-L'Alleud (B)
5 Epinal
6 Grenoble
14 Le Touquet
15 Le Mans
16 La Rochelle
18 Carcassonne

juillet
19 Vienne
20 Cannes
21 Cahors
22 Nyon (S)
23 Abbeville
29 Bollène

août
2 Sauve
3 Ramatuelle
4 Antibes
5 La Seyne/Mer
6 Béziers
7 Arles
9 Pradelles
10 Annecy

NOSTALGIE
C'est pour toujours

23 novembre Paris-Bercy COMPLET
concert supplémentaire le 22 novembre Paris-Bercy
location fnac, virgin megastore, agences, 36 15 nostalgie

10 | Choose the best answer to each question based on the advertisement you see.

1. What is being advertised here?
   a. A restaurant.
   b. A café.
   c. A dinner theater.

2. What is the name of this place?
   a. Arlequin.
   b. Trio Dany Revel.
   c. Déjeuners Musicaux.

3. What is the name of the group that is playing here from April 24 to June 26?
   a. Carte Menu.
   b. Café Arlequin.
   c. Trio Dany Revel.

4. What time is this group performing? (Times are often given using the 24-hour clock.)
   a. 12:30 — 5:00.
   b. 12:30 — 3:00.
   c. 12:30 — 2:00.

5. How much does the suggested meal cost for each person?
   a. 152 francs.
   b. 125 francs.
   c. 24 to 26 francs.

6. What telephone number do you call to make reservations?
   a. 40.68.30.85.
   b. 152.
   c. 12.30.15.

DÉJEUNERS MUSICAUX

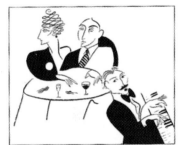

Tous les dimanches
du 24 avril au 26 juin
découvrez les déjeuners musicaux
au

Café

ARLEQUIN

ambiance musicale avec le
TRIO DANY REVEL
de 12h30 à 15h

Notre suggestion
CARTE MENU
152 Frs
(par personne)
comprenant (1 entrée, 1 plat, 1 dessert et Café)

Information - Réservation (1) 40.68.30.85

Leçon C

In this lesson you will be able to:

➤ ask for information
➤ express likes and dislikes
➤ give opinions
➤ invite

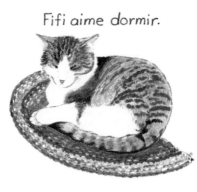

Fifi aime dormir.

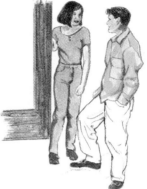

Thierry et Christine aiment sortir.

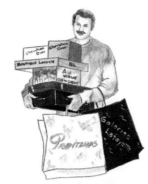

M. Delon aime faire du shopping.

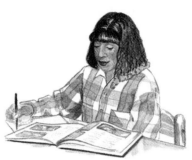

Adja aime faire les devoirs.

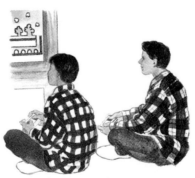

David et Mahmoud
aiment jouer aux jeux vidéo.

Mme Lafont et Delphine aiment lire.

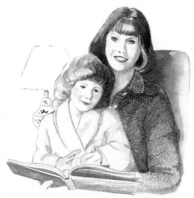

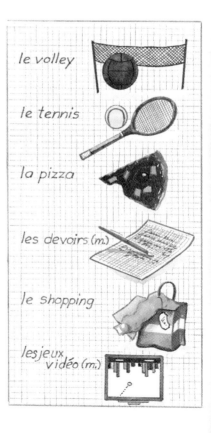

le volley

le tennis

la pizza

les devoirs (m.)

le shopping

les jeux vidéo (m.)

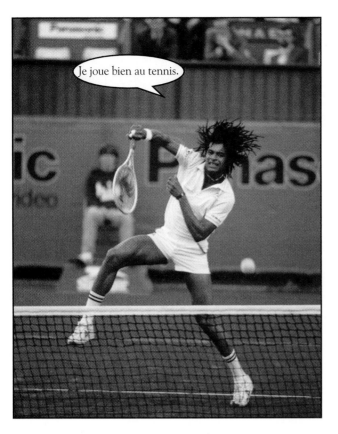

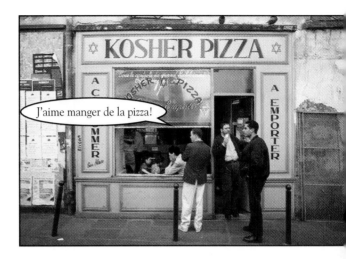

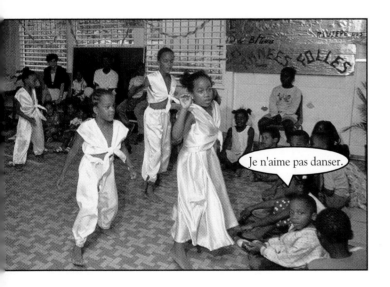

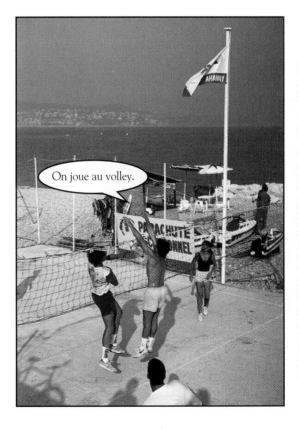

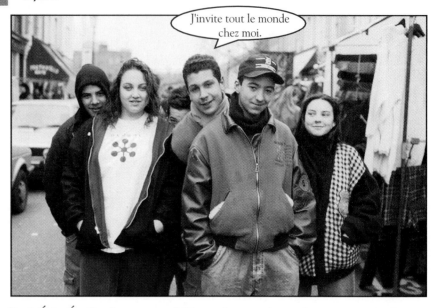

Paul, Éric, Émilie, Laurent and Chantal are making plans to get together over the weekend.

Paul: **Qui aime danser?**

Éric: **Émilie et moi, nous aimons aller en boîte. Mais Laurent et Chantal, ils n'aiment pas danser.**

Paul: **Alors, qui aime jouer au tennis?**

Chantal: **Je joue au tennis. Mais je préfère jouer au volley.**

Paul: **Bon ben, j'invite tout le monde chez moi. Tout le monde aime manger de la pizza!**

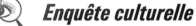

Enquête culturelle

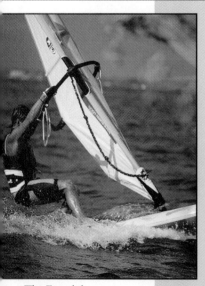

The French love windsurfing.

Since sports are not usually associated with schools in France, students often go to **le club** to exercise. Many also take private lessons there. Local communities offer opportunities for students to participate in sports and arrange competitions as well. In Canada many teenagers ski or play hockey or ringette. On the Caribbean island of Martinique they play soccer or participate in many kinds of water sports, for example, **la planche à voile** (*windsurfing*).

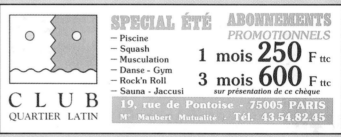

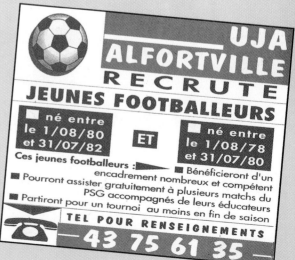

1   *Répondez en français.*

1. Émilie et Éric aiment danser?
2. Qui aime aller en boîte?
3. Qui n'aime pas danser?
4. Qui joue au tennis?
5. Qu'est-ce que Chantal préfère?
6. Qui invite tout le monde à manger de la pizza?
7. Tout le monde aime manger de la pizza?

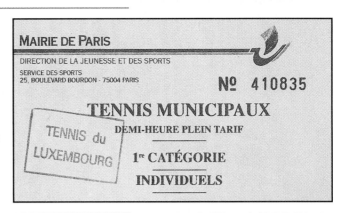

2   *Complétez le dialogue suivant.* (Complete the following dialogue.)

Aimée:	Bonjour. Ça va?
Danielle:	Ça va.... Tu aimes faire...?
Aimée:	..... Je préfère....
Danielle:	Qui aime...?
Aimée:	Moi, je n'aime pas....
Danielle:	..., à bientôt.
Aimée:	....

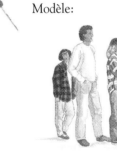

Thierry aime jouer aux jeux vidéo.

3   Say in French whether you like or don't like to do the following activities.

Modèle:

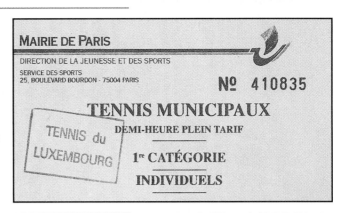

J'aime aller au cinéma.
Je n'aime pas aller au cinéma.

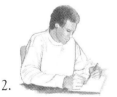

1.

4.

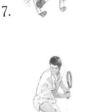

7.

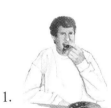

2.

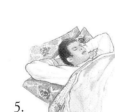

5.

8.

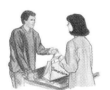

3.

6.

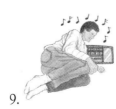

9.

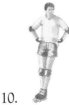

10.

Structure

Negation with *ne (n')... pas*

It takes two words to make a verb negative in French: **ne** and **pas**. Put **ne** before the verb and **pas** after it.

ne	+	verb	+	pas

Jérémy **ne** danse **pas**.   *Jérémy does not (doesn't) dance.*

Tu **ne** joues **pas** au tennis.   *You do not (don't) play tennis.*

Ne becomes **n'** before a vowel sound.

Je **n'**aime **pas** le footing.   *I do not (don't) like running.*

Vous **n'**aimez **pas** faire du shopping?   *You don't like to go shopping?*

Pratique

Modèle:

faire du shopping
André n'aime pas faire du shopping.

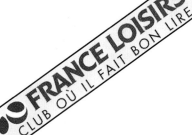

4   Although they are twins, Anne and André are very different. André likes only sports. Anne likes all activities except sports. Tell which twin doesn't like each activity.

1. jouer aux jeux vidéo
2. jouer au tennis
3. lire
4. faire du roller
5. sortir
6. dormir
7. faire les devoirs
8. skier
9. aller en boîte

Modèles:

Béatrice/jouer au volley
Béatrice aime jouer au volley.

nous/faire du footing
Nous n'aimons pas faire du footing.

5   Tell whether or not the following people like the indicated activities.

1. tu/manger de la pizza

2. vous/lire

3. Clément/téléphoner

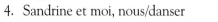

4. Sandrine et moi, nous/danser

5. je/dormir

6. M. et Mme Meunier/ faire du shopping

7. Malika/jouer au tennis

6   Your mother has called you at camp to see how you are and to find out what you and the other campers do. Answer her questions.

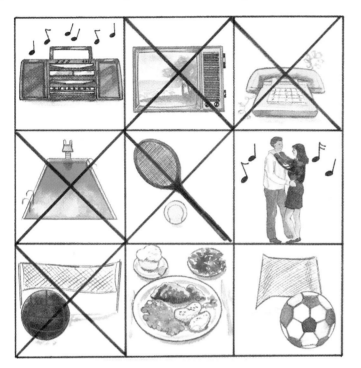

1. Vous regardez la télé?
2. Vous mangez beaucoup?
3. Vous jouez au tennis?
4. Vous écoutez de la musique?
5. Vous dansez?
6. Vous jouez au volley?
7. Vous téléphonez?

Modèles:

Vous nagez?
Non, nous ne nageons pas.

Vous jouez au foot?
Oui, nous jouons au foot.

7   Find out what you have in common with your partner. Ask each other if you participate in the indicated activities.

1. skier
2. jouer au volley
3. danser
4. étudier
5. écouter le rock
6. nager
7. jouer au basket

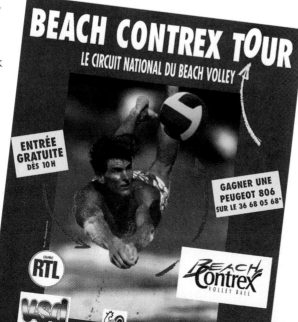

Modèle:

Stéphanie: Tu écoutes le jazz?
Daniel: Non, je n'écoute pas le jazz. Tu écoutes le jazz?
Stéphanie: Oui, j'écoute le jazz.

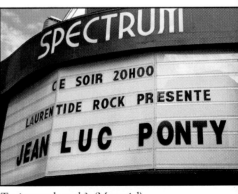

Tu écoutes le rock? (Montréal)

Communication

8 *Trouvez une personne qui....* (Find someone who . . . .) Interview your classmates to find out who participates or likes to participate in various activities. On a separate sheet of paper, number from 1 to 20. Circulate around the classroom asking your classmates one at a time the questions that follow. When someone says that he or she participates or likes to participate in a certain activity, have that person write his or her name next to the number of the appropriate question. Continue asking questions, trying to find a different person who participates or likes to participate in each activity.

Tu...

1. joues au volley?
2. préfères jouer au tennis?
3. manges de la pizza?
4. aimes beaucoup dormir?
5. aimes jouer aux jeux vidéo?
6. nages beaucoup?
7. préfères lire?
8. aimes faire du shopping?
9. écoutes le jazz?
10. danses beaucoup?
11. aimes bien le camping?
12. aimes faire du vélo?
13. skies?
14. aimes sortir?
15. aimes jouer au basket?
16. étudies?
17. joues au foot?
18. regardes la télé?
19. aimes faire les devoirs?
20. aimes beaucoup la musique?

Modèle:

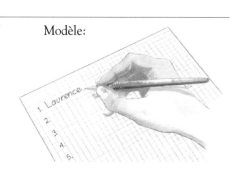

Jérémy: Tu joues au volley?
Laurence: Oui, je joue au volley.
          (Writes his name beside number 1.)

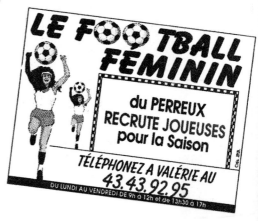

LE FOOTBALL FÉMININ
du PERREUX RECRUTE JOUEUSES pour la Saison
TÉLÉPHONEZ A VALÉRIE AU 43.43.92.95
DU LUNDI AU VENDREDI DE 9h à 12h et de 13h30 à 17h

9 You are going to write an article in French for your school newspaper in which you give the results of the survey you conducted in Activity 8. Tell what activities the students in your French class like, dislike and prefer and also which ones they do or don't participate in. To tell about one person, use that person's name and the **il** or **elle** form of the verb. To tell that you feel the same way about a certain activity that someone else does, use the **nous** form of the verb. To say that several people feel the same way, use the **ils** or **elles** form of the verb.

Modèle:

Laurence joue au volley. Jean-Claude et moi, nous ne skions pas. Nathalie et Bernard aiment sortir.

10 To make plans for the weekend, get together with four of your classmates and find out what they want to do. Everyone in the group must suggest one activity that he or she would like to do. At the end of the conversation, the group should agree on one activity that they will do together.

Tout le monde aime manger de la pizza!

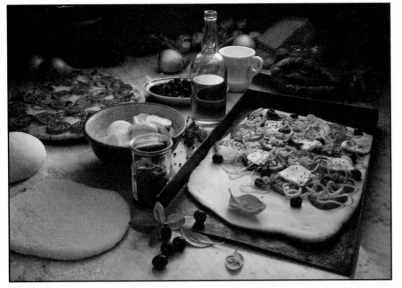

Modèle:

Karine: Qui aime faire du vélo?

Véro: J'aime beaucoup faire du vélo.

Renée: Moi, je préfère jouer au tennis.

Michel: J'aime jouer au volley. On y va?

Stéphanie: D'accord. Nous jouons au volley et j'invite tout le monde chez moi. On mange de la pizza?

Sur la bonne piste

Wouldn't it be wonderful to pick up something written in French and be able to read it as though it were in English? Have you ever asked yourself what it is that makes reading in English relatively simple? Obviously, the words themselves must be the reason for your understanding. But is it only the words? What you probably don't notice is that you take many factors into consideration that set you up for success. Look at the following paragraph:

> Why? Hello, my name is Inigo. See you later. Let's go. Homidas swims very well. I'm studying for a quiz. That's not possible.

Even though this paragraph is written in English, it makes very little sense. You may not have recognized the names that are used, but you probably knew they are names because of where they are found in the sentences. Still, there are three factors that may have made you say "Huh?" First, there is no context for the reading. Context refers to the setting or purpose of the reading. Is this part of a letter? Is this a conversation? Are the two people friends? Is the author a teenager communicating with another teenager? Second, the sentences are not in a logical order. And third, it appears that there are some sentences that are missing.

When you begin to read in another language, you are often so caught up in trying to understand the words that you skip around, trying to find anything you understand. By skipping around, you read things out of order, you miss whole sentences and you probably ignore the context. You understand very little and soon may become discouraged. Ignoring the context and skipping around lead only to frustration. Before you attempt to read something in French, look at the following suggestions.

How to approach (or sneak up on) a reading:

1. Figure out the context (setting or purpose) of the reading.
2. Look at the reading as a whole. (It's all right to skip around at this point because you are going to look at things in order in the next step.)
3. Read the sentences in order. Try to read everything in one sentence before moving on to the next one. Look for cognates, words that look the same and have the same meaning in both French and English.
4. Pick out the sentences that you don't understand and try to fit them into the rest of the reading.
5. Read the passage three times.

Here is a short essay. Using the preceding suggestions, read this account of a typical week in a student's life.

Ma Vie Hebdomadaire (A Typical Week in My Life)

Le lundi. Je salue mon amie Christine. Nous décidons d'écouter de la musique après les cours. Je préfère l'alternative, mais pas Christine. Alors, nous écoutons du reggae.

Le mardi. J'invite tout le monde chez moi. Qu'est-ce que nous aimons faire? Alors, nous jouons au volley parce qu'il fait beau.

Le mercredi. Trois heures de classe. À l'école, je dis "Bonjour" à Jean-Marc. Il demande "Tu joues au foot aujourd'hui?" Mais je refuse parce que j'ai une interro vendredi. "Non. Désolé. J'étudie pour l'interro de maths."

Le jeudi. J'adore regarder la télé lundi, mardi, mercredi, jeudi… mais c'est pas possible. J'aime aussi nager en été, skier en hiver et jouer aux jeux vidéo. Qui aime étudier? Pas moi. Mais j'ai une interro.

Le vendredi. L'interro? Pas trop difficile! Après les cours, je téléphone à Serge. Je lui demande "Qu'est-ce que tu aimes faire?" Serge aime faire du roller. Alors, nous invitons Thibaud, Karim et Nathalie aussi et nous allons faire du roller. Et comme d'habitude, j'invite tout le monde chez moi. Tout le monde arrive chez moi. "On y va?" dis-je. "D'accord. Faisons du roller!" Super!

Ça, c'est ma vie hebdomadaire.

Beginning to use approach skills:

How did you do? You probably didn't understand everything. You must learn to guess when all else fails, since you don't want to look up each word you don't know in the dictionary. Use approach skills to help you. For instance, would it have been likely to find sentences about elephants in the reading? It would have been more likely if the title were "My Day at the Zoo." The title is meant to help you understand. If a title is given, read it first! Then stop. Ask yourself "What would be some usual things that someone would write on the topic?" Also, consider the fact that "A Typical Day in My Life" would be written differently by someone else, for example, a presidential candidate. A 14-year-old may have in-line skating on his or her agenda, but it would be less likely for a 65-year-old. Continue this guessing approach, step by step, as you look at the reading again. Read the passage until your guesses seem to make sense based on the title and the context of the reading. If you spend more time when you first start reading, you will develop some reading habits that will allow you to enjoy reading. If you try to pass over the reading as quickly as possible, you will get very little out of it and feel very uncomfortable when asked about its contents.

11 Can you answer some general questions about this reading?

1. Are all the days of this person's typical week mentioned?
2. Does this person have any friends?
3. Does this person like a variety of activities? What is his or her least favorite activity?
4. Is this person a good student? How do you know?

Nathalie et Raoul

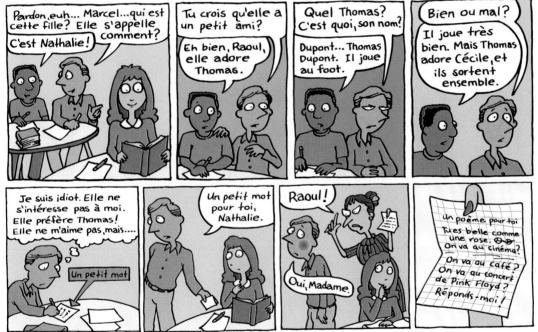

C'est à moi!

Now that you have completed this unit, take a look at what you should be able to do in French. Can you do all of these tasks?

➤ I can tell what I like and what I dislike.

➤ I can give my opinion by saying what I prefer.

➤ I can agree or disagree with someone.

➤ I can ask for information about "who," "what" and "why."

➤ I can invite someone to do something.

➤ I can refuse an invitation.

Here is a brief checkup to see how much you understand about French culture. Decide if each statement is true (**vrai**) or false (**faux**).

1. Most French teenagers don't go to school on Wednesday afternoons and spend this time at their part-time jobs.
2. Movies are a popular leisure activity for French teens.
3. High school students often dance at parties called **soirées**.
4. French teenagers limit their interest in music to **le rock** and **le funk**.
5. In France you have to be 21 years old to get a driver's license.
6. **Le Tour de France** is a 2,000-mile French bike race that takes place every summer.
7. Music in France has a multicultural influence that makes it very international.
8. Many French teens know the words to songs in English even if they don't know what the words mean.
9. Just as they do in the United States, organized sports play an important role in a French teenager's life at school.

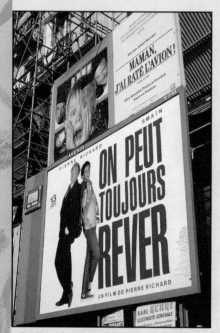

Do French teens go to the movies very often? (Paris)

Communication orale

Imagine that you have applied to be a junior counselor at a camp in France where French teenagers practice speaking English. The camp needs native speakers of English who can also communicate in French. You want to practice your French before your interview with a camp official. Have a classmate play the role of the camp official. During the course of your brief practice interview:

1. Greet each other in French and introduce yourselves.
2. Ask each other how things are going.
3. The camp official asks the student what he or she likes to do.
4. The student tells the camp official at least three activities that he or she likes to do (which are appropriate for camp) and how much he or she likes to do each one.
5. The camp official asks the student what he or she does not like to do.
6. The student tells the camp official at least one activity that he or she does not like to do.
7. The camp official asks the student if he or she likes to listen to music.

8. The student tells the camp official that he or she likes to listen to music and specifies what kinds.

9. Thank each other and tell each other good-bye.

Communication écrite

As a follow-up to your interview with the camp official for the job of junior counselor, write a letter to the director of the camp, Mr. Desrosiers, highlighting the information you supplied in your interview. Begin your letter with **Monsieur**. After you introduce yourself, tell what things you like to do and how much you like to do each one. Then name the things you don't like to do. Finally, tell what kinds of music you like and don't like to listen to. Thank the director and sign your letter.

Communication active

To say what you like, use:

J'aime le rock.	*I like rock (music).*
J'aime danser.	*I like to dance.*
J'aime aller au cinéma.	*I like to go to the movies.*
J'aime faire du sport.	*I like to play sports.*

To say what you dislike, use:

Je n'aime pas le camping.	*I don't like camping.*
Je n'aime pas étudier.	*I don't like to study.*
Je n'aime pas aller en boîte.	*I don't like to go to the dance club.*
Je n'aime pas faire du footing.	*I don't like to go running.*

To agree or disagree with someone, use:

D'accord.	*OK.*
Oui.	*Yes.*
Moi aussi.	*Me, too.*
Non.	*No.*

To give your opinion, use:

Je préfère le jazz.	*I prefer jazz.*
Je préfère jouer au volley.	*I prefer to play volleyball.*

To ask for information, use:

Qu'est-ce que tu aimes faire?	*What do you like to do?*
Qui aime skier?	*Who likes to ski?*
Pourquoi?	*Why?*

To invite someone to do something, use:

On y va?	*Shall we go (there)?*
J'invite tout le monde chez moi.	*I'm inviting everybody to my house.*

To refuse an invitation, use:

Pas possible.	*Not possible.*

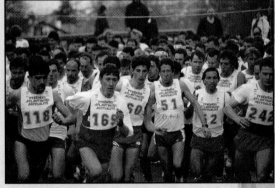

On aime faire du footing. (Bayonne)

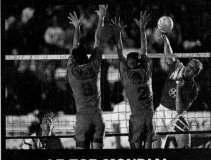

7es INTERNATIONAUX DE VOLLEY-BALL

OPEN PATRICE BEGAY

17-18 SEPTEMBRE
HALLE CARPENTIER
81, boulevard Masséna 75013 Paris

LE TOP MONDIAL
DES CLUBS

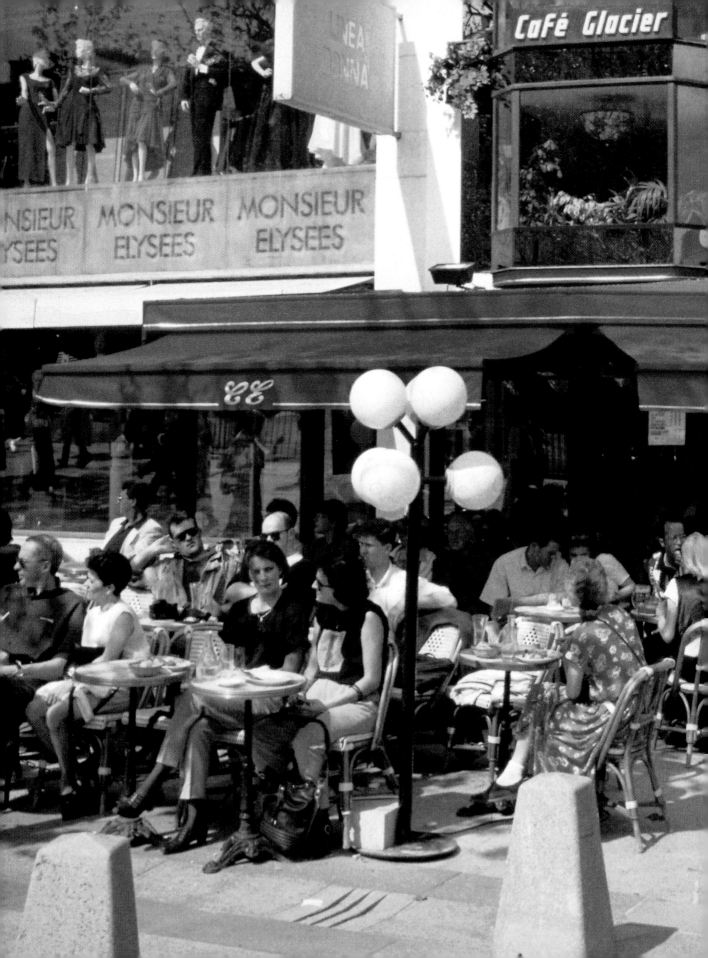

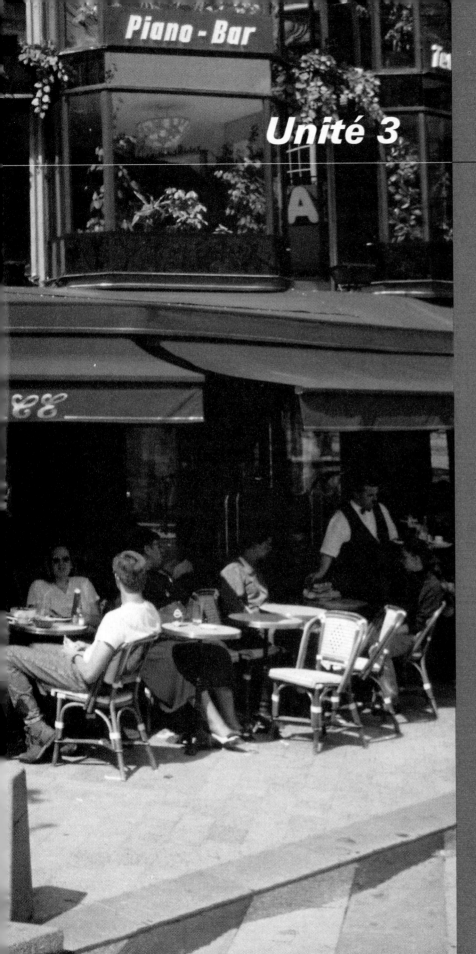

Unité 3

Au café

In this unit you will be able to:

➤ invite

➤ accept and refuse
an invitation

➤ order food and beverages

➤ ask for a price

➤ state prices

➤ ask what time it is

➤ tell time on the hour

➤ ask how someone is

➤ tell how you are

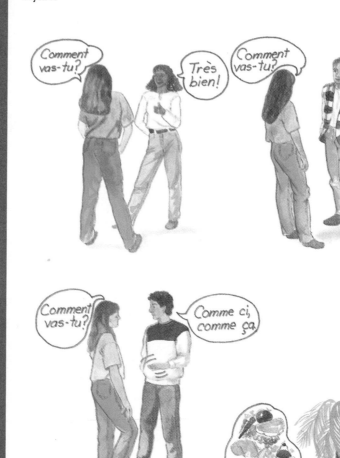

Leçon A

In this lesson you will be able to:

➤ ask how someone is

➤ tell how you are

➤ ask what time it is

➤ tell time on the hour

➤ invite

➤ accept and refuse an invitation

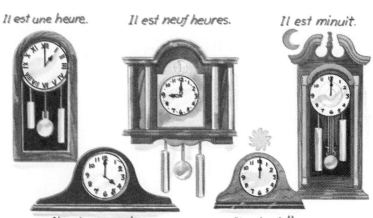

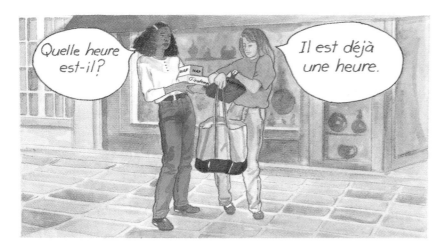

Caroline runs into her classmate Malika downtown.

Caroline: **Bonjour, Malika. Comment vas-tu?**
Malika: **Très bien, merci. Et toi?**
Caroline: **Pas mal, mais j'ai faim.**
Malika: **Moi aussi. Quelle heure est-il?**
Caroline: **Il est déjà une heure. On va au café ou au fast-food?**
Malika: **Moi, je préfère aller au fast-food.**
Caroline: **D'accord, allons-y!**

Enquête culturelle

After school or when they are out with their friends, French teenagers sometimes stop at a fast-food restaurant for something to eat. Restaurants like Quick, Free Time and Pizza del Arte serve food and beverages that many teenagers like: hamburgers, French fries, pizza, hot dogs and soft drinks. American fast-food restaurants can also be found in the French-speaking world; teenagers often eat at McDonald's, Burger King and Domino's. McDonald's, familiarly called Macdo, was the first American fast-food restaurant to cross the Atlantic.

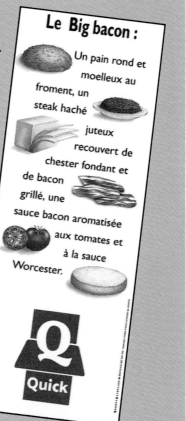

Le Big bacon : Un pain rond et moelleux au froment, un steak haché juteux recouvert de chester fondant et de bacon grillé, une sauce bacon aromatisée aux tomates et à la sauce Worcester.

Quick

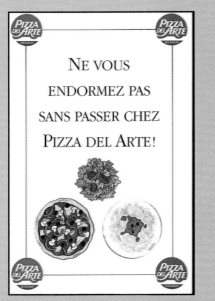

PIZZA DEL ARTE   PIZZA DEL ARTE

NE VOUS ENDORMEZ PAS SANS PASSER CHEZ PIZZA DEL ARTE!

PIZZA DEL ARTE   PIZZA DEL ARTE

It's easy to find an American-style burger in France. (Lyon)

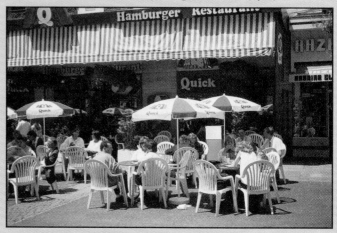

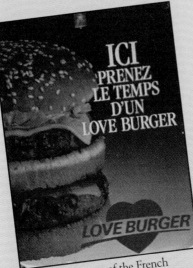

Love Burger is one of the French versions of an American fast-food restaurant. (Paris)

Approximately 300 McDonald's restaurants have opened in France since 1974. Burger King also has a large share of the fast-food business; France is Burger King's fourth-largest market in the world.

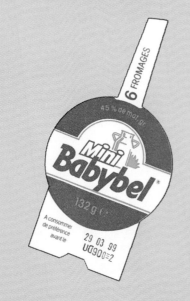

French families often end their meals with fruit and cheese.

When French families sit down for meals together at home, there is an emphasis on healthy eating and good-tasting food. Fresh bread and vegetables are frequently purchased each day. Dessert often consists of fruit, cheese or yogurt. More and more products are appearing with the expression **light** in the name. You can find **Coca-Cola light**, **ketchup light** and even **chocolat light** at supermarkets in France.

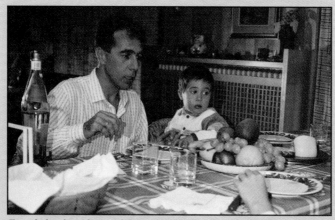

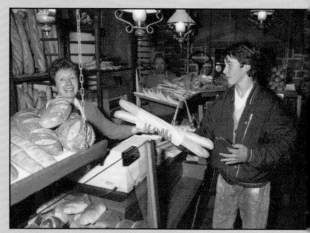

Fresh bread is no more than a few blocks from home for most peo in the city. (Bayonne)

1 How do you feel when the following things happen? Answer using **Très bien, Pas très bien** or **Comme ci, comme ça**.

1. You get an "A" on a math test.
2. It rains on the day of your trip to the amusement park.
3. You win your tennis match.
4. You have to clean your room.
5. It's the first day of school.
6. You win concert tickets from a local radio station.
7. Your date cancels at the last minute.
8. You receive an unexpected gift.

2 Based on the dialogue, match the expression on the left with whom it describes on the right.

1. Pas mal.
2. Très bien.
3. J'ai faim.
4. Elle préfère aller au fast-food.
5. On va au fast-food.

a. Malika
b. Caroline
c. Malika et Caroline

3 How do you ask your friend in French...

1. what time it is?
2. how he or she is feeling?
3. if he or she wants to go to the café?
4. what he or she likes to do?
5. if he or she likes to go to the fast-food restaurant?
6. who likes to eat pizza?

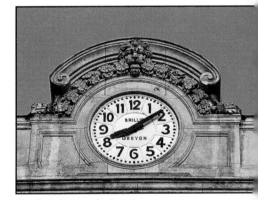

Quelle heure est-il? (Lyon)

4 *C'est à toi!*

1. Comment vas-tu?
2. Tu aimes aller au fast-food?
3. Qu'est-ce que tu préfères, Le Macdo ou Burger King?
4. Tu préfères aller au fast-food ou au café?
5. Tu aimes le Coca-Cola light?

On va au fast-food?

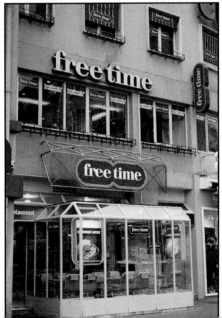

Structure

Present tense of the irregular verb *aller*

The verb **aller** (*to go*) is called an irregular verb because its forms follow an unpredictable pattern. It's the only **-er** verb that is irregular.

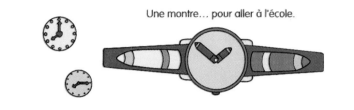

Une montre… pour aller à l'école.

	aller		
je	**vais**	Je **vais** bien.	*I'm fine.*
tu	**vas**	Comment **vas**-tu?	*How are you?*
il/elle/on	**va**	On y **va**?	*Shall we go?*
nous	**allons**	Nous **allons** au café.	*We're going to the café.*
vous	**allez**	Comment **allez**-vous?	*How are you?*
ils/elles	**vont**	Elles ne **vont** pas au cinéma.	*They're not going to the movies.*

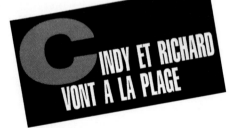

CINDY ET RICHARD VONT A LA PLAGE

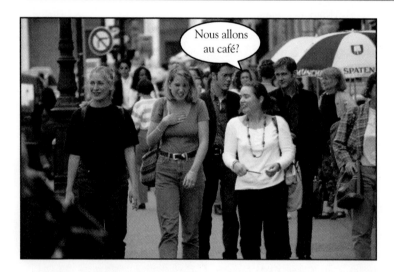

Nous allons au café?

As you can see, the verb **aller** has more than one meaning. It can be used:

1) to talk about going somewhere.
   On **va** au café.   *We're going to the café.*

2) to talk about how things are going in general.
   Ça **va**?   *How are things going?*

3) to talk about someone's health.
   Comment **vas**-tu?   *How are you?*
   Je **vais** bien, merci.   *I'm fine, thanks.*

Pratique

5 | Tell whether or not the following people are feeling fine.

1. Sylvie

2. nous

3. Vincent et Nicolas

4. je

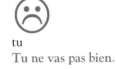

5. Marie-Christine et Laïla

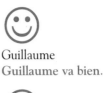

6. vous

7. Mohamed

Modèles:

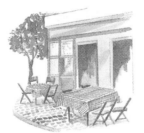

Guillaume
Guillaume va bien.

tu
Tu ne vas pas bien.

6 | It's Saturday night. Tell where the following people are going, according to the illustrations.

1. Tu....

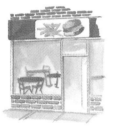

2. Tout le monde....

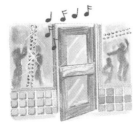

3. Théo et Martine....

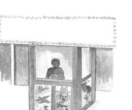

4. Vous....

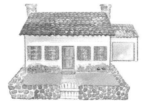

5. Je....

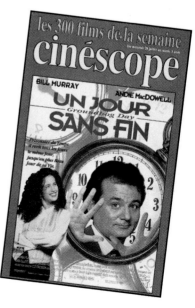

7 With a partner, play the roles of each of the following pairs of people. Student A and Student B ask and tell how they are feeling and then talk about where Student B is going.

Modèle:

Student A: **Comment vas-tu?**
Student B: **Très bien. Et toi?**
Student A: **Pas mal. Tu vas au fast-food?**
Student B: **Non, je vais en boîte.**

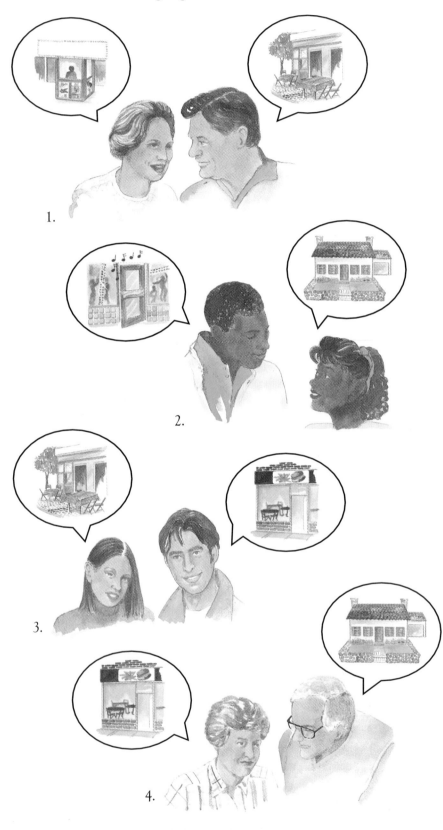

1.

2.

3.

4.

Telling time on the hour

To ask what time it is in French, say **Quelle heure est-il?** To tell what time it is, say **Il est... heure(s).** You must always use the word **heure(s)**, even though the expression "o'clock" may be omitted in English. To say that it's noon or midnight, use **Il est midi** or **Il est minuit.**

Quelle heure est-il?	*What time is it?*
Il est une heure.	*It's one (o'clock).*
Il est neuf heures.	*It's nine (o'clock).*

The abbreviation for **heure(s)** is **h**: 1h00 = 1:00.

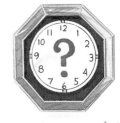

Quelle heure est-il?

Pratique

8 | Looking at each clock or watch, answer the question **Quelle heure est-il?**

1.

5.

2.

6.

3.

7.

4.

8.

Modèle:

Il est cinq heures.

9 Suzanne has made many plans for the first day of summer vacation. Looking at each illustration, tell what time it is, based on the information she has written in her daily planner.

MERCREDI 25

(6) Juin

9h00	*faire du footing*
10h00	*téléphoner à Caroline*
11h00	*faire du vélo*
12h00	*faire du shopping*
1h00	*manger au fast-food*
2h00	*jouer au tennis*
3h00	
4h00	*nager*
5h00	
6h00	
7h00	
8h00	*sortir*

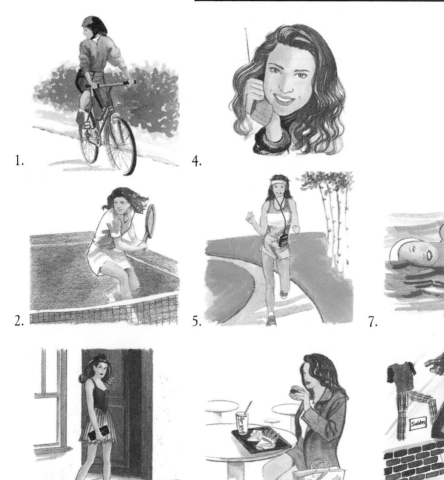

1.

4.

2.

5.

7.

3.

6.

8.

Communication

0 You meet one of your friends on the street after school. In the course of your conversation you decide to go to a café to get something to drink because you both are thirsty. With your partner:

1. Greet each other.
2. Find out how each other is feeling.
3. Student A says he or she is thirsty.
4. Student B agrees and suggests going to a fast-food restaurant.
5. Student A prefers to go to a café.
6. Student B agrees and suggests they go.

Modèle:

Student A:	Bonjour, Marie-Claire.
Student B:	Salut, Claudine. Comment vas-tu?
Student A:	Pas mal. Et toi?
Student B:	Très bien, merci.
Student A:	Dis, j'ai soif.
Student B:	Moi aussi. On va au fast-food?
Student A:	Moi, je préfère aller au café.
Student B:	D'accord, allons-y!

1 Cédric lives on the island of Martinique. His project for French class is to illustrate how he spends a typical vacation day. Help Cédric write captions to accompany his pictures, telling when he does each activity. The first caption has been done for you.

Modèle:

Il est huit heures. J'écoute de la musique.

The sound [a]

The sound of the French vowel **a** is similar to the sound of the letter "a" in the English words "calm" and "father." However, the French sound [a] is shorter than the English "a" sound. In fact, all French vowels are shorter than English vowels. Say each of these words:

mal   Malika   déjà   d'accord   allons-y   basket

The sound [i]

The sound of the French vowel **i** is similar to the sound of the letters "ee" in the English word "see." Say each of these words:

midi   merci   Christine   idée   cinéma   musique

Prononciation

Leçon B

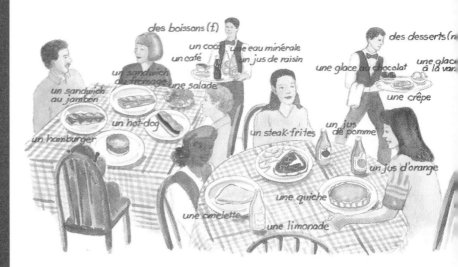

des boissons (f.)
un coca   une eau minérale
un café   un jus de raisin
un sandwich au fromage   une salade
un sandwich au jambon
un hot-dog
un hamburger
un steak-frites   un jus de pomme
des desserts (m.)
une glace au chocolat   une glace à la vanille
une crêpe
un jus d'orange
une quiche
une omelette
une limonade

In this lesson you will be able to:

➤ order food and beverages

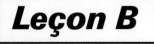

la vanille

le chocolat

le jambon

le fromage

les frites (f.)

l'orange (f.)

la pomme

les raisins (m.)

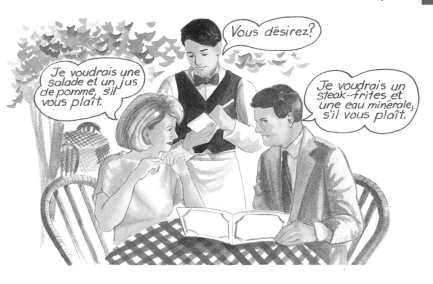

Monsieur and Madame Paganini are having lunch at a small café on **le boulevard Saint-Michel** in Paris. The server arrives to take their order.

Serveur:	**Bonjour, Messieurs-Dames. Vous désirez?**
Madame Paganini:	**Je voudrais une salade et un jus de pomme, s'il vous plaît.**
Serveur:	**Et pour vous, Monsieur?**
Monsieur Paganini:	**Je voudrais un steak-frites et une eau minérale, s'il vous plaît.**
Serveur:	**Et comme dessert?**
Monsieur Paganini:	**Je voudrais une glace au chocolat. Donnez-moi aussi un café, s'il vous plaît.**

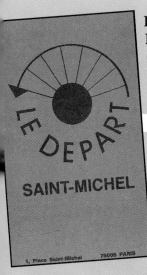

Enquête culturelle

Le boulevard Saint-Michel, often shortened to **Boul' Mich**, runs through the heart of the Latin Quarter in Paris. Located near France's most famous university, **la Sorbonne**, this street is one of the centers of student life.

Steak-frites refers to a steak that is served with French fries. French fries are also popular in Belgium, where they originated. French fry snack bars in Belgium are called **friteries**.

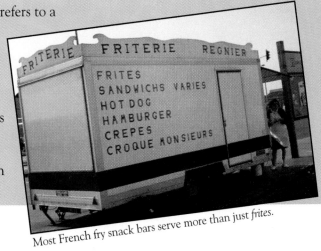

Most French fry snack bars serve more than just *frites*.

People of all ages drink mineral water. Some popular brands are Vittel, Perrier, Vichy, Contrex, Évian and Badoit. Fruit juices are not just for breakfast but are served throughout the day. Usually, only young children drink milk. **Un diabolo menthe** is a sweet drink made by mixing lemon-lime soda with mint-flavored syrup. Other drinks can be made with different flavored syrups. French speakers also buy soft drinks, such as Coke and Pepsi.

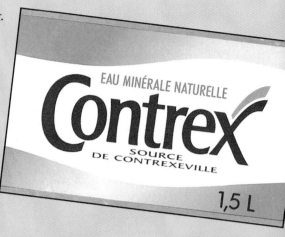

EAU MINÉRALE NATURELLE
Contrex
SOURCE DE CONTREXEVILLE
1,5 L

The French, even teenagers, have coffee at the end of a meal, rather than during it. They may order **un express** (*espresso coffee*) or **un café crème** (*coffee with cream*) during the day when at a café with their friends. Coffee is made and served one cup at a time rather than by the pot.

Students often stop with their friends at **crêperies** (*crêpe shops*), where they snack on a dessert crêpe. Resembling thin pancakes, crêpes can be

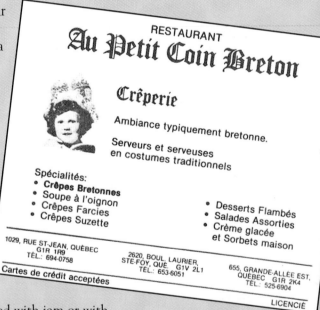

RESTAURANT
Au Petit Coin Breton

Crêperie

Ambiance typiquement bretonne.

Serveurs et serveuses en costumes traditionnels

Spécialités:
• **Crêpes Bretonnes**
• Soupe à l'oignon
• Crêpes Farcies
• Crêpes Suzette

• Desserts Flambés
• Salades Assorties
• Crème glacée et Sorbets maison

1029, RUE ST-JEAN, QUÉBEC
G1R 1R9
TÉL.: 694-0758

2620, BOUL. LAURIER,
STE-FOY, QUÉ. G1V 2L1
TÉL.: 653-6051

655, GRANDE-ALLÉE EST,
QUÉBEC G1R 2K4
TÉL.: 525-6904

Cartes de crédit acceptées

LICENCIÉ

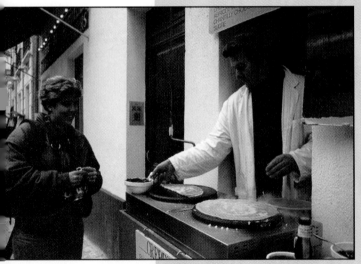

What would you like your crêpe filled with—chocolate, jam, whipped cream? (Paris)

filled with jam or with butter and sugar or even with chocolate. They originated in the province of Brittany in northwestern France but are now a popular dessert throughout the country. As a meal, these pancakes can be made with buckwheat flour. Then called **galettes**, they may be filled with ham, eggs or cheese.

1 Say in French whether you're hungry or thirsty, depending on whether you see a food or a beverage.

Modèle:

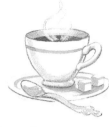

J'ai soif.

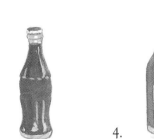

1.   4.   7.

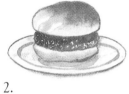 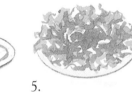 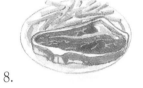

2.   5.   8.

3.   6.

2 Complete each sentence by identifying the numbered item you see in the illustration.

Modèle:
C'est une....
C'est une **omelette.**

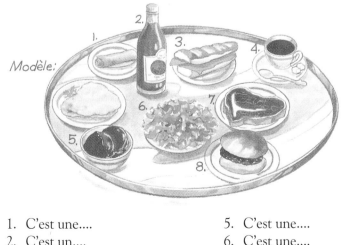

1. C'est une....
2. C'est un....
3. C'est un....
4. C'est un....

5. C'est une....
6. C'est une....
7. C'est un....
8. C'est un....

3 | If you had a choice between two items, say which one you would order.

1. Vous désirez une glace à la vanille ou une glace au chocolat?
2. Vous désirez un sandwich au fromage ou un steak-frites?
3. Vous désirez un jus de pomme ou un jus de raisin?
4. Vous désirez un coca ou une limonade?
5. Vous désirez une quiche ou une salade?
6. Vous désirez un hamburger ou un hot-dog?
7. Vous désirez une pomme ou une orange?

Modèle:

Vous désirez un café ou un jus d'orange?

Donnez-moi un jus d'orange, s'il vous plaît.

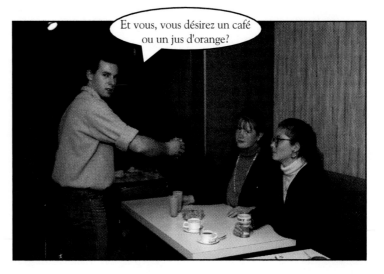

Et vous, vous désirez un café ou un jus d'orange?

Structure

Gender of nouns and indefinite articles

A noun is the name of a person, place or thing. Can you pick out the nouns in the following sentences?

1. Je voudrais une salade et un jus de pomme.
2. Donnez-moi aussi un café, s'il vous plaît.

In the first sentence the nouns are **salade** and **jus de pomme**, and in the second sentence the noun is **café**.

Unlike nouns in English, every French noun has a gender, either masculine or feminine. You will need to remember the gender of each French noun that you learn. You can usually tell if a noun is masculine or feminine by what precedes it. For example, a noun preceded by **un** is masculine, and a noun preceded by **une** is feminine. **Un** and **une**, meaning "a" or "an," are called indefinite articles. In the two sentences above, you can tell that the noun **salade** is feminine because it is preceded by **une**; the nouns **jus de pomme** and **café** are masculine because they are preceded by **un**. If you don't know whether a noun is masculine or feminine, you can find out by looking it up in the end vocabulary of this textbook.

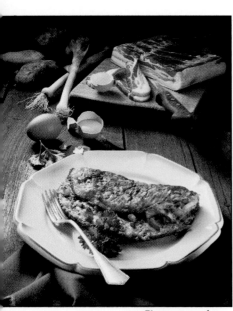

C'est une omelette.

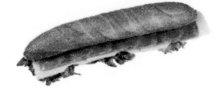

Pratique

4 Here are some café receipts. Count the number of masculine items and the number of feminine items on each one.

Café de l'Univers

	15,00
un jus de pomme	18,00
un thé	21,00
une eau minérale	27,00
une salade verte	70,00
un steak-frites	23,00
une crêpe	174,00
Total	

Café Olé

un coca	20,00
une limonade	19,00
un sandwich au jambon	28,00
un croque-monsieur	30,00
Total	97,00

Café Brocéliande

un diabolo menthe	22,00
un jus de raisin	15,00
une glace à la vanille	32,00
une glace au chocolat	32,00
Total	101,00

Café de la place de l'Horloge

	15,00
un express	18,00
un café-crème	20,00
un chocolat	27,00
une tarte aux fraises	9,00
un croissant	89,00
Total	

---

5 Using the café receipts from Activity 4, name one item you could order for each of the following prices.

1. 19,00
2. 21,00
3. 70,00
4. 23,00
5. 32,00
6. 20,00

Modèle:

18,00
un café-crème

6 With a partner, play the roles of various customers at a sidewalk café and a server. Student A orders certain things to eat and drink; Student B repeats each order to make sure everything is correct. Follow the model.

Modèle:

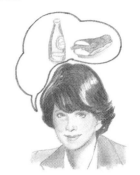

Student A: Je voudrais un sandwich au fromage et une eau minérale, s'il vous plaît.

Student B: Alors, un sandwich au fromage et une eau minérale?

Student A: Oui, Monsieur/ Madame/Mademoiselle.

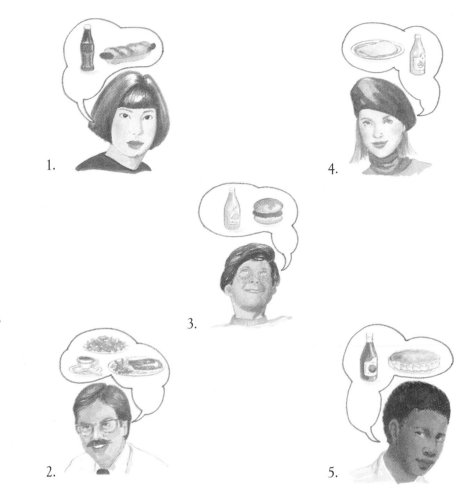

1.

2.

3.

4.

5.

Communication

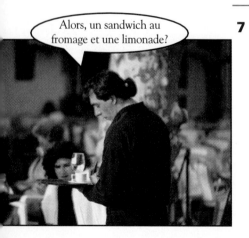

Alors, un sandwich au fromage et une limonade?

7 With two of your classmates, play the roles of two customers at a sidewalk café and the server who waits on them. The two customers are each going to order a snack and something to drink. In the course of the conversation:

1. The server and the two customers greet each other.
2. The server asks what the customers would like.
3. Each customer politely orders a snack and something to drink.
4. As the server repeats the two orders, he or she gets them mixed up, switching the beverages.
5. Each customer again says his or her order.
6. The server repeats both orders correctly.

You and your family are traveling together in France. You decide to stop at a fast-food restaurant for something to eat and drink. Since you are the only one who knows any French, you have to order for the whole family. Before you place your order, make a list in French of what everyone wants. (You should order something for yourself that no one else has ordered.) You should organize your list by categories so that you can order efficiently at the counter.

Your mother wants a salad and mineral water.

Your father wants something hot to eat and a hot drink.

Your sister wants ice cream and a cold drink.

Your brother wants a sandwich and fruit juice.

You want....

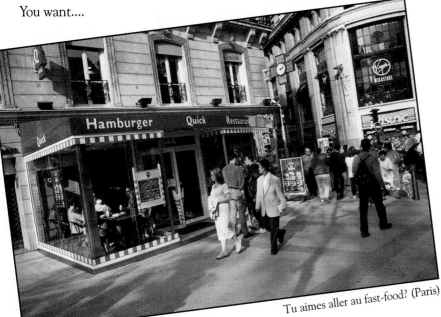

Tu aimes aller au fast-food? (Paris)

Four of your friends are coming over to your house after school today to work on a group project. You know they will all be hungry, so you decide to pick up something to eat and drink at a fast-food restaurant on your way home. Decide what you are going to order and then write it down so that you will remember everything you want when you pull up to the microphone to place your order.

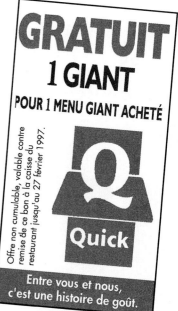

Mise au point sur... la cuisine française

When they are not enjoying meals at home with their families, French people like to eat out. French restaurants have earned the reputation of serving some of the best cuisine in the world. You can grab a sandwich from a sidewalk stand, spend some time at a café or eat a meal consisting of many courses at an elegant restaurant.

While walking downtown, people often grab a simple snack, such as a sandwich, hot dog, crêpe or slice of pizza, from a sidewalk stand. People with more time usually stop at a café where they can talk with friends, read the newspaper or watch people strolling by as they eat their food. Cafés are everywhere; you often see two or three of them in a row. Since menus are displayed outside cafés, you know in advance what is available and how much it will cost. In nice weather people usually sit on **la terrasse** (*terrace*) outside in front

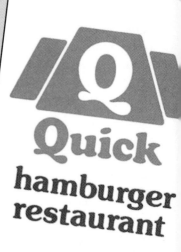

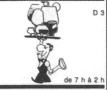

Café **LE GLOBE**
BAR - BRASSERIE - GLACIER - COCKTAIL
DANS SON NOUVEAU DÉCOR 1900
34, rue Lenepveu - 49100 ANGERS
☎ 41.88.49.95
de 7 h à 2 h
D 3

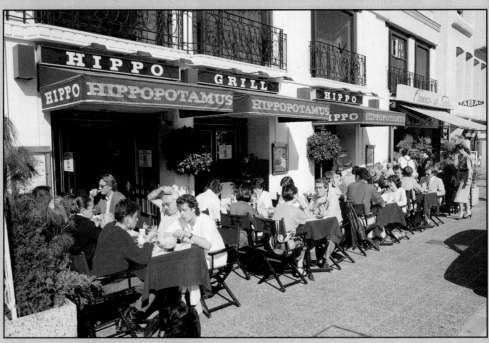

Café terraces are crowded when the weather is warm and sunny. (Nice)

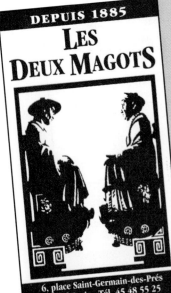

DEPUIS 1885
LES DEUX MAGOTS
6, place Saint-Germain-des-Prés
75006 Paris - Tél. 45 48 55 25

of a café. In winter most people eat inside. French cafés serve customers from early in the morning until late in the evening. In small towns, friends often gather at the local café, while tourists in Paris visit some of the world-famous cafés, such as the Deux Magots, the Café de Flore and Fouquet's.

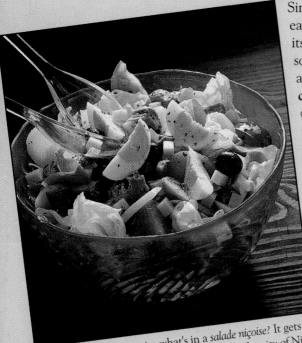

Can you recognize what's in a *salade niçoise*? It gets its name from the city of Nice.

Since each region of France and each French-speaking country has its own specialty, there is something available for every taste and budget. You can order **choucroute garnie** (*sauerkraut with meat*) from the Alsace region near Germany, a **crêpe** from Brittany or a **salade niçoise** (*salad made with lettuce, cold vegetables, hard-cooked eggs, olives, anchovies, tuna and a vinaigrette dressing*) from the city of Nice on the Riviera. Of course, each region produces

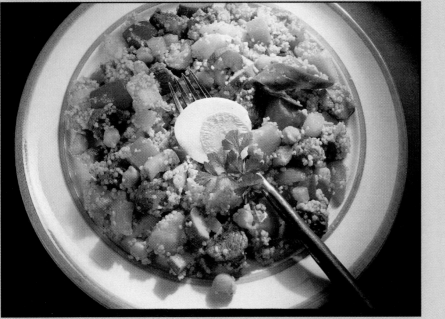

Couscous, a spicy meat stew on a bed of semolina, is a popular main course.

its own cheese, wine and even candy to share with the rest of the country. North African restaurants serve **couscous**, a dish of steamed semolina usually accompanied by a meat stew and a variety of sauces. Creole cuisine, from Martinique and Guadeloupe, is fairly spicy and uses many different fruits and seafoods. **La tourtière**, a meat potpie, originated in Quebec. Spicy Cajun cuisine from New Orleans is popular throughout the world.

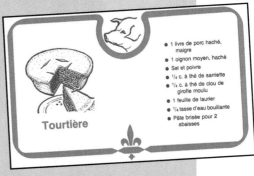

Tourtière

- 1 livre de porc haché, maigre
- 1 oignon moyen, haché
- Sel et poivre
- ¼ c. à thé de sarriette
- ¼ c. à thé de clou de girofle moulu
- 1 feuille de laurier
- ¼ tasse d'eau bouillante
- Pâte brisée pour 2 abaisses

For a meal with several courses, people may go to a restaurant. The most popular kinds of restaurants feature typical, country-style dishes which are prepared with fresh ingredients. Good restaurants are often quite small and the chef may be one of the owners. In eating formally at a

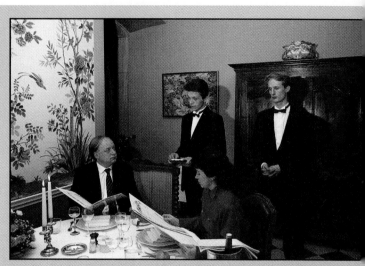

A full-course meal at a restaurant may last several hours. (Château d'Isenbour

restaurant, people can choose either certain courses from the menu or a full-course meal at a fixed price. They may eat various courses, starting with an **hors-d'œuvre**, such as **crudités** (*raw vegetables, often shredded*), then a meat and vegetable course, a salad, cheese and finally dessert. Some fixed-price meals may have only three courses. Diners eat fresh bread throughout the entire meal. A small cup of espresso is served at the end. You can expect to wait a while between courses at a French restaurant. French people do not like to eat quickly and often spend hours at the table. They take great pleasure in eating well. It is often said that a good meal is composed of three parts: good food, plenty of time and good conversation.

~ **MENU à 69 F** ~

ENTRÉE AU CHOIX

Tartine du Baptiste
Salade aux noix
Salade au bleu
Crudités du marché
Champignons à la grecque (maison)
Oeufs durs mayonnaise
Cervelas en salade
Terrine de foies de volailles
Filets de harengs
Entrée du jour..... au tableau !

PLAT AU CHOIX
(Accompagné de frites ou garniture du jour)

Brochette de boeuf grillée, sauce maison
Tranche de gigot d'agneau grillée
Steak savoyard (boeuf haché, grillé gratiné)

L'idée poisson ou L'idée du jour
(Suivant l'humeur du Chef !!!)

DESSERT AU CHOIX

Crème caramel
Mousse au chocolat
Flan à la noix de coco
Terrine de fruits, au chocolat chaud ou au coulis de framboises
Glaces ou sorbets, deux parfums au choix
(vanille, chocolat, café, coco, citron vert, cassis, poire, passion)
Coupe damnation
(crème de marrons, chocolat chaud, crème fraîche)
Tarte au citron
Dessert du jour
(Autre dessert de la carte, plus 12 F)

~ **FORMULE à 59 F** ~

Une Entrée ou un Dessert du Menu à 69 F
avec un Plat de ce même menu

Prix nets - Service compris

Carafe d'eau gratuite

0   Answer the following questions.

1. What are three types of French eating establishments?
2. What can you order to eat at a sidewalk stand?
3. Besides eating, what do people do at cafés?
4. How can you decide where you want to eat before sitting down?
5. What are two regional specialties from France?
6. What is a specialty from North Africa?
7. Where do French people go for a larger meal?
8. What are five courses a typical French restaurant serves?
9. Why may the service seem slow to an American who dines at a French restaurant?
10. For a French person, what three ingredients compose a good meal?

1   Imagine that you are a server at the restaurant called Le Rétro. You must prepare the check for your table of three customers, using the receipt from the Chez Paul restaurant as a model. Your customers at Le Rétro ordered a salad, a steak with fries, an omelette, a quiche, a cup of coffee, a bottle of Badoit mineral water and a Coke. The check you make should show the name, address and phone number of the restaurant, the number of the table you have been serving, the number of people at the table (**couverts**) and a list of the food and prices as well as the total amount to be paid.

Restaurant **LE RÉTRO**

Babeth et Roger

1, rue Paul Fort
75014 PARIS
Tél. 45 40 97 56

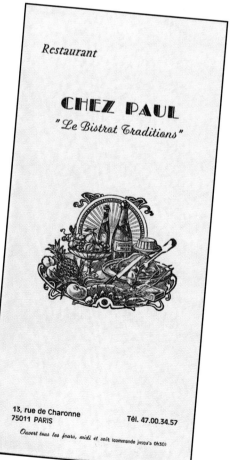

```
**********CHEZ    PAUL**********
            COMME CHEZ SOI
        13 RUE DE CHARONNE 75011
            TEL  47 00 34 57


TABLE         7

COUVERTS:   3

    1 POULET A L ESTRAGON        62.00
    1 LEGUMES SAISON             20.00
    1 ESCALOPE SAUMON            68.00
    1 SOUPE DE MELON             35.00
    1 DOUBLE CAFE                18.00
    1 BADOIT BT                  28.00
    1 PICHET 50 SAUVIGNON        36.00
    ===================================
        S/TOTAL               267.00


  *  TOTAL  *        267.00


MAISON RECOMMANDEE PAR LES GUIDES ROUGES

DIM 04  JUL 97       Garcon  *  O  *
```

Restaurant

CHEZ PAUL
"*Le Bistrot Traditions*"

13, rue de Charonne
75011 PARIS   Tél. 47.00.34.57

Ouvert tous les jours, midi et soir (commande jusqu'a 0h30)

Leçon C

In this lesson you will be able to:

➤ **ask for a price**

➤ **state prices**

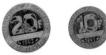

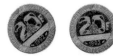

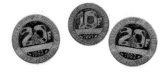

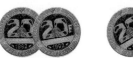

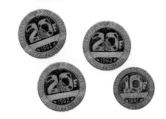

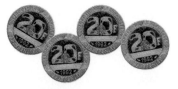

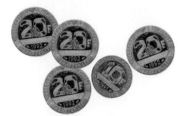

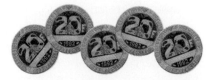

20 VINGT
21 vingt et un
22 vingt-deux
23 vingt-trois

30 TRENTE
31 trente et un
32 trente-deux
33 trente-trois

40 QUARANTE
41 quarante et un
42 quarante-deux
43 quarante-trois

50 CINQUANTE
51 cinquante et un
52 cinquante-deux
53 cinquante-trois

60 SOIXANTE
61 soixante et un
62 soixante-deux
63 soixante-trois

70 SOIXANTE-DIX
71 soixante et onze
72 soixante-douze
73 soixante-treize
74 soixante-quatorze
75 soixante-quinze
76 soixante-seize
77 soixante-dix-sept
78 soixante-dix-huit
79 soixante-dix-neuf

80 QUATRE-VINGTS
81 quatre-vingt-un
82 quatre-vingt-deux
83 quatre-vingt-trois

90 QUATRE-VINGT-DIX
91 quatre-vingt-onze
92 quatre-vingt-douze
93 quatre-vingt-treize
94 quatre-vingt-quatorze
95 quatre-vingt-quinze
96 quatre-vingt-seize
97 quatre-vingt-dix-sept
98 quatre-vingt-dix-huit
99 quatre-vingt-dix-neuf

100 CENT

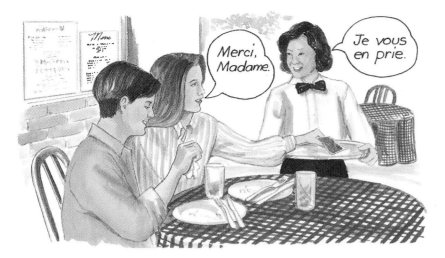

Jean-François and Myriam have just finished eating and are ready to pay the bill.

Jean-François: **Ça fait combien, Madame?**
Serveuse: **Voyons, le sandwich au jambon coûte vingt-huit francs, la quiche... trente-cinq francs, et les deux boissons... trente-quatre francs. Ça fait quatre-vingt-dix-sept francs.**
Myriam: **Voilà cent francs. Merci, Madame.**
Serveuse: **Je vous en prie.**

On a menu the words **service compris** mean that the tip (a 15% service charge) is included in the bill, but most people leave some small change as an extra tip for good service.

Enquête culturelle

Le franc is the basic unit of money in France and in many other French-speaking countries, such as Belgium, Luxembourg, Switzerland, Senegal and the Ivory Coast. In each country it has a different value. Depending on the daily exchange rate, there are usually between five and six francs to the dollar in France. French money includes bills (**les billets**) and coins (**les pièces de monnaie**). Bills are issued in denominations of 20,

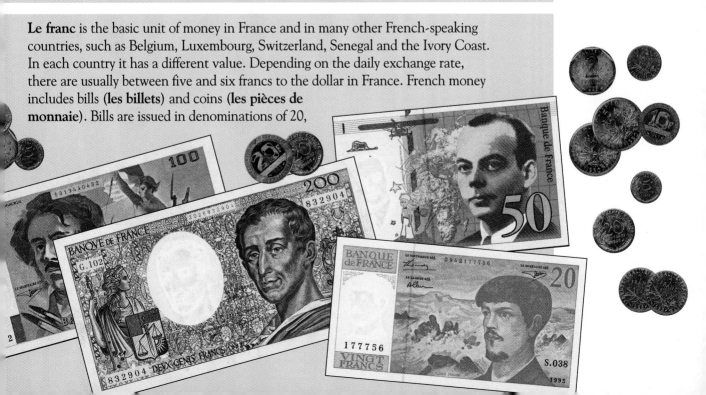

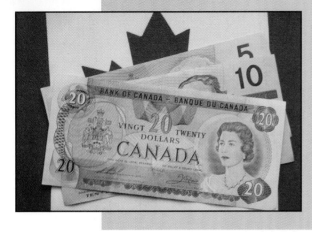

50, 100, 200 and 500 francs. Usually, the greater the value, the larger the bill. Coins are issued in denominations of 1/2, 1, 2, 5, 10 and 20 francs. The **franc** is divided into 100 **centimes**, coins that are smaller and lighter than the **franc**. In general, French money is heavier and bigger than American money. Prices in **francs** are written with an **F** and sometimes a comma (**36,50F** or **36F 50 = trente-six francs cinquante**). Some other currencies used in French-speaking countries are **le dinar** (Algeria and Tunisia), **le dirham** (Morocco) and **le dollar canadien** (Quebec).

1 Answer the following questions.

1. How do you ask in French how much something costs?
2. How do you say "You're welcome" in French?
3. What words appear on a menu to let you know that the tip is included in the bill?
4. What is the basic unit of money in France?
5. What are some other countries that use money with this name?
6. How do French coins compare to those used in the United States?
7. How do you write **dix-huit francs cinquante**?

2 *Ça fait combien? Répondez en français.*

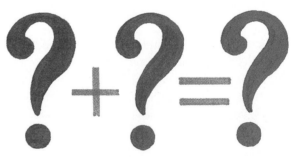

1. Douze et vingt-trois?
2. Quatorze et quarante-deux?
3. Trente-sept et vingt-huit?
4. Quarante et trente-trois?
5. Cinquante et trente?
6. Soixante et vingt et un?
7. Soixante-dix et vingt?
8. Treize et trente-quatre?

3 By looking at the menu and totaling prices, say how much the food and beverage combinations that follow cost.

sandwich au fromage	23F
steak-frites	75F
crêpe	21F
quiche	24F
omelette	28F
salade	21F
glace à la vanille	30F
eau minérale	17F
café	16F
jus d'orange	18F
jus de pomme	18F
limonade	19F
coca	20F

1. une crêpe et un jus d'orange
2. un sandwich au fromage et un jus de pomme
3. une quiche et une limonade
4. un steak-frites et un coca
5. une glace à la vanille et un café
6. une salade et une eau minérale

4 *C'est à toi!*

1. Tu aimes aller au café?
2. Qu'est-ce que tu manges au café?
3. Tu aimes beaucoup aller au fast-food?
4. Qu'est-ce que tu manges au fast-food?
5. Qu'est-ce que tu aimes comme dessert?
6. Qu'est-ce que tu aimes comme boisson?

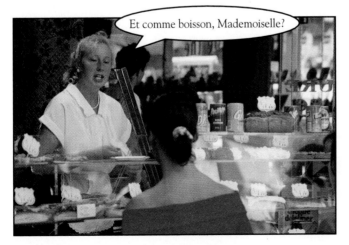

Et comme boisson, Mademoiselle?

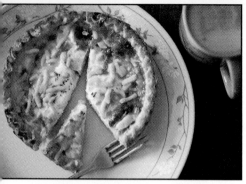

J'aime bien la quiche.

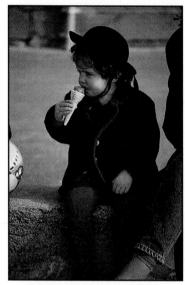

La glace est délicieuse. (Biarritz)

Structure

Definite articles

To refer to a specific person, place or thing, you use a definite article. In French the singular definite articles are **le, la** and **l'**, all meaning "the."

Le precedes a masculine word beginning with a consonant sound.

> **Le** sandwich au jambon coûte 28 francs.   *The ham sandwich costs 28 francs.*

La precedes a feminine word beginning with a consonant sound.

> **La** quiche est délicieuse.   *The quiche is delicious.*

L' is used instead of **le** or **la** before a masculine or feminine word beginning with a vowel sound.

> Je préfère **l'**eau minérale.   *I prefer mineral water.*
> **L'**omelette est pour Marie-Hélène.   *The omelette is for Marie-Hélène.*

A definite article may also designate a noun in a general sense.

> J'aime **la** glace.   *I like ice cream (in general).*

The subject pronoun **il** (*it*) may replace a masculine singular noun.

> **Le** dessert est superbe.   *The dessert is superb.*
> **Il** est superbe.   *It is superb.*

The subject pronoun **elle** (*it*) may replace a feminine singular noun.

> **La** salade est fraîche.   *The salad is fresh.*
> **Elle** est fraîche.   *It is fresh.*

Pratique

5   Tell whether or not you like the following foods and beverages.

Modèles:

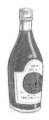

J'aime la glace à la vanille.

Je n'aime pas le jus d'orange.

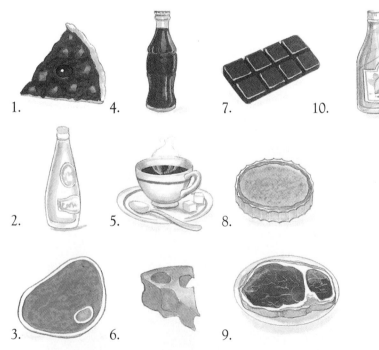

1.   4.   7.   10.

2.   5.   8.

3.   6.   9.

You and your partner are at a café. Student A, who has never been to this café before, asks how much certain things cost. Student B, who comes to this café almost every day, answers Student A's questions.

1. jus de pomme/18F
2. omelette/28F
3. steak-frites/40F
4. salade/23F
5. eau minérale/21F
6. café/19F
7. crêpe/30F
8. glace à la vanille/32F

Modèle:

sandwich au fromage/26F

Student A: Combien coûte le sandwich au fromage?

Student B: Il coûte vingt-six francs.

Plurals

The plural form of the definite articles **le, la** and **l'** is **les** (*the*).

> **Les** deux boissons coûtent 34 francs.   *The two drinks cost 34 francs.*

To form the plural of most singular nouns, add an **s**. This **s** is never pronounced. Nouns that already end in **-s** in the singular do not change in the plural.

la quiche	les quiches
le dessert	les desserts
le fast-food	les fast-foods
le jus d'orange	les jus d'orange

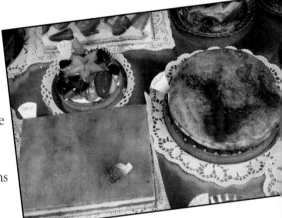

In spoken French the sound of **les** is often the only indication that the noun is plural. Always be careful to distinguish the sound of **les** from the sounds of **le** and **la**.

> Voilà **le** sandwich.   Voilà **les** sandwichs.

The subject pronoun **ils** may replace one or more masculine plural nouns or a mixed group of nouns.

> **Les deux cafés** coûtent 32 francs.   **Ils** coûtent 32 francs.
> **Le chocolat et la limonade** coûtent 38 francs.   **Ils** coûtent 38 francs.

Combien coûtent les desserts?

The subject pronoun **elles** may replace one or more feminine plural nouns.

> **Les boissons** coûtent 33 francs.   **Elles** coûtent 33 francs.

The plural form of the indefinite articles **un** and **une** is **des** (*some*).

> Vous désirez **des** frites?   *Do you want some French fries?*

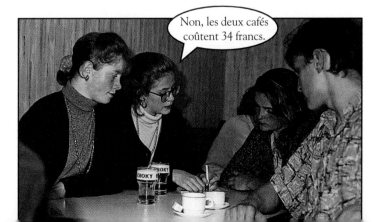

Non, les deux cafés coûtent 34 francs.

Pratique

7 Make a generalization about what each person likes.

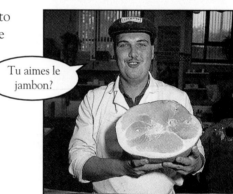

Moi? J'aime beaucoup les sports!

Modèle:

Sandrine désire une eau minérale et un café.
Elle aime les boissons.

1. André mange un sandwich au fromage et un sandwich au jambon.
2. Janine désire une glace et deux crêpes.
3. Khaled aime le jus de raisin et le coca.
4. Luc joue au foot et au tennis.
5. David aime *Aladdin* et *Dracula*.
6. Delphine n'aime pas les cafés. Elle préfère aller au Quick ou au Macdo.

8 Find out what your partner likes to eat. Ask each other if you like the indicated foods.

Tu aimes le jambon?

Modèle:

hamburgers/steak
Student A: **Tu aimes les hamburgers?**
Student B: **Oui, j'aime les hamburgers. Tu aimes le steak?**
Student A: **Non, je n'aime pas le steak.**

1. quiche/omelettes
2. sandwichs/salade
3. hot-dogs/jambon
4. pizza/frites
5. crêpes/glace
6. chocolat/raisins
7. pommes/oranges

9 With a partner, play the roles of a customer and a server at the Café Alexandre. Student A gets the receipt for the entire table. Because the receipt shows only the total price of the food and beverages ordered, Student A asks how much certain things cost. Student B answers these questions according to his or her handwritten list.

Modèle:

3 cocas
Student A: **Combien coûtent les trois cocas?**
Student B: **Ils coûtent cinquante-sept francs.**

3 cocas @ 19F	57F
2 jus de pomme @ 18F	36F
3 cafés @ 16F	48F
2 salades @ 22F	44F
2 quiches @ 21F	42F
3 sandwichs @ 23F	69F
2 crêpes @ 20F	40F
3 glaces @ 15F	45F

1. 2 jus de pomme
2. 3 cafés
3. 2 salades
4. 2 quiches
5. 3 sandwichs
6. 2 crêpes
7. 3 glaces

0 Based on their orders, tell what each pair of café customers wants to eat or drink.

1. Mme Montand: Je voudrais une glace au chocolat, s'il vous plaît.
   Mme Arnaud: Et moi, je voudrais une glace à la vanille.
2. Anne: Donnez-moi une crêpe, s'il vous plaît.
   Sara: Et pour moi, une glace.
3. Dikembe: Donnez-moi un sandwich au jambon, s'il vous plaît.
   Lamine: Et moi, je voudrais un sandwich au fromage.
4. Marie: Donnez-moi un café, s'il vous plaît.
   Daniel: Et moi, je voudrais une eau minérale.

Modèle:

Sophie: Je voudrais un coca, s'il vous plaît.
Jérémy: Donnez-moi une limonade, s'il vous plaît.
Sophie et Jérémy désirent des boissons.

Communication

1 Picture what the menu of a small neighborhood café would look like. Create this menu in French, including at least seven beverages and ten food items, each with a price indicated in francs. Give your café a French name. One idea would be to use the word **chez** (meaning "the place of") plus your French name.

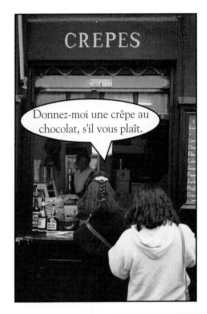

Donnez-moi une crêpe au chocolat, s'il vous plaît.

2 It's a law in France that all cafés and restaurants must post their menus outside for customers to see. You and your classmates should take the menus you made in Activity 11 and attach them to the walls in your classroom. Imagine that each menu is posted outside a different café in France. You and your partner have decided to go to a café for something to eat and drink. Walk around your classroom, noting menu prices and picking a café to eat at.

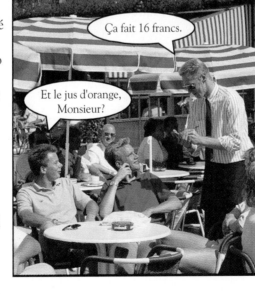

Ça fait 16 francs.

Et le jus d'orange, Monsieur?

1. Look at the menu of one of the cafés. You and your partner each name one beverage and one food item from the menu and say the prices. Do this for a total of five café menus.

Modèle:

Bruno: Voyons... la limonade - 17 francs, le sandwich au fromage - 24 francs.
Théo: Le jus d'orange - 16 francs, la glace au chocolat - 12 francs 50.
Bruno et Théo: (Name beverages, food items and their prices at four other cafés.)
Bruno: Alors, allons au café Chez Patricia!
Théo: Moi, je préfère aller au café Chez Christophe.
Bruno: D'accord. Allons-y!

2. After noting the prices at the five cafés, you and your partner each suggest one café to go to.
3. Agree on one café and go there.

Modèle:

Serveur:	Bonjour, Messieurs-Dames. Vous désirez?
Bruno:	Je voudrais une limonade et un sandwich au fromage.
Théo:	Donnez-moi un jus d'orange et une glace au chocolat, s'il vous plaît.

. . . .

Bruno:	La limonade, ça fait combien, Monsieur?
Serveur:	Ça fait 17 francs.
Théo:	Et le jus d'orange?
Serveur:	Ça fait 16 francs.
Bruno:	Voilà. Merci.
Théo:	Et voilà. Merci.
Serveur:	Je vous en prie.

13 With two of your classmates, play the roles of two customers at a sidewalk café and the server who waits on them. The server asks what the customers would like, and each one tells the server the food item and the beverage that he or she wants. After the customers finish eating, they are ready to pay, but they have some questions about the bill. In the course of the conversation:

1. The server greets the two customers and asks what they would like.
2. Each customer orders something to eat and drink.
3. After they finish eating, the customers are ready to pay their bill, but they notice that the two beverages have been omitted. Since both customers have forgotten the beverage prices, they ask the server to repeat them.
4. The server gives the price of each beverage.
5. Each customer pays his or her share of the bill and thanks the server.
6. The server says you're welcome.

Sur la bonne piste

When reading, you naturally encounter new words. As you read in French, try not to look up the words you don't know in a dictionary. Instead, try to make sense of the reading as a whole by identifying cognates. "*Cognate*" is related to the word "re*cognize*." If you recognize a word in French because there is a similar word in English, it may be a cognate. For instance, the words **invitation, table** and **café** are direct cognates; they mean the same thing in French as they do in English. For many people, the French word **préfère** looks enough like the English word "prefer" that they can quickly understand the sentence **Je préfère le chocolat**. The words **histoire** and **cours** are more or less direct cognates, although some people might not immediately recognize **histoire** as "history" or **cours** as "course." Unfortunately, there are words in French that are false cognates. A false cognate is a French word that looks like an English word but means something quite different. For example, the word **but** in French means "goal." **Chose** in French is not a verb ("to choose") but a "thing."

Here are two hints to help you make more educated guesses about possible cognates. 1) For words that contain a letter with a circumflex (^), imagine that there is an "s" that replaces or follows that letter. For example, if you add an "s" to the French word **coûter**, it starts to look like the English word "cost." 2) For French words that begin with an **é**, replace the **é** with an "s" to discover what the word means in English. For example, **école** means "school." Read the conversation that follows, remembering to pay attention to the title, the context, the order of sentences and possible cognates.

Au café

Isabelle rencontre son copain Michel à l'école.

— Salut, Michel. Ça va?
— Bien.
— Tu vas au café maintenant?

— Non, j'ai un cours.

Michel n'accepte pas l'invitation. Il va à son cours d'histoire. Isabelle a faim et elle va au café Printemps pour déjeuner.

À la terrasse du café Printemps, le serveur arrive à sa table.

— Qu'est-ce que vous désirez, Mademoiselle?

— Je ne sais pas. Qu'est-ce qu'il y a aujourd'hui?

— Des steaks-frites, des crêpes au jambon et au fromage, une belle salade niçoise, de la soupe du jour, des sandwichs....

— Combien coûtent les sandwichs?

— 25 francs.

— Je voudrais un sandwich au thon, aux œufs et au maïs, avec de la mayonnaise, s'il vous plaît. Et puis, comme j'ai soif aussi, je prendrais....

— Du thé? Du café? Du coca? Une eau minérale? Un jus d'orange?

— Je voudrais un coca, s'il vous plaît, et une glace au chocolat. Merci!

Après le déjeuner, le serveur lui apporte l'addition.

— Ça fait combien?

— Ça fait 45 francs.

— Voilà 50 francs. Merci, Monsieur.

— À votre service, Mademoiselle.

Après son cours, Michel rencontre son amie Isabelle devant le café. Quelle bonne surprise!

---

14   Make a list of all the words that you encountered in the reading that are cognates. If the French word is not spelled the same as its English counterpart, write the English word next to it.

Nathalie et Raoul

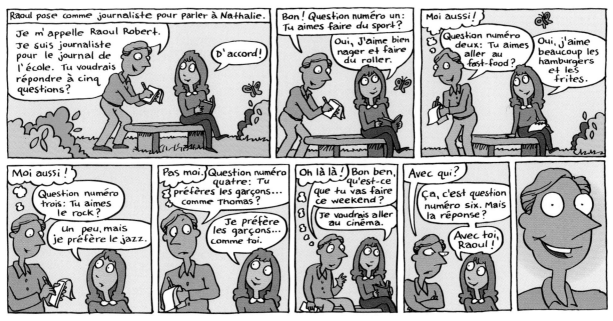

C'est à moi!

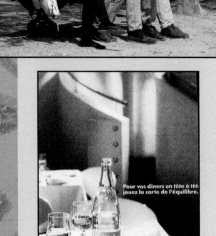

J'ai faim!

Moi, j'ai soif!

Now that you have completed this unit, take a look at what you should be able to do in French. Can you do all of these tasks?

➤ I can invite someone to do something.
➤ I can accept or refuse an invitation.
➤ I can order something to eat and drink.
➤ I can ask for and state the price of something.
➤ I can ask what time it is and tell time on the hour.
➤ I can ask people how they are and tell them how I am.
➤ I can say whether I'm hungry or thirsty.

Here is a brief checkup to see how much you understand about French culture. Decide if each statement is true (**vrai**) or false (**faux**).

1. Because France has strict rules about eating balanced meals, fast-food restaurants are not allowed in the country.
2. French families usually buy fresh bread and vegetables daily.
3. French fries originated in France.
4. Vichy, Perrier and Évian are popular brands of mineral water.
5. Crêpes resemble thin pancakes and can be filled with jam or with butter and sugar.
6. French cafés post their menus outside.
7. The French usually eat a salad before they begin their meat and vegetable course.
8. **Service compris** means that a service charge or tip is included in the price of the food and beverages.
9. **Le franc** is the basic unit of French money.

Communication orale

Imagine that the French classes in your school are planning to set up and run various French cafés for the upcoming International Day. Besides your classmates and other students, parents and community members (some of whom speak French) will also be coming to the event. You want to prepare and practice typical café conversations before the big day. With a partner, play the roles of a server and a customer. During the course of your brief practice conversation:

1. Greet each other in French.
2. Ask how each other is and respond.
3. The server asks the customer what he or she would like.
4. The customer orders something to eat and drink as well as something for dessert.
5. After the server brings the order and the customer finishes the meal, the customer asks the server how much it costs.
6. The server gives the price of each item and the total.
7. The customer says how much he or she is giving to cover the bill and tip.
8. The server thanks the customer.
9. Tell each other good-bye.

Communication écrite

To prepare for International Day and the cafés that you and other students are going to set up, divide into small groups. Each group will operate a café from one of the various regions of France. The menu of each café will reflect the types of food that are representative of that region. Begin by choosing a region of France and then, with members of your group, do research on what specific dishes come from that region. Next, determine a name for your café. Then design and write a menu that lists the food and beverages your café will serve, making the choices as authentic as you can for your region of France. Also give prices of the items in French francs. To be as realistic as possible, find the current rate of exchange for the French franc. (You can check the *Wall Street Journal* or other newspapers in your school library, or you may call a bank to learn the latest exchange rate.) Put that rate at the bottom of your menu so that your customers will be able to understand what their bill will be in dollars.

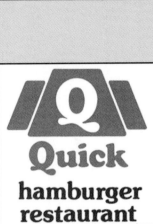

Communication active

To invite someone to do something, use:
On va au café? — *Shall we go to the café?*
Allons-y! — *Let's go (there)!*

To accept an invitation, use:
D'accord. — *OK.*

To refuse an invitation, use:
Moi, je préfère aller au fast-food. — *I prefer going to the fast-food restaurant.*

To order food and beverages, use:
Je voudrais une salade, **s'il vous plaît.** — *I would like a salad, please.*
Donnez-moi un café, **s'il vous plaît.** — *Give me (a cup of) coffee, please.*

To ask for a price, use:
Ça fait combien? — *How much is it/that?*

To state a price, use:
Ça fait vingt **francs.** — *That's/It's 20 francs.*
Ça coûte soixante **francs.** — *That costs 60 francs.*

To ask what time it is, use:
Quelle heure est-il? — *What time is it?*

To tell time on the hour, use:
Il est trois **heures.** — *It's three o'clock.*
Il est midi. — *It's noon.*
Il est minuit. — *It's midnight.*

To ask how someone is, use:
Comment vas-tu? — *How are you?*
Comment allez-vous? — *How are you?*

To tell how you are, use:
Très bien. — *Very well.*
Bien. — *Well.*
Pas mal. — *Not bad.*
Mal. — *Bad.*
Comme ci, comme ça. — *So-so.*
J'ai faim. — *I'm hungry.*
J'ai soif. — *I'm thirsty.*

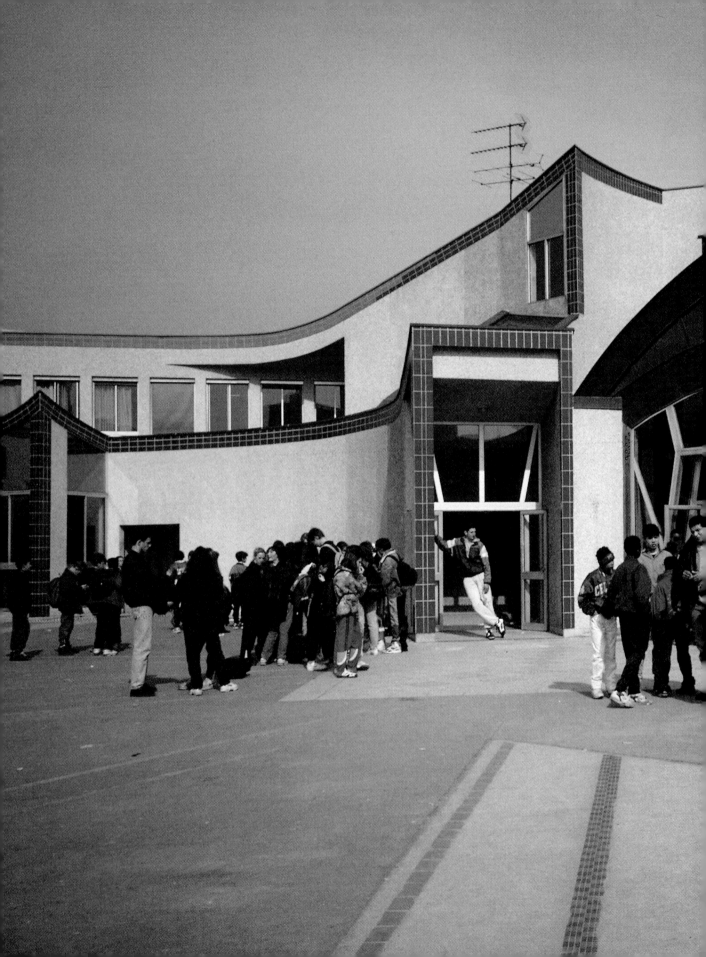

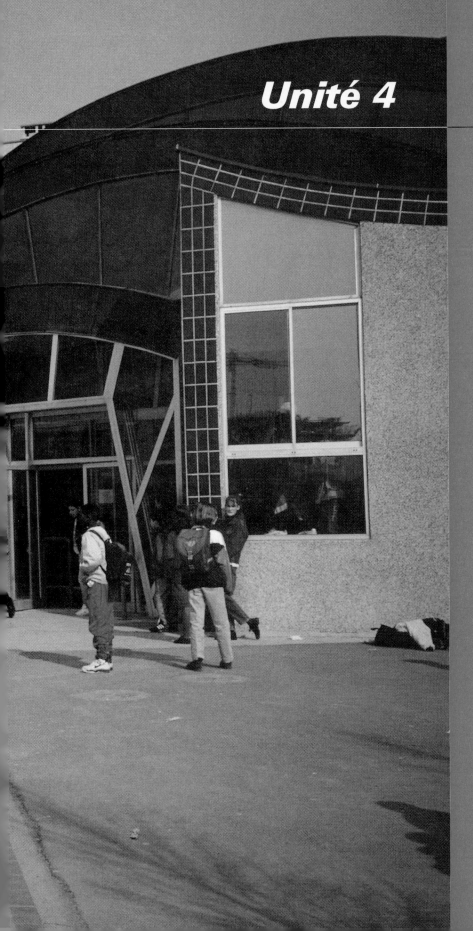

Unité 4

À l'école

In this unit you will be able to:

- ➤ express need
- ➤ ask what something is
- ➤ identify objects
- ➤ tell location
- ➤ ask for information
- ➤ give information
- ➤ agree and disagree
- ➤ express emotions
- ➤ describe daily routines
- ➤ invite
- ➤ state exact time

C'est une école.

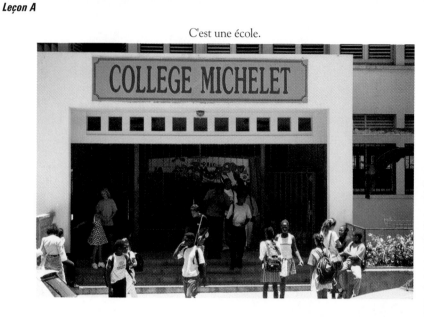

Leçon A

In this lesson you will be able to:

➤ express emotions

➤ express need

➤ ask for information

➤ tell location

➤ ask what something is

➤ identify objects

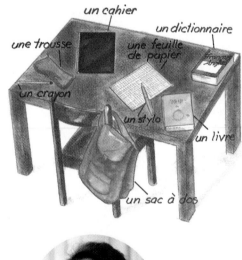

un cahier
un dictionnaire
une trousse
une feuille de papier
un crayon
un stylo
un livre
un sac à dos

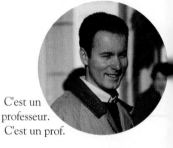

C'est un professeur.
C'est un prof.

C'est une élève.   C'est un élè

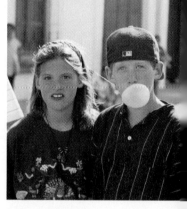

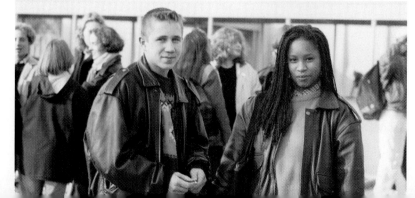

C'est un professeur.
C'est une prof.

C'est un étudiant.   C'est une étudiante.

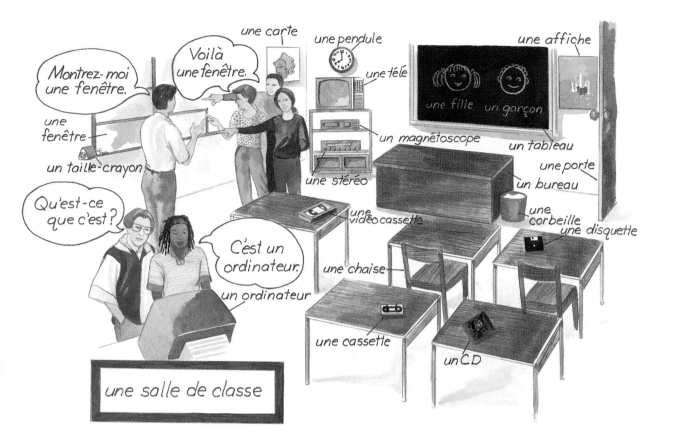

Montrez-moi une fenêtre.

Voilà une fenêtre.

une carte

une pendule

une affiche

une télé

une fenêtre

un taille-crayon

un magnétoscope

un tableau

une stéréo

une porte

un bureau

une corbeille

une disquette

Qu'est-ce que c'est ?

une vidéocassette

C'est un ordinateur.

une chaise

un ordinateur

une cassette

un CD

une salle de classe

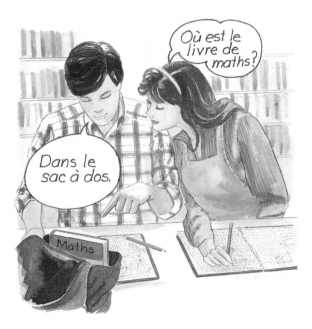

Où est le livre de maths ?

Dans le sac à dos.

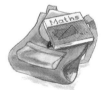

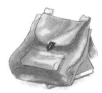

Sur le sac à dos.   Sous le sac à dos.

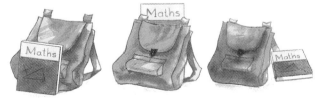

Devant le sac à dos.   Derrière le sac à dos.   Avec le sac à dos.

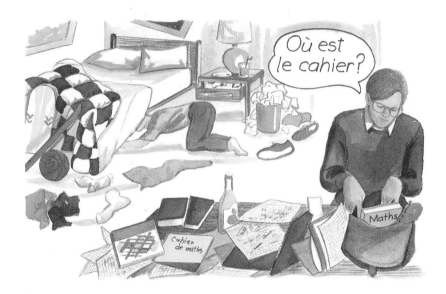

Alexandre and Louis are doing homework together.

Alexandre: **Zut! J'ai besoin d'étudier pour l'interro de maths, mais je n'ai pas le cahier. Où est le cahier de maths?**

Louis: **Dans le sac à dos?**

Alexandre: **Non, j'ai juste le livre de maths et la trousse dans le sac à dos.**

Louis: **Tiens! Qu'est-ce que c'est?**

Alexandre: **Quoi?**

Louis: **Là, devant toi, sur le bureau.**

Alexandre: **Oh, c'est le cahier de maths. Tant mieux. Bon ben, étudions!**

🔍 *Enquête culturelle*

French students often use **une trousse** to carry pens, pencils, rulers and other small school supplies. Students carry larger items in **un sac à dos**. In most French schools students do not have lockers; only teachers have a place to store their belongings.

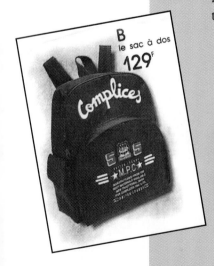

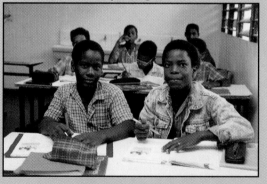

All students in Martinique bring their *trousses* to class.

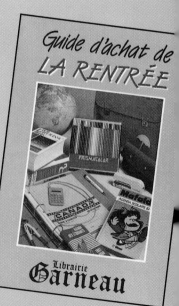

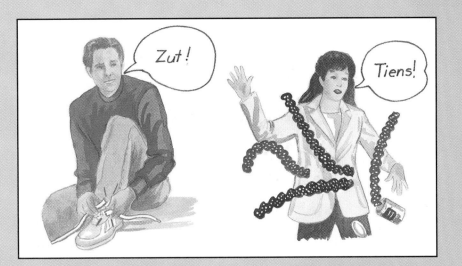

Just as you do, French speakers use short words to express strong emotion. For example, **zut!** shows disgust. You have already seen **eh!** and **tiens!** used to mean "hey!" when someone is surprised. Short French words are also used to fill pauses in conversations. For instance, **ben**, the shortened form of **bien**, means "well."

Many French schools are named after famous people, such as the rulers Charlemagne, Henri IV and Saint Louis. Although some buildings may be old, most of their facilities are very up-to-date.

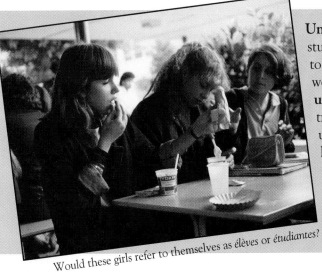

Un **élève** refers to a male student; une **élève** refers to a female student. The words **un étudiant** and **une étudiante** traditionally refer to university students, but high school students like to use these terms to refer to themselves.

Would these girls refer to themselves as *élèves* or *étudiantes*?

1 | *Répondez en français.*

1. Qui étudie avec Alexandre?
2. Alexandre étudie pour l'interro de maths?
3. Le cahier de maths est dans le sac à dos?
4. Le livre de maths est dans le sac à dos?
5. Où est la trousse?
6. Où est le cahier de maths?

2 | Identify each numbered person or object you see in the illustration.

Modèle:

C'est une pendule.

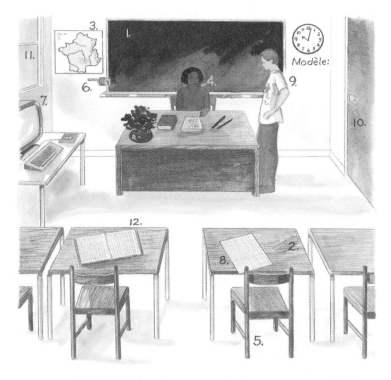

3 | A. *Où est Luc?* Say where Luc is in relation to the teacher's desk.

Modèle:

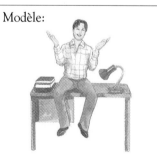

Luc est sur le bureau.

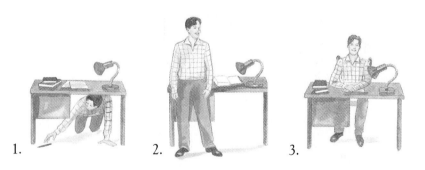

1. 2. 3.

B. *Où est la vidéocassette?* Say where the videocassette is in relation to the VCR.

Modèle:

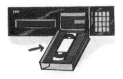

La vidéocassette est devant le magnétoscope.

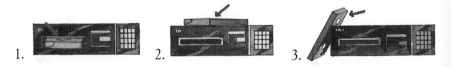

1. 2. 3.

4 | *C'est à toi!*

1. Tu étudies avec qui?
2. Tu aimes faire les devoirs?
3. Dans la salle de classe, qui est devant toi?
4. Dans la salle de classe, qui est derrière toi?
5. Qu'est-ce que tu préfères, un crayon ou un stylo?

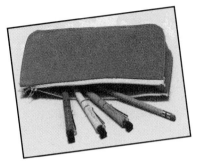

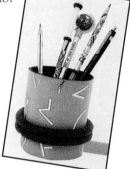

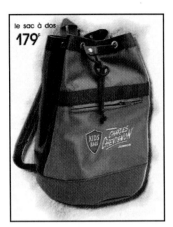

le sac à dos
179ᶠ

Structure

Present tense of the irregular verb *avoir*

The verb **avoir** (*to have*) is irregular.

avoir			
j'	**ai**	J'**ai** le cahier.	*I have the notebook.*
tu	**as**	Tu n'**as** pas la trousse?	*Don't you have the pencil case?*
il/elle/on	**a**	Luc **a** une heure de maths.	*Luc has one hour of math.*
nous	**avons**	Nous **avons** une interro.	*We have a quiz.*
vous	**avez**	Vous **avez** une feuille de papier?	*Do you have a sheet of paper?*
ils/elles	**ont**	Les Javert **ont** un ordinateur.	*The Javerts have a computer.*

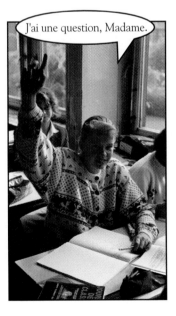

J'ai une question, Madame.

Note the sound [z] in the plural forms of **avoir: nous avons, vous avez, ils ont, elles ont.**

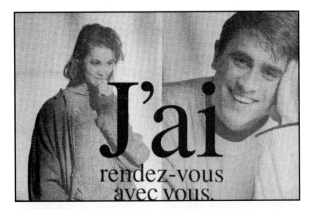

J'ai rendez-vous avec vous.

Pratique

5 | Tell whether the following students have pencils or pens in their pencil cases.

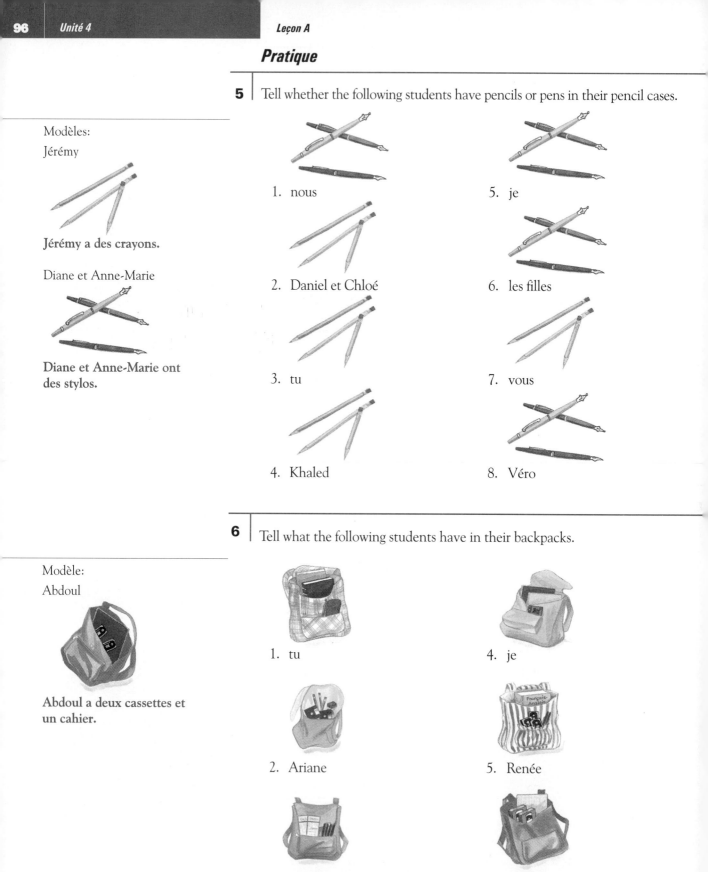

Modèles:

Jérémy

Jérémy a des crayons.

Diane et Anne-Marie

Diane et Anne-Marie ont des stylos.

1. nous

2. Daniel et Chloé

3. tu

4. Khaled

5. je

6. les filles

7. vous

8. Véro

6 | Tell what the following students have in their backpacks.

Modèle:

Abdoul

Abdoul a deux cassettes et un cahier.

1. tu

2. Ariane

3. Guillaume

4. je

5. Renée

6. Nicolas

7 | Your French class is going on a picnic today. Everyone who was supposed to bring food remembered. Unfortunately, everyone who was supposed to bring beverages forgot. Tell which people have what they were supposed to bring and which people don't.

1. Nicole et Olivier/la salade
2. vous/la limonade
3. nous/les hot-dogs
4. tu/le fromage
5. les garçons/le coca
6. je/les pommes
7. Michèle/la glace
8. le prof/l'eau minérale

Modèles:

Delphine et Saleh/les sandwichs
Delphine et Saleh ont les sandwichs.

Théo/le jus de pomme
Théo n'a pas le jus de pomme.

Expressions with *avoir*

You have already seen that forms of **avoir** are used in some French expressions where the verb "to be" is used in English. Two of these expressions are **avoir faim** (*to be hungry*) and **avoir soif** (*to be thirsty*).

J'ai faim.	*I'm hungry.*
Vous **avez soif**?	*Are you thirsty?*

To say that you need to do something or that you need something, use the expression **avoir besoin de** (*to need*). Remember that **de** becomes **d'** before a word beginning with a vowel sound.

Tu **as besoin de** téléphoner?	*Do you need to call?*
Oui, et j'**ai besoin d'**un franc.	*Yes, and I need a franc.*

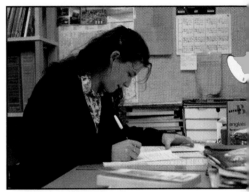

Véro a besoin d'étudier.

Pratique

8 | Tell whether the students and teachers in the school cafeteria are hungry or thirsty, based on what they have on their trays.

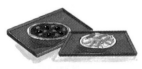

1. Théo et Nadia....

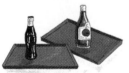

2. Nous....

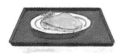

3. Monsieur Bobot....

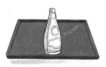

4. Yasmine....

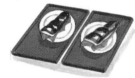

5. Vous....

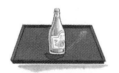

6. J'....

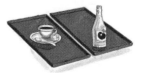

7. Les professeurs de maths....

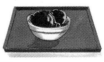

8. Tu....

9 Mme Vaillancourt's students have a test tomorrow. M. Messier's students are going on a field trip. With a partner, talk about who needs to study tonight. Student A asks questions and Student B answers them.

Modèles:

Alexandre

Student A: Alexandre a besòin d'étudier?

Student B: Oui, il a besoin d'étudier.

Sophie et Karine

Student A: Sophie et Karine ont besoin d'étudier?

Student B: Non, elles n'ont pas besoin d'étudier.

Les élèves de Mme Vaillancourt	*Les élèves de M. Messier*
Arabéa	Jean-Philippe
Charles	Fatima
Nora	Sophie
Alain	Christine
Éric	Salim
Paul	Sonia
Alexandre	Karine
Cécile	Anne

1. Salim
2. Paul et Charles
3. Nora
4. Christine et Sonia
5. Fatima
6. Éric
7. Jean-Philippe et Anne
8. Arabéa et Cécile

Communication

10 School supply stores are having their back-to-school sales. You decide to go shopping before classes begin to buy supplies that you know you will need this year. Make a list in French of what items you plan to buy.

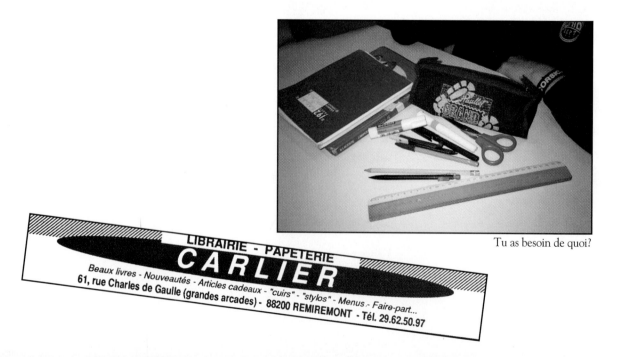

Tu as besoin de quoi?

LIBRAIRIE - PAPETERIE
CARLIER
Beaux livres - Nouveautés - Articles cadeaux - "cuirs" - "stylos" - Menus - Faire-part...
61, rue Charles de Gaulle (grandes arcades) - 88200 REMIREMONT - Tél. 29.62.50.97

11 It is early in the school year, and your French teacher has passed out a list of supplies you need to bring to class tomorrow. You have checked off what you already have. After class you get together to compare lists with a classmate who has a different French teacher. Since you plan to go shopping with your classmate, compare what each of you has and what each of you needs to buy.

Modèle:
Student A: J'ai un dictionnaire. Et toi?
Student B: Moi, j'ai besoin d'un dictionnaire.

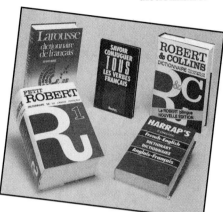

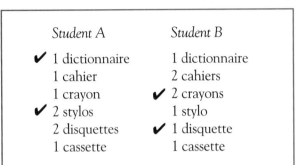

Student A	*Student B*
✔ 1 dictionnaire	1 dictionnaire
1 cahier	2 cahiers
1 crayon	✔ 2 crayons
✔ 2 stylos	1 stylo
2 disquettes	✔ 1 disquette
1 cassette	1 cassette

12 Write a paragraph in French in which you describe the people and items in your classroom and where they are located. For example, you might write **Le professeur, Madame Paquette, est devant le bureau.** Then, to check the accuracy of your description, find a partner and read your paragraphs to each other. As one of you reads, the other draws a picture illustrating the various people and items and their position in the classroom. After both of you have read your paragraphs and made sketches, compare them to see what similarities and differences you can find.

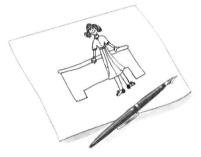

Prononciation

The sound [y]

The sound [y] of the French vowel **u** is similar, but not identical, to the sound of the first "u" in the English word "bureau." To make the sound [y], round your lips tightly and say the English sound "ew." Keep your mouth locked in one position and do not move your lips once the sound is made. Say each of these words:

étudiant   musique   salut   juste   sur   pendule

The sound [u]

The sound [u] of the letters **ou** in French is similar to the sound "oo" in the English word "moo." To make the sound [u], keep your mouth locked in the "oo" position and do not move your lips once the sound is made. Say each of these words:

jour   sous   cours   trousse   écoutons   vous

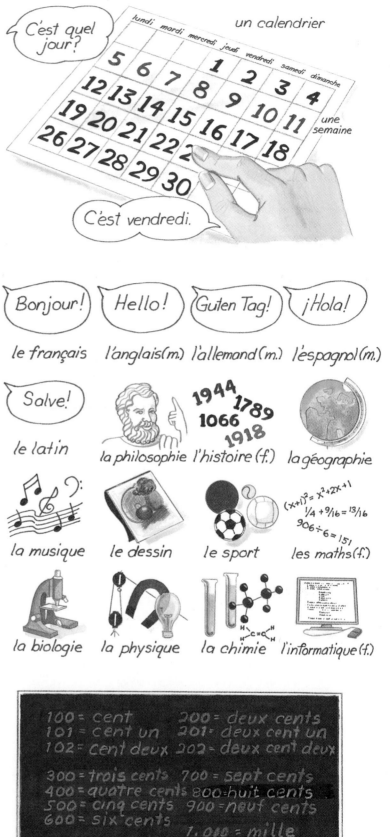

Leçon B

In this lesson you will be able to:

➤ **express emotions**

➤ **describe daily routines**

➤ **agree and disagree**

➤ **ask for information**

➤ **give information**

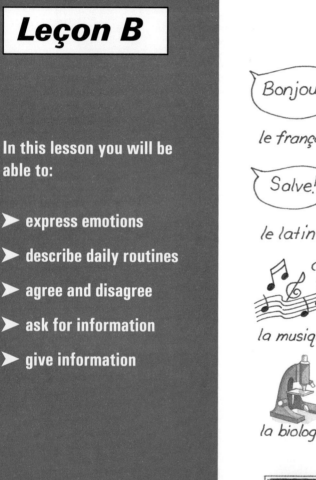

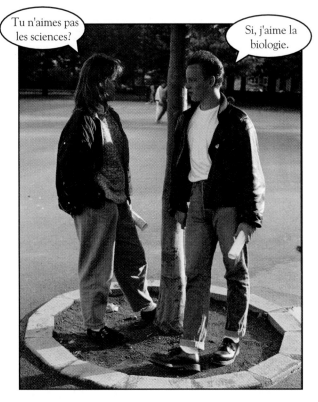

David is talking to Béatrice about his school schedule before their class begins.

David: **J'en ai marre! J'ai une heure de chimie le lundi, deux heures de physique le mardi et deux heures de biologie le samedi. Ça fait deux cent quarante minutes de sciences par semaine!**

Béatrice: **Tu n'aimes pas les sciences?**

David: **Si, j'aime la biologie, mais je n'aime pas la chimie.**

Béatrice: **Tiens, tu as juste un cours le mercredi?**

David: **Oui, géographie, de 9h00 à 10h00.**

Béatrice: **Tu finis à 10h00 le mercredi? Moi aussi.**

J'en ai marre! is a slang expression for "I'm sick of it!" or "I've had it!" Young French speakers frequently use slang when talking to friends and classmates.

Enquête culturelle 🔍

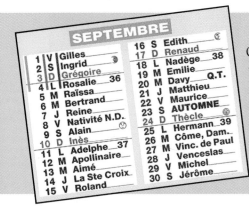

On French calendars the week traditionally begins with Monday. However, in Canada, Sunday is the first day of the week, just as it is in the United States. In French the names of days of the week usually are not capitalized.

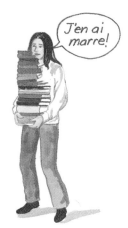

French high school students take certain required courses and some electives which relate to their specific area of study. Unlike most students in the United States, French students may take three courses in one subject area at the same time, for example, **la biologie, la chimie** and **la physique.** French students also study **la philosophie** and **la géographie,** subjects which are seldom offered in American high schools.

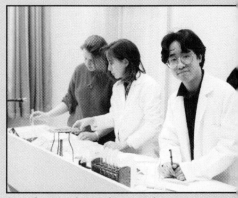

Jiro's favorite class is chemistry, but he also takes biology and physics.

In Canada, where people communicate in both French and English, the number of immersion schools grows steadily. Teachers conduct most or all classes in these schools in the language the student is learning. Immersion schools, in part, account for why many Canadians are bilingual.

1 | *Répondez en français.*

1. Où est le garçon?
2. David est avec qui?
3. David a combien de minutes de chimie par semaine?
4. Il a combien d'heures de biologie le samedi?
5. David aime les sciences?
6. David a trois cours le mercredi?

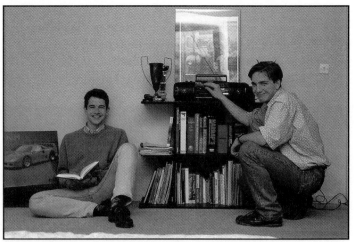

Serge et Daniel n'ont pas cours le mercredi.

2 | Say what day of the week follows the one you see.

1. dimanche
2. vendredi
3. mercredi
4. lundi
5. jeudi
6. samedi

Modèle:

mardi
C'est mercredi.

3 | Marie-Ève is a 15-year-old girl who lives in France. Look at her **emploi du temps** (*schedule*) and then write the appropriate day (or days) of the week that matches each description.

Modèle:

Elle a musique.
le vendredi

EMPLOI DU TEMPS

heures	LUNDI	MARDI	MERCREDI	JEUDI	VENDREDI	SAMEDI
8 h. - 9 h.	Allemand	Géographie		Français	Sciences Naturelles	Latin (option)
9 h. - 10 h.	Fra / E. E.	Mathématiques		Français	Etude	Mathématiques
10 h. - 11 h.	Mathématiques	Technologie		Latin (option)	Mathématiques	Sciences Physiques
11 h. - 12 h.	Français	Etude		Etude	Anglais	Anglais
12 h. - 13 h 30	Repas	Repas		Repas	Repas	
13 h 30 - 14 h 30	Etude	Allemand		Sciences Physiques	Allemand	
14 h 30 - 15 h 30	Sport	Anglais		Latin (option)	Musique	
15 h 30 - 16 h 30	Histoire	Français		Histoire	Sport	
16 h 30 - 17 h 30	Dessin					

1. Elle a juste quatre cours.
2. Elle a sport.
3. Elle n'a pas cours.
4. Elle a allemand.
5. Elle a histoire.
6. Elle n'a pas maths.
7. Elle a géographie.
8. Elle a anglais.
9. Elle a deux heures de français et deux heures de latin.

4 | *C'est à toi!*

1. Tu préfères quel jour de la semaine?
2. Tu as combien d'heures de sciences par semaine?
3. Tu aimes un peu ou beaucoup les sciences?
4. Tu as combien de minutes de français par jour?
5. Tu as combien de cours le mercredi?

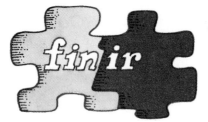

Structure

Present tense of regular verbs ending in *-ir*

The infinitives of many French verbs end in **-ir**. Most of these verbs, such as **finir** (*to finish*), are regular because their forms follow a predictable pattern. To form the present tense of a regular **-ir** verb, first find the stem of the verb by removing the **-ir** ending from its infinitive.

Now add the endings (**-is, -is, -it, -issons, -issez, -issent**) to the stem of the verb depending on the corresponding subject pronouns.

<table>
<tr><th colspan="4">finir</th></tr>
<tr><td>je</td><td>finis</td><td>Je finis le livre.</td><td>I'm finishing the book.</td></tr>
<tr><td>tu</td><td>finis</td><td>Tu finis à 10h00?</td><td>Do you finish at 10:00?</td></tr>
<tr><td>il/elle/on</td><td>finit</td><td>Le cours finit à midi.</td><td>The class ends at noon.</td></tr>
<tr><td>nous</td><td>finissons</td><td>Nous finissons les devoirs.</td><td>We're finishing the homework.</td></tr>
<tr><td>vous</td><td>finissez</td><td>Vous finissez à quelle heure?</td><td>At what time do you finish?</td></tr>
<tr><td>ils/elles</td><td>finissent</td><td>Les élèves ne finissent pas l'interro.</td><td>The students don't finish the quiz.</td></tr>
</table>

The final consonant of each form of **finir** is silent.

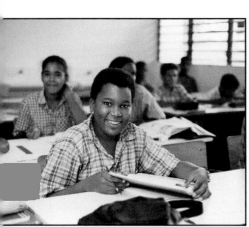

François finit les devoirs. (Martinique)

Pratique

Modèle:

le steak/la salade
Student A: Tu finis le steak?
Student B: Oui, je finis le steak. Tu finis la salade?
Student A: Non, je ne finis pas la salade.

5   Because you and your partner are the last two people to arrive for dinner, there is only a little bit of each type of food left. Student A likes only fruits and desserts. Student B likes everything but fruits and desserts. Determine who will finish what.

1. la glace/les frites
2. la quiche/les raisins
3. le chocolat/les pommes
4. le jambon/le fromage

Diane finit le sandwich au fromage?

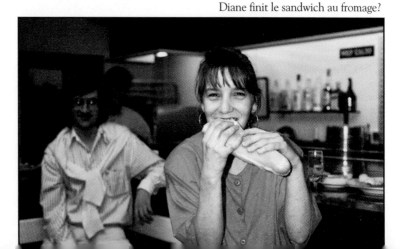

6 A group of friends from school is meeting at a café at 3h30. David asks you who is going. Knowing that only those people who finish their last class of the day before 3h30 can go, answer his questions.

1. Et Catherine va au café? (5h00)
2. Et Laïla et toi, vous allez au café? (3h00)
3. Et Florence et Sabrina vont au café? (4h00)
4. Et Daniel va au café? (2h00)
5. Et André et Nicole vont au café? (3h00)
6. Et Max et moi, nous allons au café? (6h00)

Modèles:

Assane va au café? (2h00)
Oui, il finit à deux heures.

Et Élisabeth et Louis vont au café? (4h00)
Non, ils finissent à quatre heures.

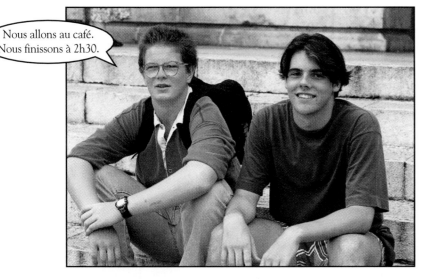

Nous allons au café.
Nous finissons à 2h30.

Communication

7 You want to know how much your classmates like various school subjects. Draw a grid like the one that follows. In the grid write the names in French of five common subjects. Then poll ten of your classmates to determine how much they like each subject. In your survey:

1. Ask each classmate if he or she likes each subject a lot, a little or not at all.
2. As each classmate answers your question, make a check by the appropriate response.
3. After you have finished asking questions, count how many people like each subject a lot, a little or not at all and be ready to share your findings with the rest of the class.

Modèle:

| Henri: | Tu aimes l'histoire? |
| Marie-Claire: | J'aime beaucoup l'histoire. |

. . . .

Henri: Six élèves aiment beaucoup l'histoire, trois élèves aiment un peu l'histoire et un élève n'aime pas l'histoire.

	beaucoup	un peu	ne...pas
Tu aimes l'histoire?	✔✔✔✔✔	✔✔✔	✔
Tu aimes...?			
Tu aimes...?			
Tu aimes...?			
Tu aimes...?			

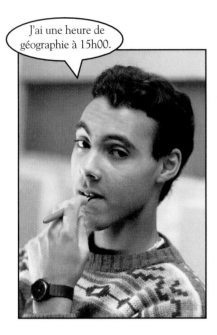

J'ai une heure de géographie à 15h00.

8 You just received a letter from your French pen pal, Pierre-Jean, in which he describes his weekly class schedule. After reading his description, create on a separate sheet of paper his **emploi du temps** to show to your classmates and teacher. Here is the part of his letter in which he talks about his schedule.

J'ai dix cours différents par semaine. J'ai une heure de chimie le lundi à 10h00, de 10h00 à 12h00 le mardi et le jeudi, et de 9h00 à 10h00 le vendredi. Le lundi, le mardi, le mercredi, le jeudi et le samedi, j'ai une heure de maths à 9h00. Le français est de 14h00 à 15h00 le lundi et de 15h00 à 17h00 le jeudi. Le lundi, le mardi et le vendredi, j'ai une heure de géographie à 15h00. J'ai sport le mercredi de 14h00 à 17h00. J'aime beaucoup le sport! J'ai anglais de 10h00 à 11h00 le mercredi, le vendredi et le samedi, et j'ai une heure d'allemand le lundi et le mercredi à 11h00 et de 14h00 à 15h00 le vendredi. Le samedi à 11h00 j'ai une heure de musique. J'ai une heure de philosophie à 14h00 le mardi et le jeudi, et j'ai une heure d'histoire à 13h00 le lundi et à 11h00 le vendredi. Je finis à 12h00 le samedi.

9 Referring to the schedule you created in Activity 8, list in French the ten classes that Pierre-Jean has each week. Then figure out how many minutes he spends in each class and write this number in French words beside the appropriate class. Finally, write the total number of minutes he spends in class each week.

Modèle:

la chimie - trois cents minutes par semaine

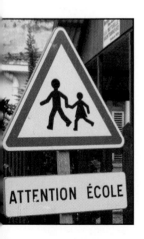

Mise au point sur... l'enseignement secondaire en France

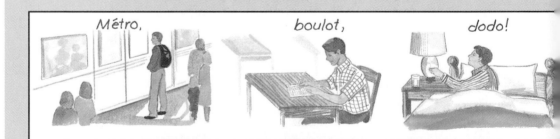

Métro,   boulot,   dodo!

"Métro, boulot, dodo!" This expression sums up how people who live in Paris describe their daily routine of taking the subway, going to work and then going to bed. This rhyme also describes the busy schedule of students, since education is a full-time job for French teenagers.

Secondary education begins when 11-year-olds enter **le collège**, or **C.E.S. (Collège d'Enseignement Secondaire)**. They stay here for four years: **sixième (6ème)**, **cinquième (5ème)**, **quatrième (4ème)** and **troisième (3ème)**. These years correspond to junior high school or middle school in the United States. (Note that the way of labeling school years is the opposite of the American system.)

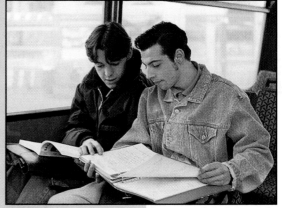

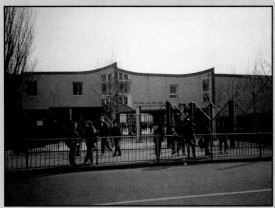

Le collège begins with *sixième* and ends with *troisième*. Then students may go on to *le lycée*. (Créteil)

Since the public educational system is the same all over the country, all French students use similar textbooks, follow similar course schedules and take the same major tests. Students spend up to ten hours a day at school, since classes begin as early as 8:00 A.M. and sometimes continue as late as 6:00 P.M. However, all classes do not meet every day. For example, one day a student may have six classes, and another day just two; he or she may have history twice a week, French three times a week, and drawing once a week. Students have Wednesday afternoons off to study, play sports or meet friends. Some classes are held on Saturday mornings. Students must take a second language. They begin learning their first foreign language, usually English or German, in **sixième** and then add a second language a few years later. Teenagers usually have hours of homework to do every night.

At the end of **troisième**, students take their first big exam, **le brevet des collèges**. The results of this test do not affect entrance into high school (**le lycée**), but a high grade is naturally a morale boost. After four years at **le collège**, some students choose to go to a vocational school, while others who are academically inclined attend **le lycée**.

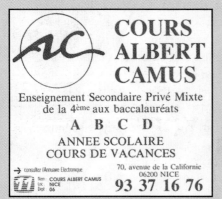

Laurent and André even do their homework on the bus.

Students go to **le lycée** in **seconde (2ème)**, **première (1ère)** and **terminale**. Here they choose a major area of study in preparation for **le baccalauréat (bac)**, the national exam which usually determines whether or not students may continue their studies at a university. In **première**, students take the first part of **le bac**, which concentrates on the French language. The second half of **le bac**, given in **terminale**, focuses on each student's area of concentration.

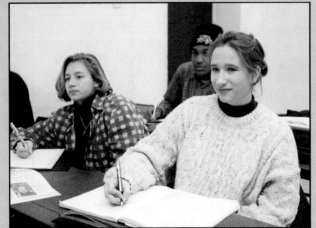

Different classes are often taught in the same classroom, so many rooms have bare walls.

A typical French **lycée** classroom is sparsely decorated. Students sit at tables instead of desks. Classroom instruction focuses on the teacher and textbook, with few of the visual aids seen on the walls of many American classrooms. Likewise, the relationship between teacher and students, which is often personal in the United States, is more formal in France.

As for grades, the French use a point system, with 20 points being the top score. Instead of an "A," a student might receive 18 out of 20. Teachers grade strictly and students are often happy when they get a score of 12 out of 20. Students need to have an overall average of 10 out of 20 to pass to the next grade, otherwise they must repeat it. Repeating a grade is fairly common in France: over half of the students in **le lycée** repeat at least one year of school. They may take **le bac** over if they don't pass it the first time, but if they fail a second time, they must repeat the whole school year.

During the school day, students meet in the school courtyard or at lunch to talk with friends. A long lunch period in **la cantine** or **la caféteria** usually breaks up the school day. However, many students choose to leave the school grounds to have lunch in a café or at home. After school, teenagers may stop for **un goûter** (*afternoon snack*) at a sidewalk stand or for a beverage at a local café. Cocurricular activities generally take place away from school in France, and organized sports are less important in French **lycées** than they are in American high schools. Secondary schools are viewed as places to study and learn, and education is as important to teenagers as a job is to their parents.

SYNTHESE		
NOMS	Moyenne Géné / Fut	classent
GRANDJEAN Geoffroy	11,3	12e
HUSSON Gabrielle	13,4	1e
JOJOVIC Milan	11,8	7e
LEUVREY Christelle	11,8	7e
MANGEL Karine	12	4e

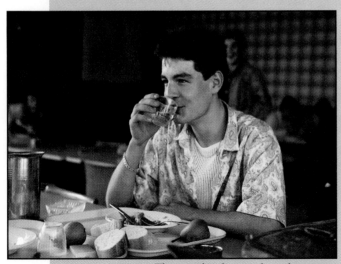

Théo eats lunch every day in *la cantine.*

0 Answer the following questions.

1. What is junior high school called in France?
2. What is one similarity between French and American secondary schools?
3. What is one difference between French and American secondary schools?
4. What is the name of the test that students take at the end of **le collège**?
5. What is senior high school called in France?
6. What may French students do instead of attending a **lycée**?
7. Why is **le baccalauréat** so important?
8. What is one difference between French and American classrooms?
9. What overall score do students need to pass to the next grade?
10. Where might students go to eat lunch during the school day?

1 Michel goes to the **Collège Mongazon** in Angers. Look at his **bulletin de notes** (*report card*) for a three-week period and answer the questions that follow.

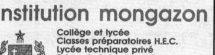

Institution mongazon

Collège et lycée
Classes préparatoires H.E.C.
Lycée technique privé
Externat et demi-pension
Internat : filles et garçons

1, rue du Colombier
49000 ANGERS   **41 66 41 33**

1. How many different courses did Michel take?
2. In what class did Michel receive the highest grade?
3. What were Michel's three scores in French composition?
4. What four languages did he take?
5. How many periods of science did Michel have?
6. What grade did Michel receive for his **leçons** (*lessons*) in art?
7. How many teachers signed the report card?
8. Was Michel an honor student?
9. The **appréciations** (*comments*), such as **très bien, bien, assez bien** (*fairly well*) and **vous pouvez mieux faire** (*you can do better*), show the teachers' opinions of Michel's efforts. What would your French teacher write about your efforts in class?
10. In what class did Michel do **assez bien**?

PÉRIODE DU			AU	
Composition française	Leçons	Devoirs de contrôle	Autres devoirs	APPRÉCIATIONS
Composition française	14	16	15	
Orthographe Grammaire	17	17,5	18	C'est bien, Continuez.
Récitations	18	16	17	
Mathématiques	17,5	15,5	16	Bien, vous pouvez mieux faire.
Langue vivante I Anglais Allemand	17	19	18,5	Très bien.
Langue vivante II Anglais Allemand Espagnol	15,5	16	17,5	Bien, vous avez fourni des efforts.
Latin ou Grec ou langue renforcée	15	14,5	16	Bien, Continuez
Histoire Géographie	16	16	17	C'est bien. Apprenez plus la Géographie.
Biologie Géologie	17,5	15,5	16	C'est bien. Travaillez encore la Géologie
Sciences Physiques	18	15	17,5	Très bien.
Technologie	18	18	18	Très bien.
Dessin	17,5	17	17	
Musique	17	15,5	16	Assez bien
Education Physique	17	15	16	Continuez
Le Professeur Principal				

Pr. De la Bastelle

TABLEAU D'HONNEUR   ENCOURAGEMENT

Les Parents

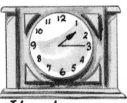

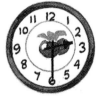

Il est une heure et quart.

Il est deux heures et demie.

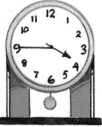

Il est quatre heures moins le quart.

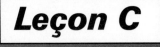

Leçon C

In this lesson you will be able to:

➤ **invite**

➤ **describe daily routines**

➤ **state exact time**

On finit à 12h40.

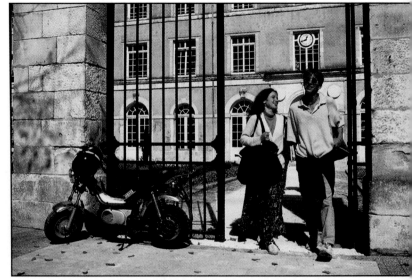

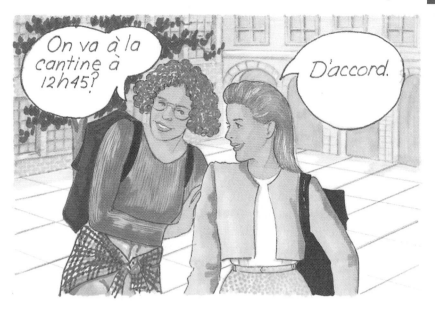

Nora and Patricia meet in the courtyard before school.

Nora: **On mange ensemble?**

Patricia: **Voyons, c'est vendredi. J'ai trois cours - musique, dessin et philosophie. Je finis à 12h30. On va à la cantine à 12h45?**

Nora: **D'accord. Tu as un bon emploi du temps.**

Patricia: **Mais c'est vendredi. Le lundi je commence à 8h00 et je finis à 17h30.**

Enquête culturelle

Many French-speaking countries use the 24-hour clock to give the times for TV programs, films, plays, sporting events, class schedules, plane and train schedules, etc.). This 24-hour system eliminates the need for specifying A.M. or P.M. To convert the P.M. system to the 24-hour system, add 12 hours. For example, 3:00 P.M. is the same as 15h00. Conversely, to convert the 24-hour system to the P.M. system, subtract 12 hours.

France 3 DIMANCHE	**13 mars**

7.15	**Bonjour les petits loups** Les petits malins - **7.40** Les histoires du Père Castor - **7.55** Les aventures de Tintin : L'oreille cassée (4).
8.00	**Les Minikeums** Le cristal magique - **8.25** Lucky Luke - **8.55** Les mondes fantastiques - **9.25** Les inventures des Minikeums - **9.35** Microkids.
10.05	**C'est pas sorcier** Drôles de savants et drôles de machines, avec Dominique Girard.
10.30	**D'un soleil à l'autre** L'agriculture en Allemagne.
11.00	**Mascarines** Présenté par **Gladys Says**. **12.00** Flash 3 - Météo.
12.05	**Programme régional**
12.45	**Le journal**
13.00	**Musicales** Elle s'appelle Anne Gastinel. La violoncelliste interprète *Concerto pour violoncelle et orchestre en la mineur opus 129* de Schumann.
14.05	**La croisière s'amuse** Série américaine. Rediffusion. L'amour de ses rêves.
14.55	**Sport 3 dimanche** **15.05** Tiercé en direct d'Auteuil. **15.25** Cyclisme : Paris-Saint-Etienne-Nice, 8e et dernière étape - **16.35** Escrime : Challenge BNP, finale - **16.55** Athlétisme : Championnats d'Europe à Paris-Bercy.
17.50	**Un commissaire à Rome** Série italienne inédite (2/9). Avec Nino Manfredi, Françoise Fabian, Dario Cantarelli, Sophie Carle. Secrets de bureau.
19.00	**19-20** **19.10** Le journal de la région.
20.05	**Yacapa** Avec Carlos, Annie Cordy, Brigitte Lahaie, Cendrine Dominguez, Georges Beller. XVII

To clarify the difference between A.M. and P.M., the French say **du matin** (*in the morning*), **de l'après-midi** (*in the afternoon*) and **du soir** (*in the evening*).

SAMEDI 1 OCT 20H30 **DIMANCHE 2 OCT** 17H

THÉÂTRE — LE GRAND SUCCÈS DU PALAIS ROYAL **"Une Folie"** une comédie de Sacha Guitry

1 | *Répondez en français.*

    1. C'est quel jour?
    2. Patricia a combien de cours?
    3. Patricia finit à quelle heure?
    4. Nora et Patricia vont manger où?
    5. Patricia commence à quelle heure le lundi?
    6. Patricia finit à quelle heure le lundi?

2 | Write your weekly **emploi du temps** in French. You may want to follow the format of the schedule that appears on page 103. If you have courses for which you don't know the French terms, ask your teacher or consult a French dictionary.

3 | *C'est à toi!*

    1. Qu'est-ce que tu étudies à 9h00?
    2. Tu manges avec qui à midi?
    3. Tu manges à l'école?
    4. Tu as combien de cours le vendredi?
    5. Tu finis à 12h30 le vendredi?
    6. Qu'est-ce que tu aimes faire à 17h00?

Structure

Telling exact time

You have already learned how to ask what time it is and to tell time on the hour in French.

    Quelle heure est-il?   *What time is it?*
    Il est dix heures.   *It's 10:00.*

To tell that it's quarter after the hour, add **et quart** or **quinze.**

    Il est huit heures **et quart.**
    Il est huit heures **quinze.**   *It's 8:15.*

To tell that it's half past the hour, add **et demi(e)** or **trente**.

    Il est midi **et demi.**   *It's 12:30.*

    Il est trois heures **et demie.**
    Il est trois heures **trente.**   *It's 3:30.*

To tell that it's quarter to the hour, add **moins le quart** before the next hour or **quarante-cinq** after the hour.

    Il est **six heures moins le quart.**
    Il est **cinq heures quarante-cinq.**   *It's 5:45.*

To tell that it's minutes after the hour but before the half hour, say the number of minutes after the hour.

    Il est quinze heures **vingt.**   *It's 3:20 P.M.*

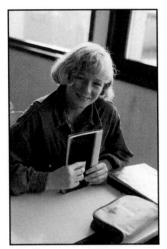

Sandrine étudie le français à 9h00.

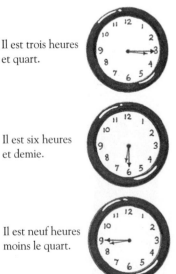

Il est trois heures et quart.

Il est six heures et demie.

Il est neuf heures moins le quart.

To tell that it's minutes before the hour, say either **moins** and the number of minutes subtracted from the next hour or say the number of minutes after the hour. (With the increased use of digital clocks, it is becoming more and more common to express the time with minutes after the hour.)

> Il est **quatre heures moins cinq.**
> Il est **trois heures cinquante-cinq.** } *It's 3:55.*

To ask at what time something happens, use **à quelle heure.**

> On mange **à quelle heure**?   *At what time are we eating?*

Pratique

4   For each clock or watch, answer the question **Quelle heure est-il**?

1.

2.

3.

4.

5.

6.

7.

5   Because there is an assembly this afternoon, your school is on a special schedule. You and your partner have all the same classes. Student A, who doesn't know the special schedule, asks Student B if each class starts at a certain time. Student B, who *does* know today's schedule, answers.

1. le cours de biologie (8h30/8h40)
2. le cours de géographie (9h15/9h30)
3. le cours d'histoire (9h50/10h20)
4. le cours d'informatique (10h45/11h10)
5. le cours de maths (13h00/12h45)
6. le cours de français (13h25/13h35)

Modèle:

le cours d'anglais (8h00/7h50)
Student A: Le cours d'anglais commence à huit heures?
Student B: Non, il commence à huit heures moins dix.

6 | *C'est à toi!*

1. Tu arrives à l'école à quelle heure?
2. Tu as anglais à quelle heure?
3. Le cours d'anglais finit à quelle heure?
4. Tu vas à la cantine à quelle heure?
5. Tu finis à quelle heure le vendredi?
6. Tu préfères faire les devoirs à quelle heure?

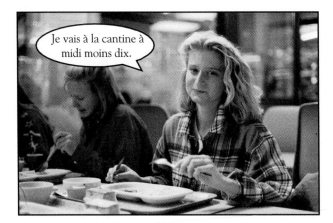

Communication

7 | Anne Khoury, a classmate's French pen pal, has just faxed your class her school schedule. With a partner, look at this schedule and talk about what courses she takes, when they are, etc. Then compare Anne's weekly **emploi du temps** with your own. Take turns making a comment about one of Anne's courses and asking your partner if his or her schedule is the same.

Modèles:

Student A: Anne a deux cours de maths le lundi. Et toi?

Student B: Moi, j'ai juste un cours de maths le lundi.

Student B: Anne a latin le mardi de 8h00 à 9h00. Et toi?

Student A: Moi, je n'ai pas latin.

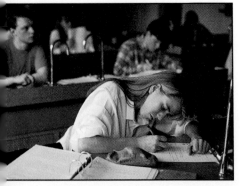

EMPLOI DU TEMPS

heures	LUNDI	MARDI	MERCREDI	JEUDI	VENDREDI	SAMEDI
8 à 9 h.	Histoire-Géo	Latin	Mathématiques	Mathématiques	Latin	Physique
9 à 10 h.	Histoire-Géo	Mathématiques	Mathématiques	Mathématiques	Anglais	
10 à 11 h.	Mathématiques	Mathématiques	Sport	Anglais	Physique	Sciences Naturelles
11 à 12 h.	Latin	Sciences Naturelles	Sport	Physique	Philosophie	
12 à 13 h.						
13 à 14 h.	Mathématiques				Espagnol	Mathématiques
14 à 15 h.	Philosophie	Physique				Espagnol
15 à 16 h.	Philosophie	Physique			Histoire-Géo	Mathématiques
16 à 17 h.	Espagnol					

Anne a physique le mardi de 14h00 à 16h00, le vendredi de 10h00 à 11h00 et le samedi de 8h00 à 9h00.

3   You observe various signs in French-speaking countries that tell when places open and close, when trains or planes arrive and leave, etc. These times are usually given using the 24-hour system. Match each sign you see with the letter of its 12-hour system description.

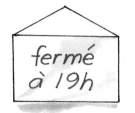

1.

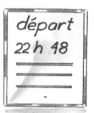

2.

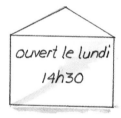

3.

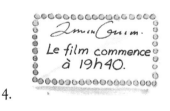

4.

Les cours finissent à 16h15.

5.

Lycée Curie 10h- 17h45

6.

message téléphone a 15h55

7.

arrivée à 18h05

8.

a. quatre heures et quart
b. dix heures à six heures moins le quart
c. huit heures moins vingt
d. deux heures et demie

e. six heures cinq
f. sept heures
g. quatre heures moins cinq
h. onze heures moins douze

9 | Here is a program listing for a French TV channel. You want to set your VCR to record specific programs. Using the 24-hour system, write the time in words to show when you will begin recording each program.

Modèle:

"RAVEN"
dix-neuf heures

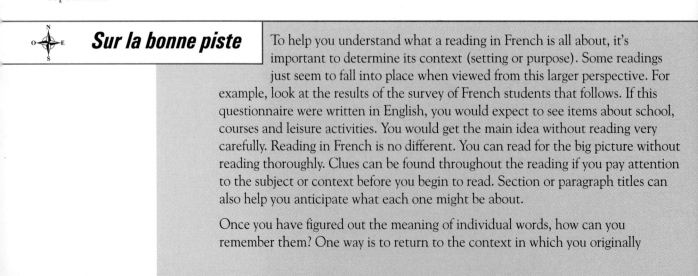

22 septembre VENDREDI M6		
REDIFFUSIONS Ⓡ		
5.45	**Boulevard des clips** 7.00 M6 Express.	
7.05	**Matin Express** Présenté par **Emmanuelle Gaume.** Avec à **8.00** et **9.00** M6 Express.	
9.05	**M6 Boutique**	
9.35	**Boulevard des clips** Avec à **10.00** et **11.00** M6 Express - **10.55** Info-conso - **11.10** Passé simple.	
11.20	**Les années coup de cœur** Chocolat et sympathie. **11.50** M6 Express - Météo.	
12.00	**Ma sorcière bien-aimée** Sur deux notes.	
12.30	**La petite maison dans la prairie** Promesses (2).	

13.25	**Les rues de San Francisco** Une collection d'aigles. Un trafiquant de pièces de monnaies de collection se fait piéger par la police à cause d'un simple oubli.
14.20	**Wolff, police criminelle** Coup monté.
15.15	**Boulevard des clips**
17.00	**Hit machine** Animé par **Yves Noël** et **Ophélie Winter.**
17.30	**Classe mannequin** Un K de force majeure.
18.00	**Highlander** Jeux dangereux. Richie, le jeune protégé de Duncan, est à la recherche de sa famille qu'il n'a jamais connue. Enquêtant sur son passé, il apprend qu'il était un immortel et que son père naturel a stoppé son évolution.
19.00	**Raven** Apprenti cambrioleur. Engagé par la séduisante Erin Stuckey pour vérifier les systèmes de sécurité d'un musée, Ski finit par convaincre Raven de voler une ancienne statue en or. **19.54** 6 minutes - Météo.
20.00	**Le grand zap** Divertissement présenté par **Olivier Carreras.** **20.35** Décrochages info ou Ciné 6.

1. "LA PETITE MAISON DANS LA PRAIRIE"
2. "LE GRAND ZAP"
3. "WOLFF, POLICE CRIMINELLE"
4. "HIGHLANDER"
5. "HIT MACHINE"
6. "LES RUES DE SAN FRANCISCO"
7. "MA SORCIÈRE BIEN-AIMÉE"

10 | Do Activity 9 again, this time giving answers using the 12-hour system.

Modèle:

"RAVEN"
sept heures

Sur la bonne piste

To help you understand what a reading in French is all about, it's important to determine its context (setting or purpose). Some readings just seem to fall into place when viewed from this larger perspective. For example, look at the results of the survey of French students that follows. If this questionnaire were written in English, you would expect to see items about school, courses and leisure activities. You would get the main idea without reading very carefully. Reading in French is no different. You can read for the big picture without reading thoroughly. Clues can be found throughout the reading if you pay attention to the subject or context before you begin to read. Section or paragraph titles can also help you anticipate what each one might be about.

Once you have figured out the meaning of individual words, how can you remember them? One way is to return to the context in which you originally encountered a word. For instance, if you read about attitudes toward school, let the reading set a scene in your mind and give you a feeling of what school or student life is like. It is better to think back on the context of what you read rather than simply repeating vocabulary words in English over and over again. Another way to remember vocabulary is to create mental images. Try to recall what you read by forming a picture in your mind of the what, who, where, when and why of the reading. Then try to label your mental pictures of things, people or activities in French while you review what you read. You will be surprised at what you can remember! More importantly, the words will start to come back to you in French rather than in English.

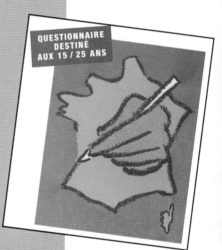

QUESTIONNAIRE
DESTINÉ
AUX 15 / 25 ANS

Voici un questionnaire distribué à quelques élèves âgés de 15 ans dans un collège à Tours en France.

Les réponses: 1 = Oui, tout à fait d'accord.
                2 = Plutôt d'accord.
                3 = Plutôt pas d'accord.
                4 = Non, pas du tout d'accord.

Mon opinion sur l'école et les études:	La moyenne des résultats:
J'ai besoin d'étudier pour l'école.	1,7
J'utilise un agenda.	1,2
J'ai beaucoup de devoirs.	1,0
J'en ai marre de l'école.	1,6
Je préfère:	
les maths.	3,2
les langues.	2,0
la littérature.	3,0
la biologie.	2,7
le dessin.	1,6

Mon opinion sur les sports et les loisirs:	
J'aime manger au resto.	2,5
J'aime aller au café.	1,2
J'aime sortir avec mes ami(e)s.	1,1
J'aime:	
le tennis.	2,0
le foot.	1,6
le basket.	2,0
le volley.	1,4
Je vais souvent au cinéma.	2,0
J'écoute de la musique.	1,2
Je skie souvent.	3,3
Je téléphone souvent.	2,4

11 Everyone knows that opinions are subjective: the answers to a questionnaire are valid only for those students who are interviewed. The opinions expressed in the preceding questionnaire are not necessarily the same for students from all French-speaking areas. However, the statements that follow are generally correct or incorrect, according to the opinions expressed by the teenagers (**les adolescents**) surveyed in Tours. If a sentence is correct, write **vrai**. If not, write **faux**.

1. Les ados aiment sortir avec leurs ami(e)s.
2. Les ados aiment les sports.
3. Les ados vont souvent au ciné.
4. Les ados écoutent de la musique.
5. Les ados téléphonent souvent.
6. Les ados n'ont pas besoin d'un calendrier.
7. Les ados ont beaucoup de devoirs.
8. Les ados en ont marre de l'école.
9. Les ados préfèrent les maths et la biologie.
10. Les ados préfèrent les langues et le dessin.

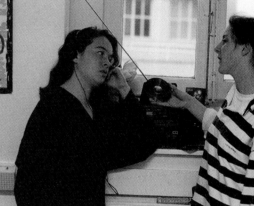

Sylvie et Myriam écoutent souvent de la musique

Nathalie et Raoul

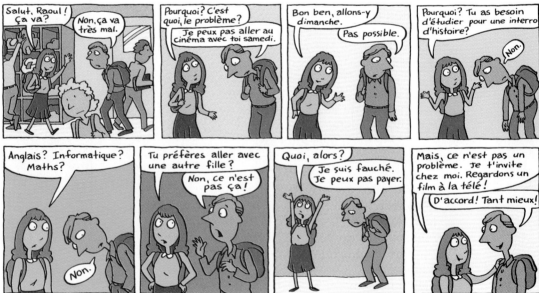

C'est à moi!

Now that you have completed this unit, take a look at what you should be able to do in French. Can you do all of these tasks?

➤ I can say what I need.

➤ I can ask what something is.

➤ I can identify school objects.

➤ I can tell where people or things are.

➤ I can ask for information about "where" and "what."

➤ I can describe my school schedule.

➤ I can disagree with someone.

➤ I can express emotions.

➤ I can invite someone to do something.

➤ I can tell exact time.

Here is a brief checkup to see how much you understand about French culture. Decide if each statement is **vrai** or **faux**.

1. Students in French schools store their belongings in lockers, just as American students do.
2. French students often use slang expressions, such as **J'en ai marre!**, when they greet their teachers as they enter class each day.
3. French students study **la philosophie** and **la géographie**, subjects which are not always offered in high schools in the United States.
4. An 11-year-old French student enters **le collège** to begin a six-year university program.
5. French students usually don't have classes on Wednesday and Saturday afternoons.

French students often play sports on days when they don't have school. (Verneuil-sur-Seine)

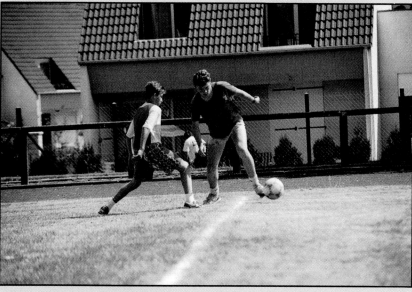

6. The exam which decides whether French students may go on to a university is called the **terminale**.
7. The walls of classrooms in French high schools are filled with examples of students' work, pictures, posters, etc., and look similar to those of American classrooms.
8. French students are often happy with a score of 12 out of 20.
9. Time in France is always expressed according to the 24-hour clock.
10. If you use the 24-hour clock, you don't need to specify A.M. or P.M.

Communication orale

A French exchange student is spending the year at your school. With a partner, play the roles of a student in your school and the visiting French student. Exchange information about daily schedules, what courses you're both taking and what school supplies you need. During the course of your conversation:

1. Greet each other in French and introduce yourselves.
2. Ask each other how things are going and respond.
3. Ask and tell each other several courses that you are taking now.
4. Ask and tell each other the teacher's name for each of these courses.
5. Ask and tell each other when each of these classes begins.
6. Ask and tell each other which courses you like.
7. Ask and tell each other what supplies you need.
8. Tell each other good-bye and say that you'll see each other soon.

Communication écrite

As a follow-up to your conversation, write a paragraph telling what you have discovered about your partner's daily schedule, courses and needed school supplies. You might begin to organize your thoughts by writing lists that have the following headings: **les cours, les profs, les heures, il/elle aime..., il/elle a besoin de...**. Use the information from your lists to write your paragraph.

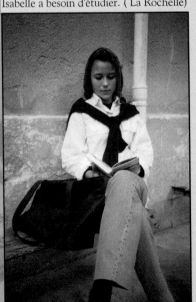

Isabelle a besoin d'étudier. (La Rochelle)

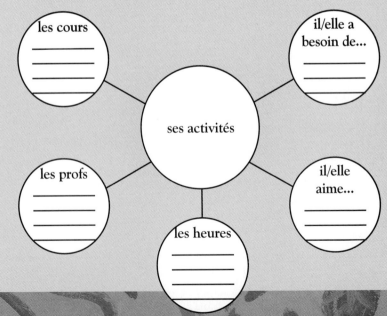

les cours

il/elle a besoin de...

les profs

ses activités

il/elle aime...

les heures

Communication active

To express need, use:

J'ai besoin de dormir.	*I need to sleep.*
J'ai besoin d'étudier.	*I need to study.*

To ask what something is, use:

Qu'est-ce que c'est?	*What is it/this?*

To identify something, use:

C'est le cahier de maths.	*This is the math notebook.*

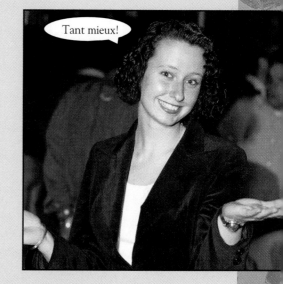

Tant mieux!

To tell location, use:

Il/Elle est devant le café.	*It's in front of the café.*
Il/Elle est derrière la chaise.	*It's behind the chair.*
Il/Elle est sur le bureau.	*It's on the desk.*
Il/Elle est sous le sac à dos.	*It's under the backpack.*
Il/Elle est dans la trousse.	*It's in the pencil case.*
Il/Elle est avec le stylo.	*It's with the pen.*
Il/Elle est là.	*It's there/here.*

To ask for information, use:

Où est la trousse?	*Where is the pencil case?*
Quoi?	*What?*
Tu as juste un cours le mercredi?	*Do you have just one class on Wednesday?*

To give information, use:

Je finis à 10h00.	*I finish at 10:00.*

To disagree with someone, use:

Si, j'aime la biologie.	*Yes (on the contrary), I like biology.*

To express emotions, use:

Tant mieux.	*That's great.*
J'en ai marre!	*I'm sick of it! I've had it!*
Zut!	*Darn!*

To describe daily routines, use:

J'ai une heure de chimie.	*I have one hour of chemistry.*
J'ai trois **cours.**	*I have three classes.*
Je commence à 8h00.	*I begin at 8:00.*
Je finis à 17h30.	*I finish at 5:30.*

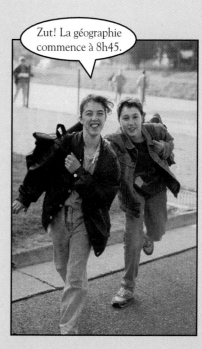

Zut! La géographie commence à 8h45.

To invite someone to do something, use:

On mange **ensemble?**	*Shall we eat together?*

To state exact time, use:

Il est deux heures **et quart.**	*It's 2:15.*
Il est deux heures **quinze.**	*It's 2:15.*
Il est quatre heures **et demie.**	*It's 4:30.*
Il est quatre heures **trente.**	*It's 4:30.*
Il est six heures **moins le quart.**	*It's 5:45.*
Il est cinq heures **quarante-cinq.**	*It's 5:45.*
Il est sept heures **dix.**	*It's 7:10.*
Il est neuf heures **moins vingt.**	*It's 8:40.*
Il est huit heures **quarante.**	*It's 8:40.*

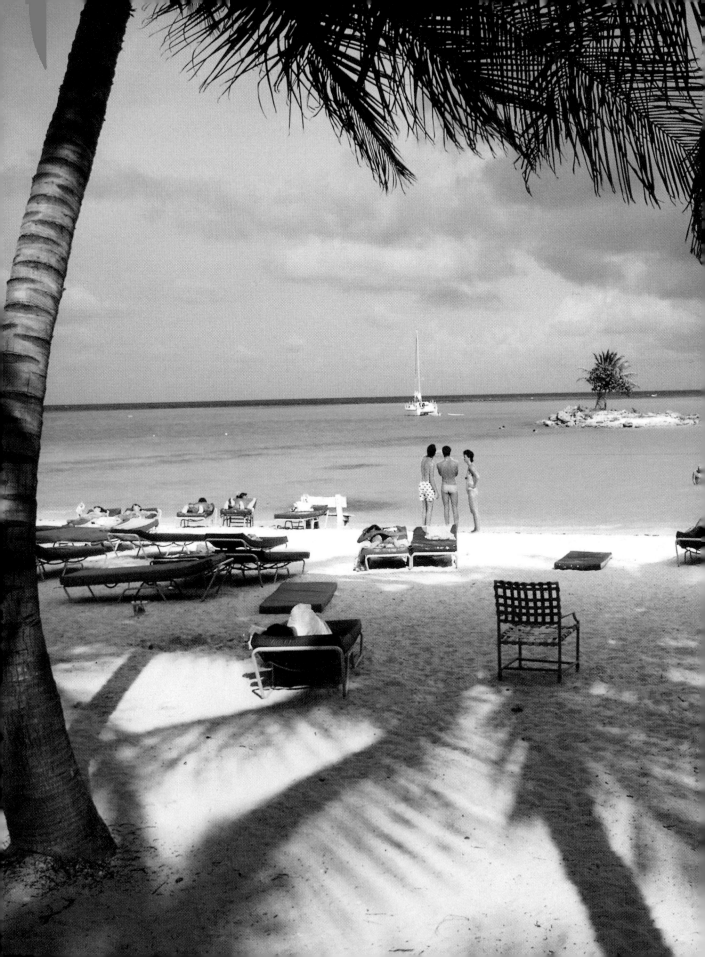

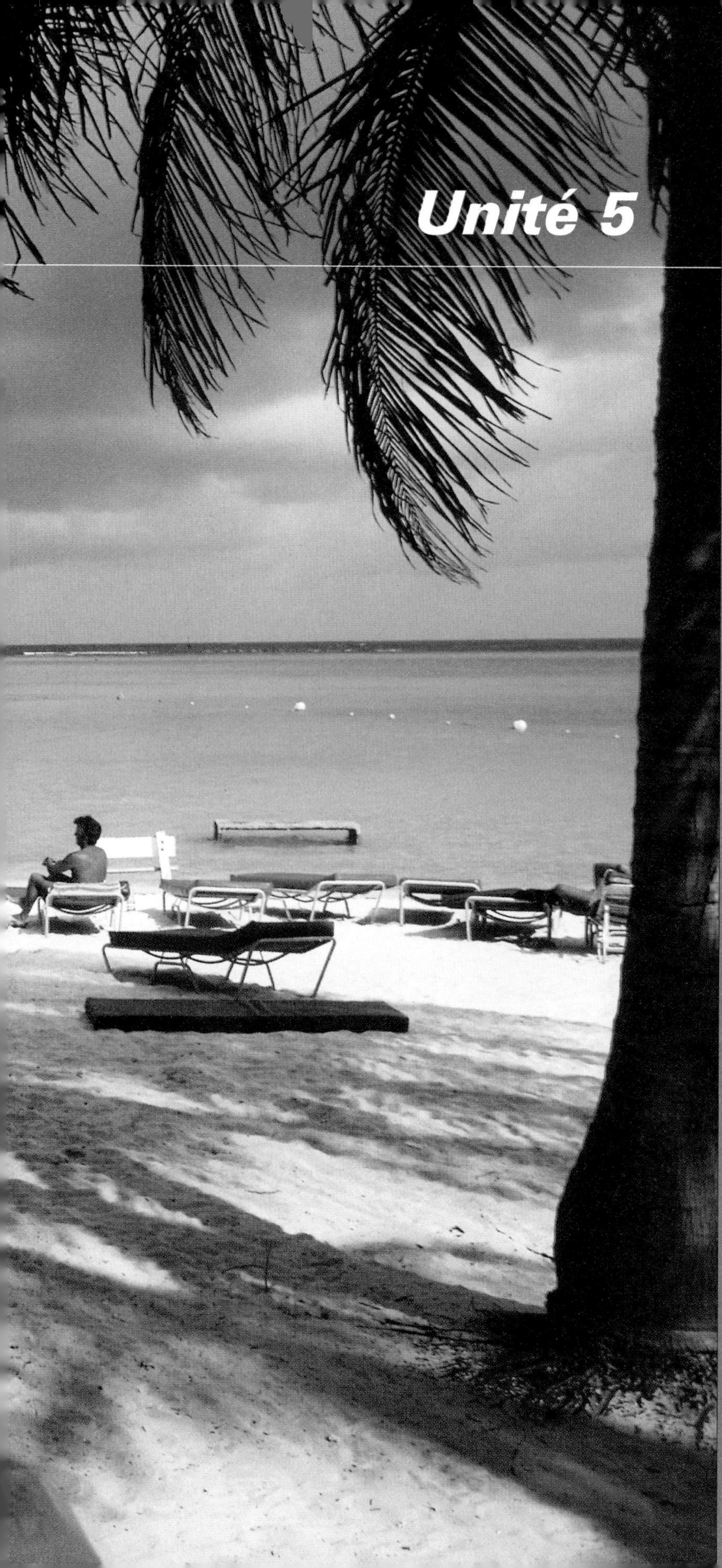

Unité 5

En famille

In this unit you will be able to:

➤ **ask for information**

➤ **give information**

➤ **explain something**

➤ **point out family members**

➤ **describe physical traits**

➤ **describe character**

➤ **express emotions**

➤ **ask and tell how old someone is**

➤ **ask and tell what the date is**

➤ **tell when someone's birthday is**

➤ **tell location**

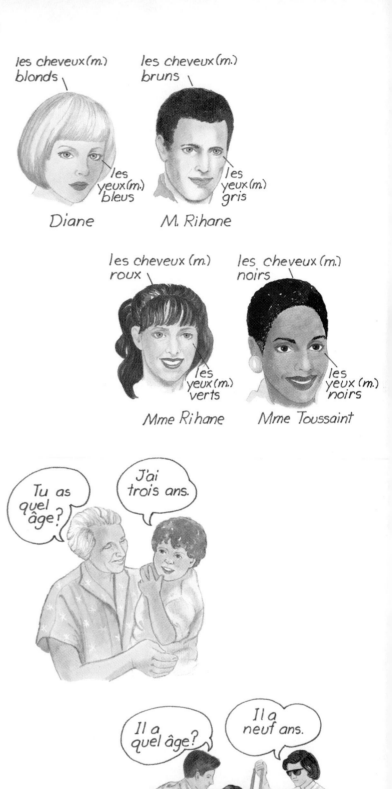

Leçon A

In this lesson you will be able to:

➤ ask for information

➤ give information

➤ point out family members

➤ ask and tell how old someone is

➤ describe physical traits

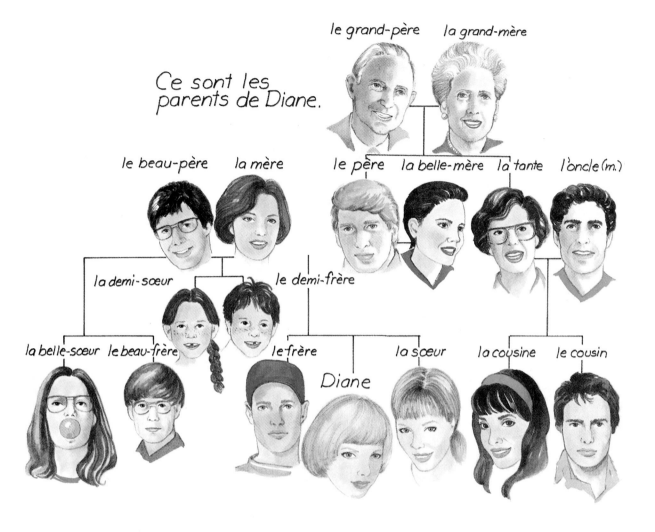

le grand-père   la grand-mère

Ce sont les parents de Diane.

le beau-père   la mère   le père   la belle-mère   la tante   l'oncle (m.)

la demi-sœur   le demi-frère

la belle-sœur   le beau-frère   le frère   Diane   la sœur   la cousine   le cousin

Ce sont les parents de M. Rihane.

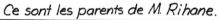
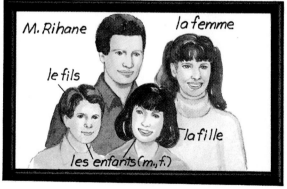

M. Rihane   la femme

le fils

la fille

les enfants (m., f.)

Ce sont les parents de Mme Toussaint.

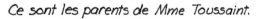
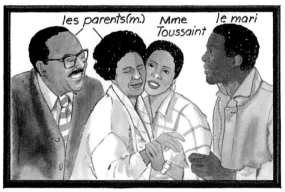

les parents (m.)   Mme Toussaint   le mari

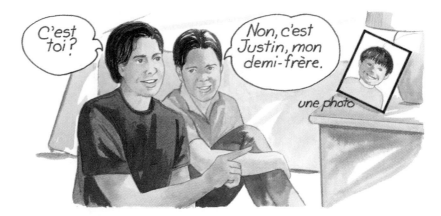

Max is looking at a photo of a young boy in Thierry's room.

Max: **C'est toi?**
Thierry: **Non, c'est Justin, mon demi-frère. Il a deux ans. C'est le fils de mon père et de ma belle-mère.**
Max: **Il a tes yeux bleus et tes cheveux bruns.**
Thierry: **Il est beau comme moi, n'est-ce pas? Nous ressemblons tous les deux à notre père.**

🔍 *Enquête culturelle*

Proverbs demonstrate certain values or point out people's attitudes. The French proverb **Tel père, tel fils** means "Like father, like son." This proverb emphasizes the traditional belief that sons look and act like their fathers, follow in their father's footsteps by entering the same profession or carrying on the family business, and tend to marry women similar to the ones their fathers married.

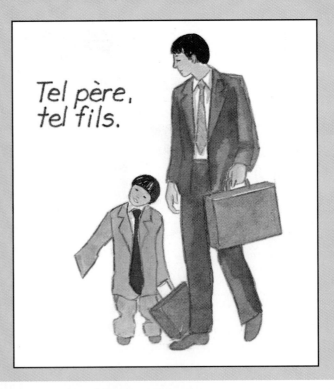

The French use the same prefix, **beau-** or **belle-**, for members of stepfamilies and in-laws. For example, the word **beau-frère** means both "stepbrother" and "brother-in-law."

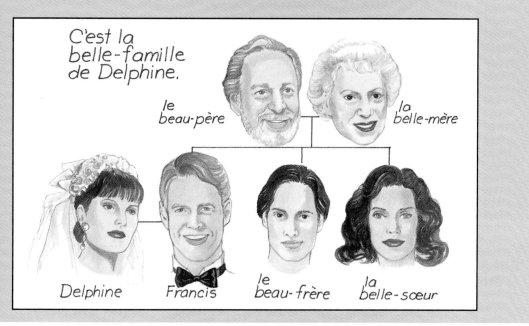

C'est la belle-famille de Delphine.

le beau-père — la belle-mère

Delphine — Francis — le beau-frère — la belle-sœur

Répondez en français.

1. Qui est avec Thierry?
2. C'est une photo de Thierry?
3. Qui est Justin?
4. Justin a quel âge?
5. Qui a les yeux bleus et les cheveux bruns?
6. Le père de Thierry a aussi les yeux bleus?

Trouvez dans la liste suivante le mot qui complète correctement chaque phrase.
(In the following list find the word that correctly completes each sentence.)

| grand-père | verts | sœur | âge | ressemble |
| belle-sœur | blonds | oncle |

1. Pierre a les yeux....
2. Le frère de ma mère est mon....
3. J'ai les yeux gris et les cheveux blonds. Mon père a aussi les yeux gris et les cheveux blonds. Je... à mon père.
4. Tu as quel...?
5. Nicole a les cheveux....
6. Le père de ma mère est mon....
7. La fille de mon père est ma....
8. La femme de mon frère est ma....

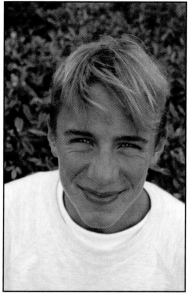

Bernard a les cheveux blonds.

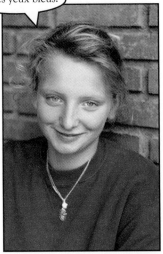

J'ai les yeux bleus.

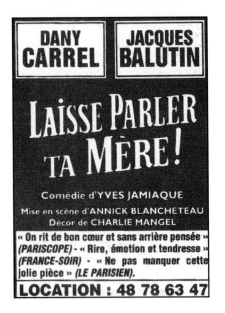

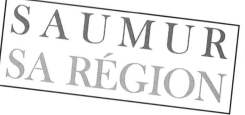

SAUMUR SA RÉGION

3 | *C'est à toi!*

1. Tu as quel âge?
2. Tu ressembles à qui?
3. Tu as les cheveux blonds, bruns, noirs ou roux?
4. Tu as les yeux noirs, gris, verts ou bleus?
5. Tu as combien de cousins?

Structure

Possessive adjectives

Possessive adjectives show ownership or relationship, for example, "my" computer or "his" sister. In French, possessive adjectives have different forms depending on the nouns they describe. Note how possessive adjectives agree in gender (masculine or feminine) and in number (singular or plural) with the nouns that follow them.

	Singular		Plural
	Masculine	Feminine before a Consonant Sound	
my	mon	ma	mes
your	ton	ta	tes
his, her, one's, its	son	sa	ses
our	notre	notre	nos
your	votre	votre	vos
their	leur	leur	leurs

(frère)   (sœur)   (parents)

The possessive adjective agrees with the noun that follows it, not with the owner.

C'est une photo de **mes** cousins et de **ma** tante.   *This is a picture of my cousins and my aunt.*

Leur père est très beau.   *Their father is very handsome.*

Son, sa and **ses** may mean "his," "her," "its" or "one's," depending on the gender of the owner.

Luc aime bien **sa** belle-mère.   *Luc really likes his stepmother.*
Claire et **son** frère étudient ensemble.   *Claire and her brother are studying together.*

Before a feminine singular word beginning with a vowel sound, **ma, ta** and **sa** become **mon, ton** and **son**, respectively.

Ton interro est demain?   *Is your test tomorrow?*
Ma sœur, Renée, a **mon** affiche.   *My sister, Renée, has my poster.*

Pratique

Answer the questions about Sabrina's relatives, according to the family tree.

Modèles:

Nadine est la tante de Sabrina?
Oui, Nadine est sa tante.

Pierre est le père de Sabrina?
Non, Pierre est son grand-père.

1. Max est le frère de Sabrina?
2. Éric est le beau-père de Sabrina?
3. Cécile est la grand-mère de Sabrina?
4. Isabelle est la cousine de Sabrina?
5. Vincent est l'oncle de Sabrina?
6. David est le cousin de Sabrina?
7. Diane est la mère de Sabrina?
8. Alain est le père de Sabrina?
9. Sylvie est la sœur de Sabrina?

Modèle:

Benjamin

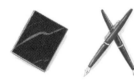

Benjamin a son cahier et ses stylos. Il n'a pas sa photo.

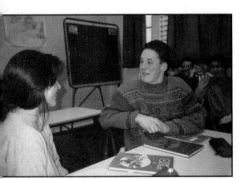

Philippe a ses livres et sa trousse. Il n'a pas son cahier. (Chelles)

5 Your teacher told you and your classmates to bring a picture of your family, a notebook and two pens to class today. Tell which people have what they were supposed to bring and which people don't.

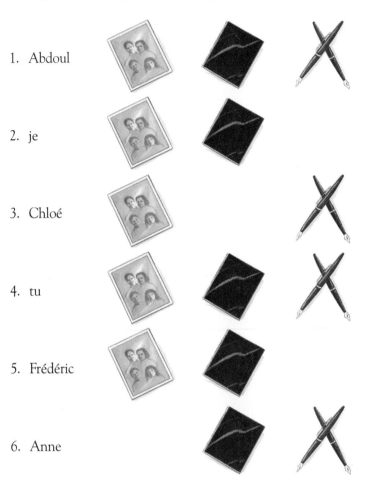

1. Abdoul

2. je

3. Chloé

4. tu

5. Frédéric

6. Anne

---

6 Tell which family members are going to the café with the following people.

1. je (parents/grand-père)
2. Monsieur Eberhardt (femme/enfants)
3. vous (père/belles-sœurs)
4. Sophie et Ariane (beau-père/frères)
5. Manu et Christophe (belle-mère/sœurs)
6. Madame Magouet (mari/fille)
7. nous (mère/cousins)

Modèle:

Luc (mère/frère)
Luc va au café avec sa mère et son frère.

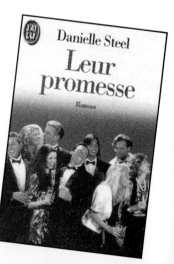

7 Tell how much the following people look like their relatives. Complete each sentence with the appropriate form of the possessive adjective.

1. Je ressemble beaucoup à... cousins. Je ressemble un peu à... mère. Je ne ressemble pas à... oncle.
2. Michel et Karine ressemblent beaucoup à... demi-sœur. Ils ressemblent un peu à... père. Ils ne ressemblent pas à... cousins.

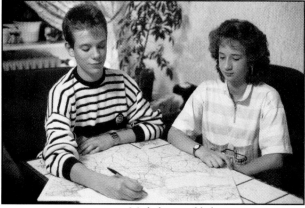

Michel ressemble beaucoup à sa sœur.

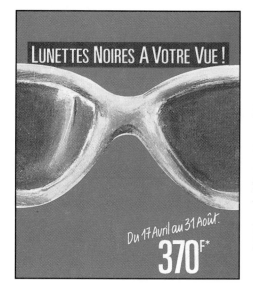

LUNETTES NOIRES A VOTRE VUE !

Du 17 Avril au 31 Août.

370^{F*}

3. Vous ressemblez beaucoup à... grand-père. Vous ressemblez un peu à... parents. Vous ne ressemblez pas à... sœur.
4. Ahmed ressemble beaucoup à... mère. Il ressemble un peu à... sœurs. Il ne ressemble pas à... demi-frère.
5. Tu ressembles beaucoup à... frère. Tu ressembles un peu à... cousins. Tu ne ressembles pas à... tante.
6. Nous ressemblons beaucoup à... père. Nous ressemblons un peu à... grand-mère. Nous ne ressemblons pas à... cousins.

Expressions with *avoir*

You have already learned several expressions where the verb "to be" is used in English but forms of **avoir** are used in French. Two more of these expressions are **avoir quel âge** to ask someone's age and **avoir... an(s)** to tell someone's age.

Tu **as quel âge**?   *How old are you?*
J'**ai** quatorze **ans**.   *I'm fourteen (years old).*

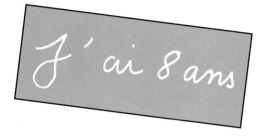

J'ai 8 ans

J'ai quinze ans.

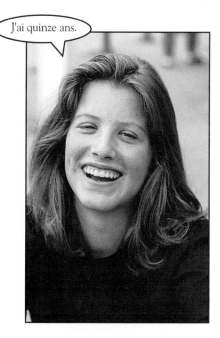

Pratique

8 With a partner, take turns asking and telling how old certain people are.

Modèle:

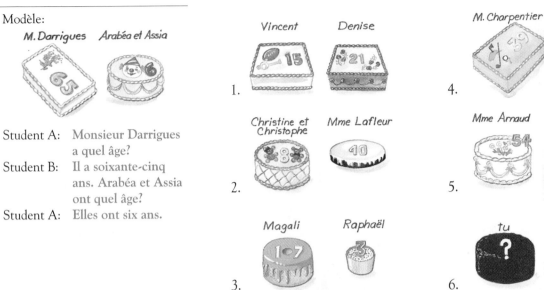

M. Darrigues   Arabéa et Assia

Student A:	Monsieur Darrigues a quel âge?
Student B:	Il a soixante-cinq ans. Arabéa et Assia ont quel âge?
Student A:	Elles ont six ans.

Vincent   Denise

1.

Christine et Christophe   Mme Lafleur

2.

Magali   Raphaël

3.

M. Charpentier   Marie-Alix

4.

Mme Arnaud   Théo et Thierry

5.

tu   tu

6.

Communication

9 You gave your friend a new photo album for her birthday. Help her organize some of her family pictures and their labels. Match each photo with the appropriate label. The first one has been done for you.

Modèle:

C'est ma sœur Claire. Elle a 6 ans.

g

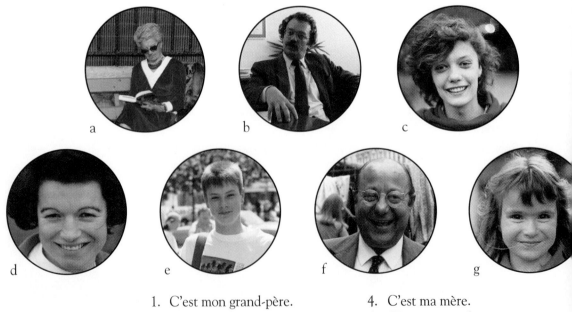

a   b   c

d   e   f   g

1. C'est mon grand-père.
2. C'est mon beau-père.
3. C'est mon frère, Alexandre.
4. C'est ma mère.
5. C'est ma grand-mère.
6. C'est ma sœur Anne. Elle a 19 ans.

10 The pictures that follow show some of the members of your imaginary family. Choose any two of these pictures, and write three sentences for each one on a separate sheet of paper. In each set of sentences, the first one should tell how this person is related to you; the second one should tell this person's approximate age; the third one should tell what color eyes and hair this person has. After you finish writing your descriptions, leave them on your desk, choose a partner and switch seats. Read the two sets of sentences on your partner's desk, and then write the letter of the appropriate picture next to each description. When you return to your seat, see if your partner correctly identified the two people you described.

Modèle:
C'est mon cousin.
Il a douze ans.
Il a les cheveux roux et les yeux verts.

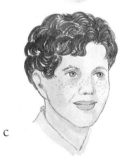

a

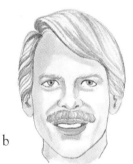

b

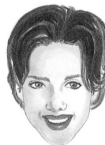

c

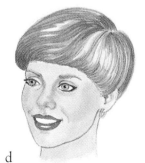

d

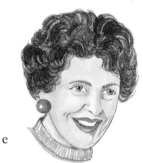

e

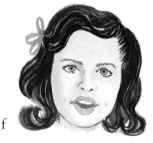

f

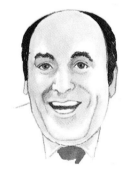

g

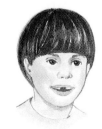

h

Modèle:

Moi, je m'appelle Derrick. J'ai 15 ans. Ma mère s'appelle Cynthia. Elle a 43 ans. Mon père s'appelle Glen. Il a 41 ans. Ma sœur s'appelle Ashley. Elle a 17 ans.

11 Write a brief description of each member of your real or imaginary family in which you tell each person's name, relationship to you and age. Then, with a partner, take turns reading your description aloud. While you listen to your partner's description, draw his or her family tree and label each person by name, family relationship and age, beginning with your partner.

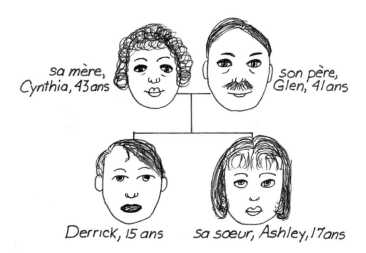

sa mère, Cynthia, 43 ans   son père, Glen, 41 ans

Derrick, 15 ans   sa sœur, Ashley, 17 ans

Prononciation

Liaison

You have already seen examples of liaison (linking of sounds) after some possessive adjectives when the next word begins with a vowel sound.

Leurs enfants ont faim.   Ton oncle s'appelle Michel.

  [z]   [n]

In general, final consonants in French are silent. However, there is liaison between two words when the second one begins with a vowel sound: **a, e, i, o, u** and sometimes **h** and **y**. The final consonant of the first word is pronounced as though it were the first sound of the second word. Say each of these expressions:

les ordinateurs   On y va?

   [z]   [n]

deux élèves   neuf ans

   [z]   [v]

cinq heures   Il est au café.

   [k]   [t]

les mois (m.)

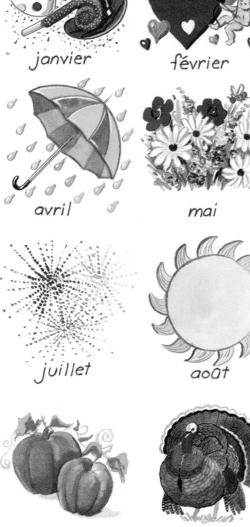

janvier

février

mars

avril

mai

juin

juillet

août

septembre

octobre

novembre

décembre

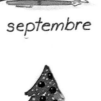

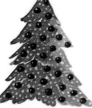

Leçon B

In this lesson you will be able to:

➤ ask and tell what the date is

➤ tell location

➤ point out family members

1.000 = mille

1.001 = mille un

1.002 = mille deux

2.000 = deux mille

3.000 = trois mille

1.000.000 = un million

2.000.000 = deux millions

3.000.000 = trois millions

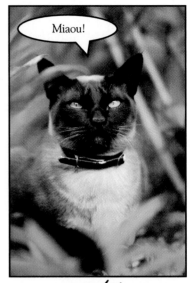

Miaou!

un chat

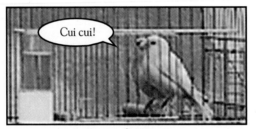

Cui cui!

un oiseau

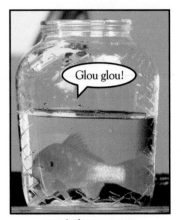

Glou glou!

un poisson rouge

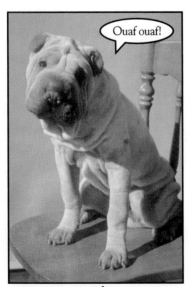

Ouaf ouaf!

un chien

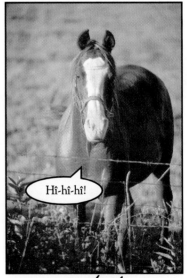

Hî-hî-hî!

un cheval

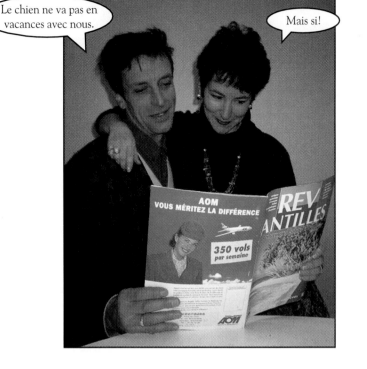

Monsieur and Madame Lévesque from Nantes are deciding where to go for their summer vacation.

Monsieur Lévesque:	**C'est quelle date?**
Madame Lévesque:	**C'est le 25 avril. Nous sommes jeudi. Pourquoi?**
Monsieur Lévesque:	**Nous allons en vacances dans trois mois, le 1ᵉʳ août.**
Madame Lévesque:	**Nous allons où? À Fort-de-France? À Pointe-à-Pitre?**
Monsieur Lévesque:	**Mais, la Martinique et la Guadeloupe sont à 7.000 kilomètres de Nantes. Le chien ne va pas en vacances avec nous?**
Madame Lévesque:	**Mais si! Milou est un membre de la famille.**

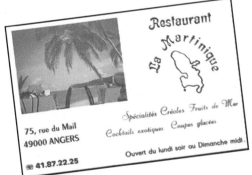

Enquête culturelle

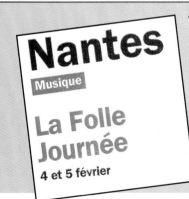

The Lévesque family is from Nantes, a port city on the western coast of France near the mouth of the Loire River.

Nantes was the site of the signing in 1598 of the Edict of Nantes, which gave French Protestants, called Huguenots, some religious freedoms. However, it was revoked by Louis XIV in 1685; consequently, about 200,000 Huguenots left France.

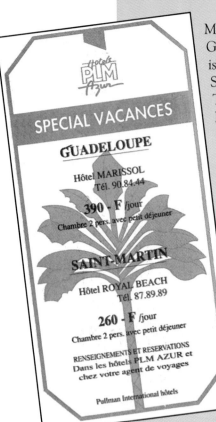

Martinique and Guadeloupe, two tropical islands in the Caribbean Sea, belong to France. The capitals of these two French overseas departments (**Départements d'Outre-Mer**) are Fort-de-France and Basse-Terre, respectively. Joséphine, the wife of Napoléon I (1769-1821), was born in Martinique.

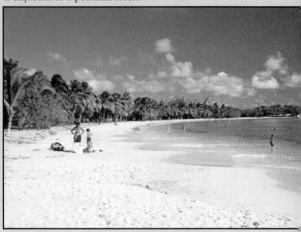

Les Salines, the most beautiful beach on Martinique, is adjacent to a petrified forest.

The French use the metric system of measurement, developed by a commission of French scientists in the 1790s. In the metric system distance is measured in **kilomètres** instead of in miles. One kilometer equals .62 miles.

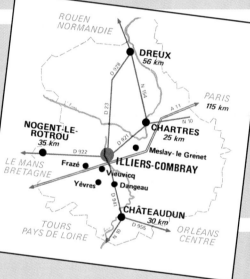

Most French workers get six weeks of paid vacation each year. Many families spend the entire month of July or August on vacation.

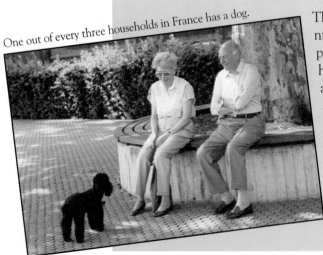

One out of every three households in France has a dog.

There are 35 million pets in France, more than double the number of French children! France has more dogs per person than any other country in western Europe. Paris has 40 animal clinics open day and night, animal ambulances, a therapy center for dogs and dog-sitter agencies. By law, the French must clean up after their pets. **Caninettes**, bright green motorbikes with rotating brushes and suction hoses, keep the city's sidewalks spotless.

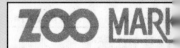

Usually trained to behave very well, French dogs are welcome in hotels, stores and even the fanciest restaurants, where they may be served food prepared by the chef. They are often treated as part of the family and given affectionate nicknames. Some common names for dogs include Médor, Rex, Reine, Fidèle and Fifi. Pedigreed dogs born in a particular year must all have a name starting with a certain letter of the alphabet. In one recent year, the names of all pedigreed dogs began with the letter "H"; names such as Hercule and Hortensia were very popular.

1 | *Répondez en français.*

1. C'est le 20 avril?
2. Les vacances de M. et Mme Lévesque, elles commencent le 25 avril?
3. Les Lévesque vont où en vacances?
4. Où sont la Martinique et la Guadeloupe?
5. Qui est Milou?
6. Qui va en vacances avec M. et Mme Lévesque? Pourquoi?

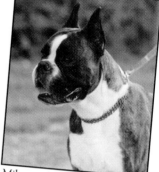

Milou est le chien de la famille Lévesque.

2 | Using the information in the illustrations, answer the questions about these people and their pets.

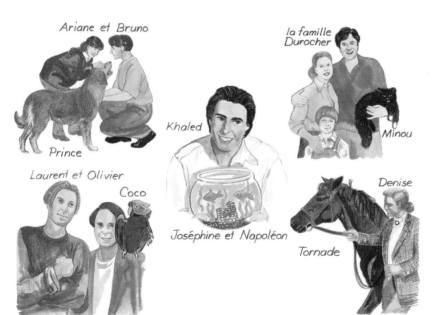

Ariane et Bruno

Prince

la famille Durocher

Minou

Khaled

Laurent et Olivier

Coco

Joséphine et Napoléon

Denise

Tornade

Modèle:

Le chat de la famille Durocher s'appelle comment?
Leur chat s'appelle Minou.

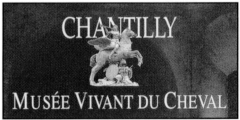

CHANTILLY

MUSÉE VIVANT DU CHEVAL

1. Qui a un cheval?
2. Combien de poissons rouges a Khaled?
3. La famille Durocher a un chien?
4. L'oiseau de Laurent et Olivier s'appelle comment?
5. Ariane et Bruno ont un chat?
6. Combien de chats a la famille Durocher?
7. Le cheval de Denise s'appelle Napoléon?
8. Qui a un chien?

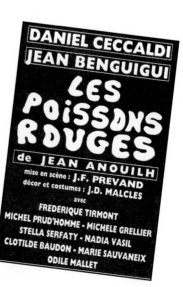

DANIEL CECCALDI
JEAN BENGUIGUI
LES POISSONS ROUGES
de JEAN ANOUILH
mise en scène : J.F. PREVAND
décor et costumes : J.D. MALCLES
avec
FREDERIQUE TIRMONT
MICHEL PRUD'HOMME - MICHELE GRELLIER
STELLA SERFATY - NADIA VASIL
CLOTILDE BAUDON - MARIE SAUVANEIX
ODILE MALLET

3 | *C'est à toi!*

1. Tu préfères quel mois?
2. Tu vas où en vacances?
3. Tu vas en vacances avec qui?
4. Qu'est-ce que tu aimes faire en vacances?
5. Tu préfères les chats ou les chiens?
6. Qui sont les membres de ta famille?

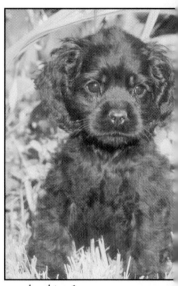

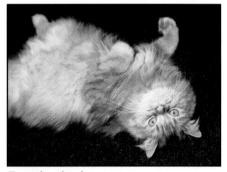

Tu préfères les chats...   ...ou les chiens?

Structure

Present tense of the irregular verb *être*

The verb **être** (*to be*) is irregular.

être			
je	**suis**	Je **suis** intelligent.	*I am intelligent.*
tu	**es**	Tu n'**es** pas timide.	*You aren't timid.*
il/elle/on	**est**	Il **est** beau.	*He's handsome.*
nous	**sommes**	Nous **sommes** au café.	*We're at the café.*
vous	**êtes**	Vous **êtes** ensemble?	*Are you together?*
ils/elles	**sont**	Elles **sont** à l'école.	*They are at school.*

Note that the **s** in **vous** is pronounced [z] before **êtes**:
Vous êtes professeur?
　　[z]

Elle est belle...

Les filles sont ensemble. (Angers)

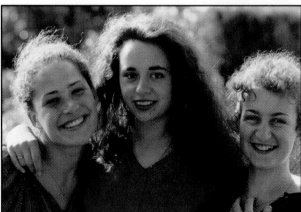

Pratique

4 | Tell whether or not you think the following people are on vacation.

Modèles:

Karine

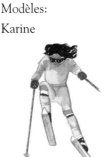

Karine est en vacances.

Luc et Ousmane

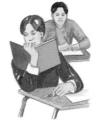

Luc et Ousmane ne sont pas en vacances.

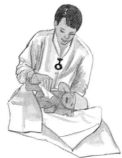

1. M. Simon

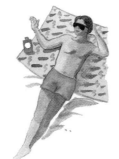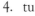

4. tu

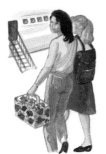

2. Delphine et sa sœur

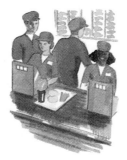

5. vous

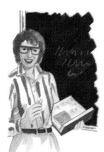

3. la prof de français

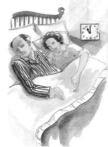

6. M. et Mme Dupont

5 | Complete each short dialogue with the appropriate forms of the verb **être**.

1. C'... quelle date?
   C'... le 20 décembre. Nous... mercredi.
2. Tes chiens... en vacances avec toi?
   Oui, Rex et Reine... des membres de la famille.
3. Tu... avec Étienne?
   Oui, nous... ensemble.
4. C'... ton frère?
   Oui, il... beau comme moi.
5. Tu... à l'école?
   Non, je... au café.
6. Vous... les sœurs de Catherine?
   Non, nous... ses cousines.
7. Vous... de Nantes?
   Non, je... de Paris.

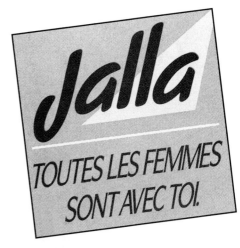

6 | Use appropriate forms of the verb **être** and the listed locations to tell where everyone is.

| à l'école | au café | au cinéma | au fast-food |

1. Les Maurel mangent des hamburgers et des frites.
   Ils....
2. J'écoute le professeur de biologie.
   Je....
3. Christine mange une quiche et une crêpe.
   Elle....
4. Nous étudions.
   Nous....
5. Tu es serveur.
   Tu....
6. Jeanne et toi, vous avez une interro.
   Vous....
7. Alain regarde un film.
   Il....

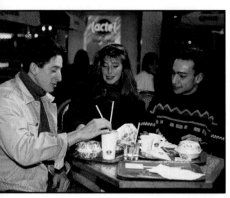

Ils sont au fast-food.

Dates

To express the date in French, follow this pattern:

> **le** + number + month

C'est le 12 décembre.
Nous sommes le 12 décembre. $\Big\}$ *It's December 12.*

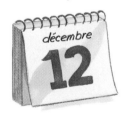

An exception to this rule is "the first" of any month. Use **le premier** before the name of a month.

C'est le premier mai.
C'est le 1ᵉʳ mai. $\Big\}$ *It's May first.*

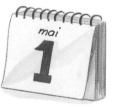

When a date is abbreviated, note that the day precedes the month: 12/7 is July 12.

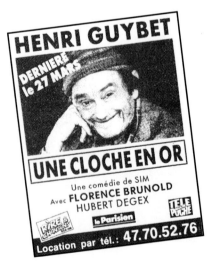

HENRI GUYBET

DERNIÈRE le 27 MARS

UNE CLOCHE EN OR

Une comédie de SIM
Avec **FLORENCE BRUNOLD**
HUBERT DEGEX

le Parisien

Location par tél.: 47.70.52.76

Pratique

7 The French teacher at the Lycée Carnot is very organized. She has already posted the dates of all the tests she will give throughout the school year. Give each date on the list in French.

Modèle:
3.11
le trois novembre

Dates des interros
10.12
18.1
23.2
15.3
1.4
12.5
9.6

8 Give the date of each of the following holidays and events in French.

1. your birthday
2. Valentine's Day
3. New Year's Day
4. April Fools' Day
5. New Year's Eve
6. Saint Patrick's Day
7. Independence Day (U.S.)
8. Halloween
9. the last day of the school year

Modèle:
Christmas
C'est le 25 décembre.

9 With a partner, take turns asking and telling who is performing at the Zénith in Paris on certain dates. Follow the model.

Modèle:
4.6/1.10
Student A: Qui est au Zénith le 4 juin?
Student B: Alain Chamfort. Qui est au Zénith le premier octobre?
Student A: Khaled.

Au Zénith...

18.1	DANY BRILLANT
13.2	VANESSA PARADIS
28.4	NEIL YOUNG
3.5	ALAIN SOUCHON
4.6	ALAIN CHAMFORT
30.7	JORDY
22.8	PATRICIA KAAS
26.9	TINA TURNER
1.10	KHALED
7.12	LITTLE BOB

1. 7.12/30.7
2. 28.4/18.1
3. 3.5/26.9
4. 22.8/13.2

Communication

10 When you were at your grandparents' house, you looked through an old scrapbook and found some birth annoucements. Based on these announcements, answer the questions that follow.

naissances

Nicole et Daniel VANNIER
sont heureux d'annoncer
la naissance
de leur fils

Étienne

le 11 janvier
mil neuf cent dix-huit
23, rue Montpensier, 75001 Paris.

naissances

Sabine GIÉ et François AHMEL
sont heureux d'annoncer
la naissance
de leur fille

Malika

le 21 août
mil neuf cent soixante et un
15, avenue des Roses, Dakar,
Sénégal.

naissances

M. et Mme AUBRUN
sont heureux d'annoncer
la naissance
de leur fille

Françoise

le 6 février
mil neuf cent quarante-sept
20, boulevard Bérenger, 37000 Tours.

1. How many couples had daughters?
2. What is the baby boy's name?
3. What is Malika's mother's name?
4. What is Étienne's last name?
5. Which of the three children is the oldest?
6. Which of the three children is the youngest?
7. Which child was not born in France?
8. Which person's birthday is celebrated first each year?
9. Which person's birthday is in the summer?

1 Your mother was sent to Aix-en-Provence in southern France on business for the month of July. Since you had vacation at the same time, you went along with her. Your mother traveled to many cities while she was based in Aix-en-Provence. Help her complete her mileage report for the month by telling the number of kilometers she traveled between Aix-en-Provence and each of the cities listed. (Note that the chart gives only one-way distances from Aix-en-Provence to each city.) Then give the total number of kilometers she traveled during the month. Follow the model.

Modèle:

Lyon
six cents kilomètres

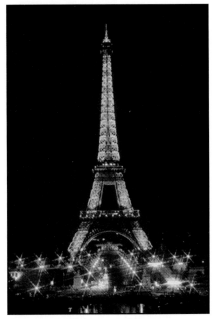

Paris est à 765 kilomètres d'Aix-en-Provence.

> ### Distances kilométriques d'Aix-en-Provence à:
>
> | | | | |
> |---|---|---|---|
> | Antibes | 165 | Marseille | 30 |
> | Arles | 75 | Montpellier | 145 |
> | Avignon | 75 | Nice | 190 |
> | Bordeaux | 645 | Orange | 100 |
> | Cannes | 155 | Paris | 765 |
> | Genève | 430 | Saint-Tropez | 150 |
> | Grenoble | 290 | Toulon | 80 |
> | Lyon | 300 | | |

Orange   Genève   Arles   Marseille   Montpellier
        Nice   Paris   Cannes

2 While reading the French newspaper *Le Parisien*, you find the lost and found section (**Perdu - Trouvé**) in the classified ads. Read the three ads about lost pets so that, if you spot one of them, you can call its owner. Answer the questions that follow.

> Perdu le 3/4, chien noir et brun, yeux gris.
> S'appelle Hugo. Contacter le 44.56.70.91.
> Forte récompense.

> Perdu le 31/3, grand chat gris, yeux verts.
> S'appelle César. Tél: 42.09.23.18.

> Perdu le 1/4, chien noir et brun, yeux
> noirs. S'appelle Rex. Porte un large collier
> noir. Contacter le 43.98.45.23.

1. What two kinds of pets are lost?
2. Which pet has been lost the longest?
3. What are the names of the other two animals?
4. In what way are the two dogs similar?
5. What is one difference in the appearance of the two dogs?
6. For which animal is there a reward?
7. Which animal is wearing a black collar?

Mise au point sur... les familles françaises

When Americans talk about their families, they usually mean their immediate families: parents, children, brothers and sisters. In France, the term **la famille** is used to refer to the extended family, including grandparents, uncles, aunts, nephews, nieces and cousins. In the past, whole families often lived in the same town. They gathered together for Sunday dinners, important holidays and special events. The mother usually stayed at home to raise the children and take care of the household. But with today's ever-changing family structure, it has become more and more difficult to define the word **famille**.

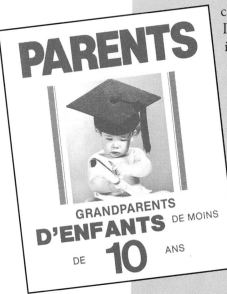

PARENTS
D'ENFANTS DE MOINS DE **10** ANS
GRANDPARENTS

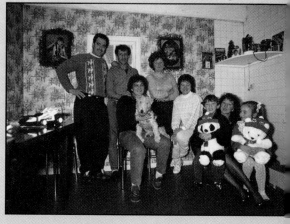

Extended families still get together for important holidays.

The changing family structure is reflected by the decrease in the birth rate in France. In order to maintain the population at its current level, the French government gives money to families upon the birth of each child after the first two. French children often make adult decisions at a younger age than their parents did. Much advertising is aimed at teenagers, because they often help their families decide what cars, clothes, food, computers, etc., to buy.

In most cases today, family members don't all live in the same town, but they still enjoy getting together to celebrate special occasions, especially weddings. In France, couples often have two wedding ceremonies. First, there is a required official ceremony at **la mairie** (*town hall*). Instead of choosing a maid or matron of honor and a best man, the bride and groom select two or more witnesses to listen to their vows. Other family members and friends also attend this civil ceremony. A second, optional ceremony takes place at the couple's place of worship. The entire wedding celebration may last for several days and include dancing, singing and lots of good food. Couples with more modest tastes simply invite their friends and family to a restaurant for a special dinner afterward.

Madame Joseph Ri...
Monsieur et Madame Jean-Pier...
Jourd...
sont heureux de vous faire part ...
mariage de le...
petite-fille et fille *Frédérique*, ave...
Monsieu...
Sébastien Martel...

En vous prient d'assister ou de vous unir
d'intention à la Cérémonie Religieuse qui
sera célébrée le
Samedi 19 Décembre 1998, à 15 h. 30,
en l'Église de
Saint-Suliac (Ille-et-Vilaine).

Un Cocktail sera servi à l'issue de la
Cérémonie.

9, rue du Moulin aux Pauvres
35300 Fougères

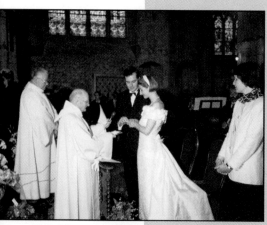

To celebrate a wedding in France, there are usually two ceremonies. The one at the church is optional.

In France, young women must be 15 years old (with parental permission) to marry; young men must be 18 years old. After her marriage, a woman may choose to keep her maiden name or to take the surname of her husband. She may also hyphenate her name, i.e., Martin-Dubois. But the legal name of a woman remains the name that she was given at birth.

French families don't need special occasions in order to get together. Some families have **une maison de campagne** (*country home*) to go to when they want to get away from the stress of city life. They often personalize this home with a name, such as **Mon Repos** (*My Place to Relax*).

Families usually spend a month-long summer vacation together. During July or August they head for their country home, go camping, travel, rent a home by the sea or visit relatives.

Reflecting both a gradually changing structure and a desire to preserve time-honored traditions, the family remains an important social institution in France.

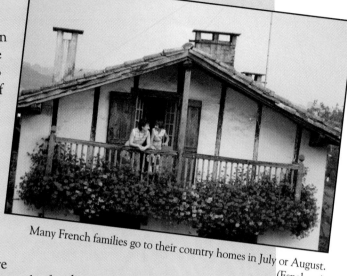

Many French families go to their country homes in July or August. (Espelette)

---

13 Answer the following questions.

1. When Americans talk about their family, whom do they include?
2. When the French talk about their family, whom do they include?
3. Why does the French government give money to families upon the birth of each child after the first two?
4. Why is much advertising aimed at teenagers?
5. How are wedding ceremonies in France and in the United States similar?
6. How are they different?
7. How old must French people be in order to marry?
8. Where do French families go when they want to escape the stress of city life?

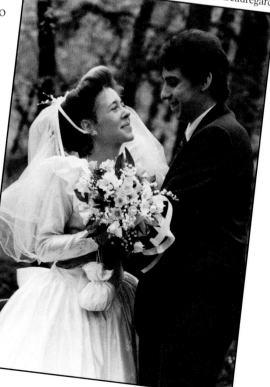

Francis and Isabelle Cazette were married in Beauregard.

14 Here is a French wedding invitation. The bride's family is listed on the left side of the invitation; the groom's family is listed on the right side. The names of the grandparents come before the names of the parents. The parents' addresses are given at the bottom of the invitation. Answer the questions that follow about Anne and Frédéric's wedding.

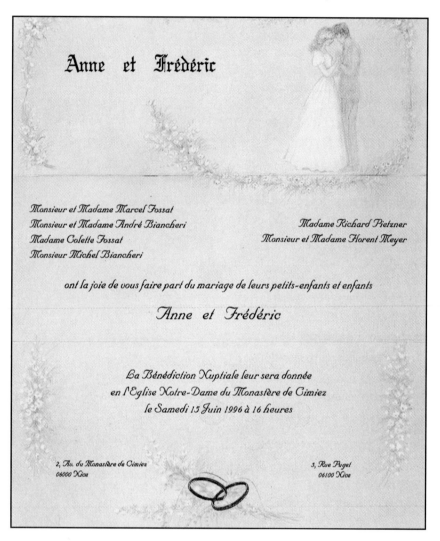

Anne et Frédéric

Monsieur et Madame Marcel Fossat
Monsieur et Madame André Biancheri
Madame Colette Fossat
Monsieur Michel Biancheri

Madame Richard Pietzner
Monsieur et Madame Florent Meyer

ont la joie de vous faire part du mariage de leurs petits-enfants et enfants

Anne et Frédéric

La Bénédiction Nuptiale leur sera donnée
en l'Eglise Notre-Dame du Monastère de Cimiez
le Samedi 15 Juin 1996 à 16 heures

2, Av. du Monastère de Cimiez
06000 Nice

5, Rue Pagel
06100 Nice

1. What is Frédéric's last name?
2. What is Anne's last name?
3. Who are Colette and Michel?
4. How many of Frédéric's grandparents will be at the wedding?
5. What is the name of the church where Anne and Frédéric will be married?
6. What is the date of the wedding?
7. At what time does the wedding begin?
8. Who lives on the street where the church is located?
9. In what city do Anne and Frédéric's parents live?
10. Where is the zip code placed in relation to the name of the city in a French address?

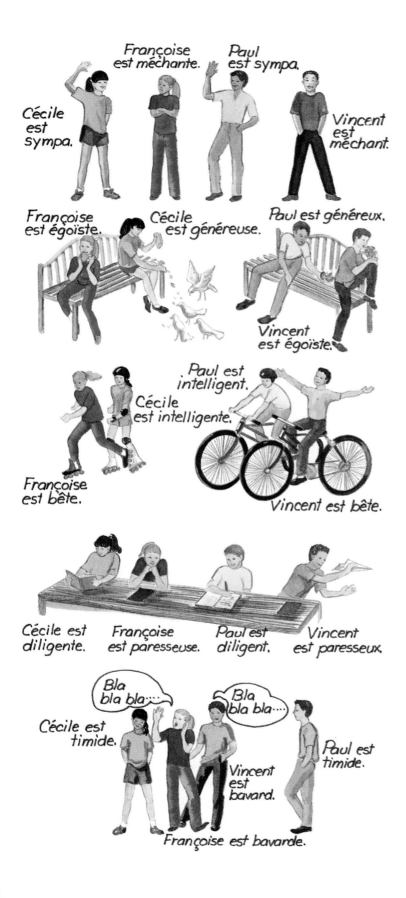

Françoise est méchante.

Paul est sympa.

Cécile est sympa.

Vincent est méchant.

Françoise est égoïste.

Cécile est généreuse.

Paul est généreux.

Vincent est égoïste.

Paul est intelligent.

Cécile est intelligente.

Françoise est bête.

Vincent est bête.

Cécile est diligente.

Françoise est paresseuse.

Paul est diligent.

Vincent est paresseux.

Cécile est timide.

Bla bla bla...

Bla bla bla...

Vincent est bavard.

Paul est timide.

Françoise est bavarde.

Leçon C

In this lesson you will be able to:

➤ **explain something**

➤ **tell when someone's birthday is**

➤ **express emotions**

➤ **describe character**

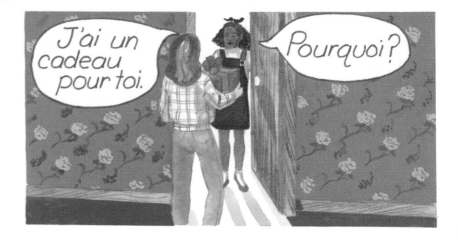

Sandrine brings her friend Jamila a gift.

Sandrine: **J'ai un cadeau pour toi.**
Jamila: **Pourquoi?**
Sandrine: **Parce que c'est le 26 octobre. C'est ton anniversaire.**
Jamila: **Mais mon anniversaire est le 26 novembre.**
Sandrine: **Que je suis bête!**
Jamila: **Non, tu es généreuse.**

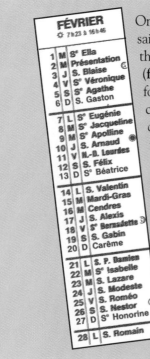

Enquête culturelle

Joyeux anniversaire, Julien!

The French often celebrate birthdays with a cake topped with candles, just as Americans do. To wish someone a happy birthday, they say **Joyeux anniversaire** or **Bon anniversaire**.

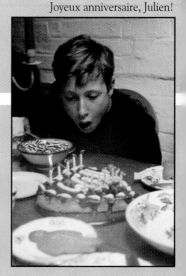

On French calendars the name of a saint is usually listed for each day, that particular saint's feast day (**fête**). Some French parents still follow the tradition of naming their child after the saint on whose feast day he or she was born. However, if the child is named after a saint whose feast day doesn't fall on the child's date of birth, he or she can celebrate twice each year. For example, a girl named Véronique who was born on May 14 may celebrate on that day and again on February 4, her saint's day. Children may receive a small gift from their family on their saint's day, while adults wish each other **Bonne fête** and may exchange cards.

1 Answer the following questions.

1. What is one similarity between French and American birthday celebrations?
2. How do the French wish each other a happy birthday?
3. Where are **fête** days listed?
4. Why may people named after saints celebrate twice each year?
5. When does a girl named Isabelle celebrate her **fête** day?
6. What do children receive on their **fête** day?
7. How do people wish each other a happy **fête** day?

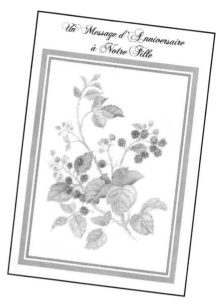

2 *Répondez en français.*

1. Qui a un cadeau?
2. Pour qui est le cadeau?
3. C'est l'anniversaire de Sandrine ou de Jamila?
4. Quelle est la date?
5. Quelle est la date de l'anniversaire de Jamila?
6. Sandrine, elle est bête ou généreuse?

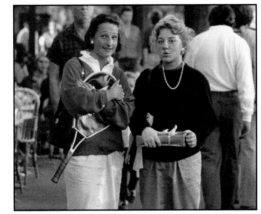

Béatrice a un cadeau pour qui?

3 On a sheet of paper write the names of five of your family members. They may be members of your immediate family as well as distant relatives. Then write a sentence that tells how each person is related to you. Finally, describe each relative using an adjective from the list. Pick an adjective from the left-hand column for a male; pick one from the right-hand column for a female.

Modèle:

Robert
C'est mon grand-père.
Il est timide.

beau	belle
généreux	généreuse
intelligent	intelligente
timide	timide
bavard	bavarde
super	super
sympa	sympa
égoïste	égoïste
bête	bête
paresseux	paresseuse
diligent	diligente
méchant	méchante

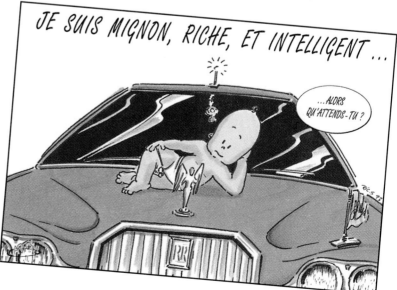

4 | *C'est à toi!*

1. Quelle est la date de ton anniversaire?
2. Qu'est-ce que tu aimes faire pour ton anniversaire?
3. Tu es timide?
4. Ta grand-mère, elle est généreuse ou égoïste?
5. Ton professeur de français est sympa?

Structure

Agreement of adjectives

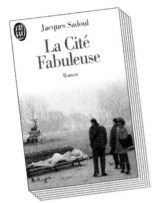

Adjectives, words that describe nouns and pronouns, are either masculine or feminine, singular or plural. Masculine adjectives are used with masculine nouns and pronouns; feminine adjectives are used with feminine nouns and pronouns. In French, adjectives usually follow the nouns they describe.

> M. Blot est un prof **intelligent**.   Mme Thibault est une prof **intelligente**.

Most feminine adjectives are formed by adding an **e** to masculine adjectives.

> masculine adjective + **e** = feminine adjective

> Thierry est un élève **diligent**.   Latifa est une élève **diligente**.

If a masculine adjective ends in **-e**, the feminine adjective is identical.

> Mon frère est **timide**.   Ma sœur est **timide** aussi.

If a masculine adjective ends in **-eux,** the feminine adjective ends in **-euse.**

> Sébastien est **généreux**.   Sandrine est **généreuse** aussi.

Some common adjectives, like **beau**, precede the nouns they describe. The masculine adjective **beau** has an irregular feminine form, **belle**. Before a masculine noun beginning with a vowel sound, use **bel**.

> Voilà un **beau** garçon.
> Voilà un **bel** étudiant.
> Voilà une **belle** fille.

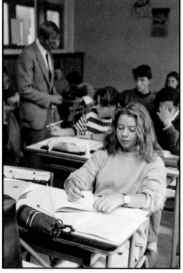

Stéphanie est une élève diligente.

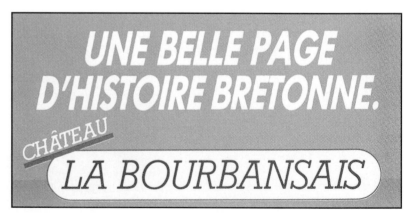

If an adjective describes a plural noun, the adjective must be plural also. To form the plural of most adjectives, add an **s** to singular adjectives.

> singular adjective + **s** = plural adjective

Ton cousin est bavard.	Mes cousins sont bavards aussi.
Ma sœur est paresseuse.	Ses sœurs sont paresseuses aussi.

If a masculine singular adjective ends in **-s**, the masculine plural adjective is identical.

Le chat est gris.	Les chiens sont gris aussi.

The masculine singular adjective **beau** has an irregular plural form, **beaux.**

> Jérémy a deux beaux chiens.

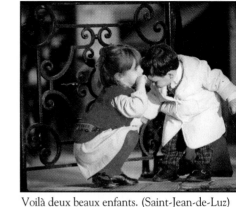

Voilà deux beaux enfants. (Saint-Jean-de-Luz)

Pratique

5 | Describe some of the people in your classroom. Use a different adjective to describe each one.

Modèle:

Jamila est bavarde.

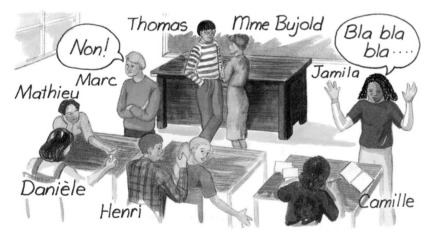

6 | Brothers and sisters sometimes are very different. Say that these brothers and sisters are the opposites of their siblings.

1. Paul et Pierre sont bavards. Et Patricia et Pauline?
2. Judith et Claudette sont généreuses. Et Jean?
3. Myriam est intelligente. Et Max et Michel?
4. Fayçal est méchant. Et Fatima?
5. Anne-Marie et Ariane sont bêtes. Et Alexandre?
6. Christophe est égoïste. Et Christine et Chloé?
7. Florence est timide. Et Fred et Fabrice?
8. Delphine et Denise sont diligentes. Et David et Daniel?

Modèle:

Charles est paresseux. Et Caroline et Catherine?
Caroline et Catherine ne sont pas paresseuses. Elles sont diligentes.

7 Flatter M. Diouf by telling him that his family members and pets are beautiful or handsome.

1. une femme
2. un cheval
3. trois chiens
4. un oiseau
5. deux filles
6. un fils
7. quatre poissons rouges

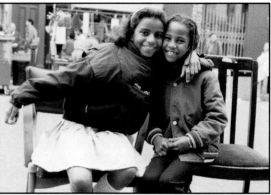

Monsieur Diouf, vous avez deux belles filles!

Communication

8 Your French teacher wants to know the birthdays of all the students in class in order to send birthday cards to everyone on the appropriate date. To make your teacher's job easier, ask your classmates their dates of birth in French and then arrange yourselves in a line in chronological order from left to right according to the information you obtain. Ask as many classmates as possible their dates of birth in order to know if you should stand to the right or left of them. When everyone is in the correct birth order, go down the line, one by one, saying your date of birth.

9 To get to know some of your classmates better, interview five of them, asking them their name, age, birthday and what they're like. To help you organize the information you gather, make a "sun" for each student you interview.

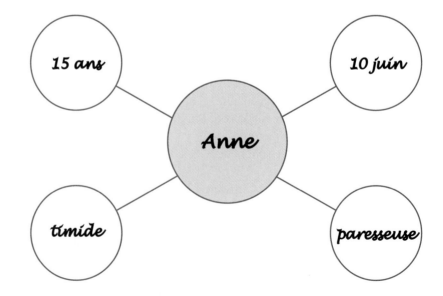

10 Your French pen pal, Jérémy, sent you a picture of his family. Describe each person in the picture as completely as you can, mentioning a physical trait and a character trait.

Modèle:

Le grand-père de Jérémy a les cheveux noirs. Il est méchant.

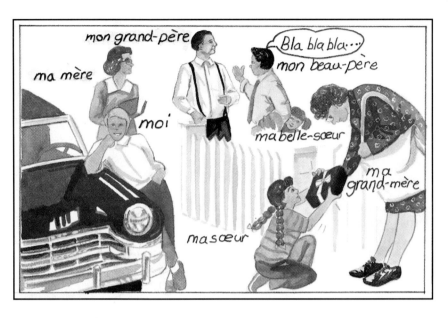

Sur la bonne piste

When reading something, you naturally form mental pictures based on your own cultural viewpoint. If you are an American, this means that you "see" the reading through the eyes of an American: what's true or common in the United States seems like it should be true elsewhere in the world. Furthermore, your mind has a limited capacity and doesn't consider all the different possible definitions of a word. Instead, your mind tries to save thinking space by forming a very brief picture of what that word means and skipping by many other possible interpretations. The information that "slips by" may be important to other people, especially those from a different culture.

For example, when you see **une maison**, the French word for "house," you might picture a little white house with a garden, perhaps out in the country. You probably save the picture of an inner-city dwelling for the word "apartment." But many French people live in apartments and call them **une maison**. For another example, when you look at the number sequence 11-3-97 in English, it represents November 3, 1997. However, you already know that the French write 3.11.97 to represent this date. If you weren't aware of this, it's possible you could order tickets to the theater for the wrong night or wait for a train on the wrong day. You might ask "Why don't the French write the date the 'right' way?" The French believe they do, sequencing the date from the shortest period of time (the day) to the longest (the year).

In Marie-Claire's letter to her pen pal that follows, she tells about where she lives and gives the date. As you read her letter, remember that some words and ideas can be interpreted in more than one way. Writers give you many clues that can tell you whether or not you're on the right track. Keeping the context of the reading in mind will help guide you as you encounter events that are different in another culture.

En famille

Marie-Claire va recevoir une jeune fille canadienne, Gilberte, pendant trois semaines en décembre. Gilberte fait partie d'un programme d'échanges. Voici la lettre de Marie-Claire à Gilberte.

12.7.97

Chère Gilberte,

Je suis très contente que tu viennes chez moi en décembre. J'ai 15 ans et je vais à l'école à Tours. Mes parents sont divorcés. J'habite dans une maison avec ma mère et mon beau-père. Ma mère est blonde aux yeux bleus. Demain c'est son anniversaire. Elle va avoir 42 ans. C'est aussi la fête de mon père. Quelle coïncidence, n'est-ce pas? Mon père est brun, grand et intelligent.

J'ai une sœur, Danielle. Elle a 21 ans. En ce moment, elle est à l'Université de Nantes. J'ai aussi un demi-frère. Il s'appelle Patrick et il a 9 ans.

J'adore les animaux. J'ai un chat, un chien et un canari chez ma belle-mère et mon père.

J'ai hâte de faire ta connaissance. Tu vas être comme un membre de la famille.

À bientôt,
Marie-Claire

11 Answer the following questions.

1. When did Marie-Claire write this letter?
2. When will Gilberte's visit take place?
3. How many cats does Marie-Claire have?
4. What is Marie-Claire's sister like?
5. Why is Marie-Claire writing to Gilberte?
6. Marie-Claire bought gifts for certain members of her family. For whom does she have gifts and why?

Nathalie et Raoul

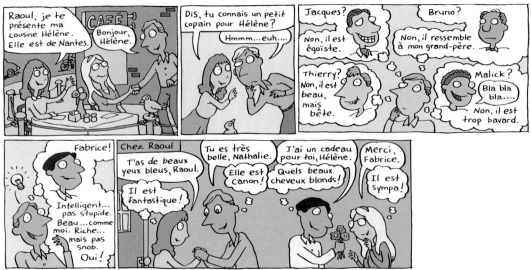

C'est à moi!

Now that you have completed this unit, take a look at what you should be able to do in French. Can you do all of these tasks?

➤ I can ask for and give information about who someone is.

➤ I can identify family members, including pets.

➤ I can ask and tell how old someone is.

➤ I can describe someone's physical and character traits.

➤ I can express emotions.

➤ I can ask and tell what the date is.

➤ I can say when someone's birthday is.

➤ I can explain why.

➤ I can tell where places are located.

Here is a brief checkup to see how much you understand about French culture. Decide if each statement is **vrai** or **faux**.

1. The French word **beau-père** is used for both "father-in-law" and "stepfather."
2. Martinique and Guadeloupe are both located in French-speaking Canada.
3. Huguenots are the only French workers who get one month's paid vacation each year.
4. There are more pets than children in France.
5. French people usually have well-mannered dogs that are accepted even in hotels and restaurants.
6. Extended families in France live in the same towns or cities and get together every Sunday.

Why do extended families get together so often in France? ((Dinard)

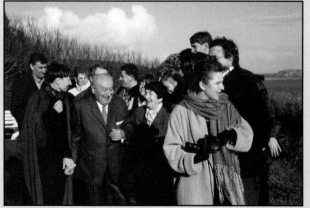

7. French parents receive money from the government upon the birth of each child.
8. Couples in France must get married at **la mairie**.
9. The French often celebrate birthdays with cakes topped with candles.
10. Besides celebrating the day on which they were born, the French also celebrate their saint's feast day.

Communication orale

Modèle:

Student A: Qu'est-ce que le prof d'anglais donne à l'école?

Student B: Le prof d'anglais donne un dictionnaire et des stylos. Il est généreux.

Imagine that a school in Martinique was recently destroyed by a hurricane. Your school's student government is collecting school supplies to send to the students and teachers there. They need everything from pens and pencils to VCRs and TVs. With a partner, ask and tell what various students and teachers, as well as your family members, are donating to this cause. As you take turns with your partner naming people who are contributing, give one more piece of information about each person, for example, a character trait. Follow the model.

Communication écrite

As a follow-up to your conversation with your partner about contributing to the relief fund for the school in Martinique, write a memo to your French teacher. Begin your memo with today's date. Then, based on your conversation, mention who is giving what to the students and teachers whose school was destroyed and tell something about each donor. Finally, ask your teacher what he or she is giving.

Communication active

To ask for information, use:

C'est toi? — *Is this you?*

Il est beau comme moi, **n'est-ce pas?** — *He's handsome like I am, isn't that so?*

To give information, use:

C'est Justin. — *It's Justin.*

To point out family members, use:

C'est mon père. — *This is my father.*

C'est ma mère. — *This is my mother.*

Ce sont mes parents. — *These are my parents.*

Milou **est un membre de la famille.** — *Milou is a member of the family.*

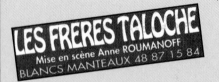

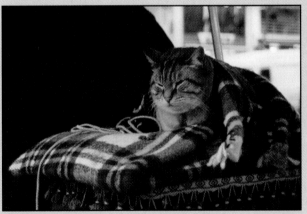

Mistigris est aussi un membre de la famille. (Paris)

To ask how old someone is, use:
    Tu as quel âge?   *How old are you?*

To tell how old someone is, use:
    Il/Elle a quinze **an(s).**   *He/She is fifteen years old.*

To describe physical traits, use:
    J'ai les cheveux blonds.   *I have blond hair.*
    J'ai les yeux bleus.   *I have blue eyes.*

To describe character, use:
    Je suis généreux/généreuse.   *I'm generous.*

To express emotions, use:
    Que je suis bête!   *How stupid I am!*

To ask what the date is, use:
    C'est quelle date?   *What's the date?*

To tell what the date is, use:
    Nous sommes le 25 avril.   *It's April 25.*
    C'est le 1er août.   *It's August 1.*

To tell when someone's birthday is, use:
    Son anniversaire est le   *His/Her birthday is October 26.*
    vingt-six octobre.

To explain something, use:
    Parce que c'est ton anniversaire.   *Because it's your birthday.*

To tell location, use:
    C'est **à** 7.000 **kilomètres**   *It's 7,000 kilometers from Nantes.*
    de Nantes.

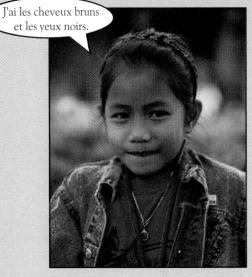

J'ai les cheveux bruns
et les yeux noirs.

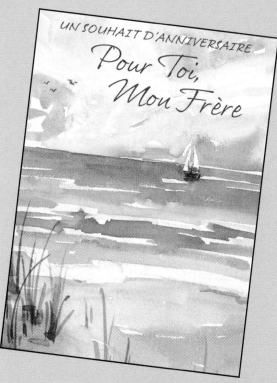

UN SOUHAIT D'ANNIVERSAIRE
Pour Toi,
Mon Frère

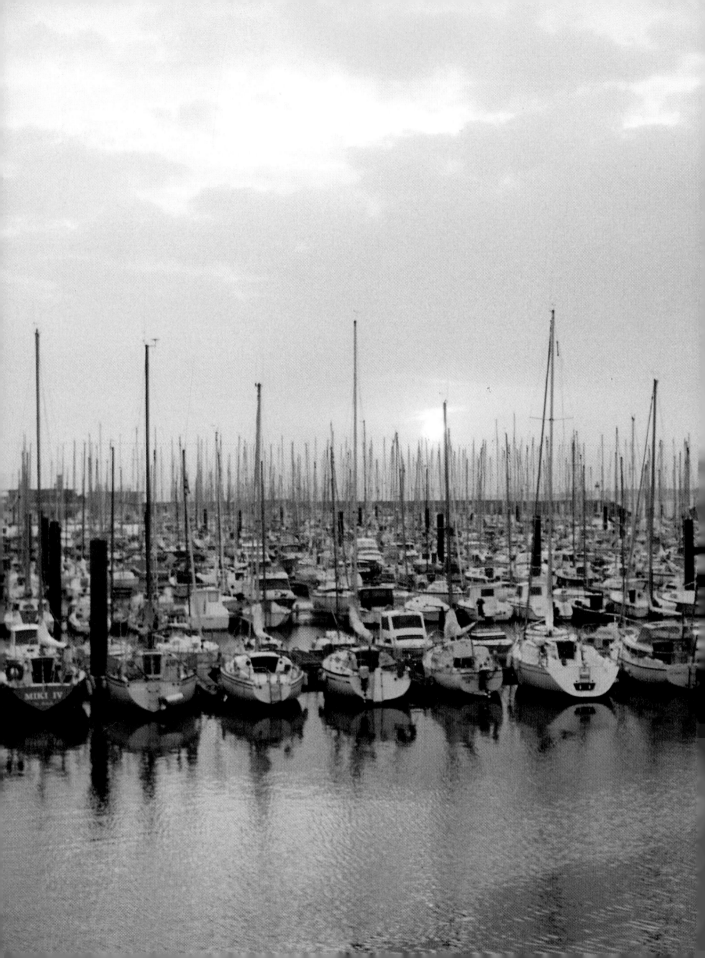

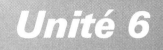

Unité 6

Tu viens d'où?

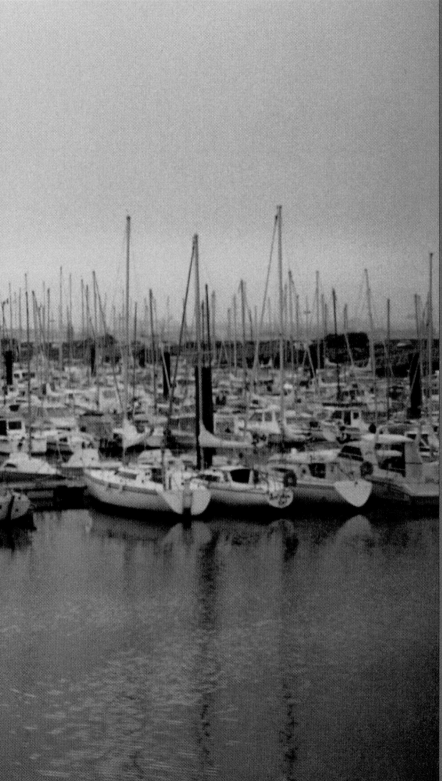

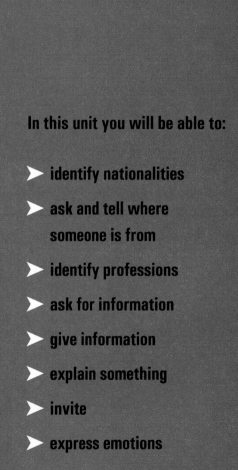

In this unit you will be able to:

- ➤ identify nationalities
- ➤ ask and tell where someone is from
- ➤ identify professions
- ➤ ask for information
- ➤ give information
- ➤ explain something
- ➤ invite
- ➤ express emotions

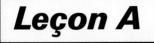

Leçon A

In this lesson you will be able to:

➤ ask for information

➤ ask and tell where someone is from

➤ identify nationalities

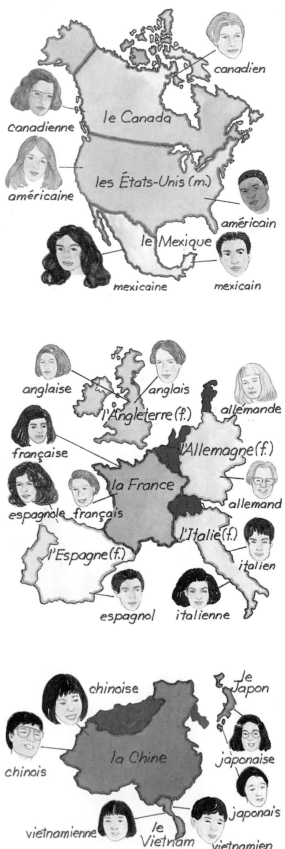

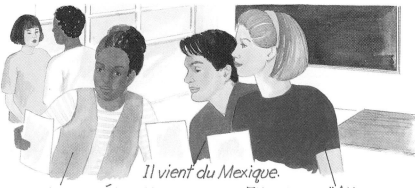

Ils viennent d'où?

Elle vient des États-Unis.

Il vient du Mexique.

Elle vient d'Allemagne.

It's the beginning of the school year in Tours. At a meeting of international exchange students, Petra, Sandy and José are showing each other pictures of their families.

Sandy: **C'est qui sur la photo?**

José: **C'est ma famille... mon père et ma belle-mère.**

Petra: **Vous venez d'où?**

José: **Nous venons du Mexique. Mon père et moi, nous sommes mexicains, et ma belle-mère est japonaise. Et toi, Petra, tu viens d'où? Est-ce que tu es allemande?**

Petra: **Oui, je viens d'Allemagne. Voilà ma famille.**

Sandy: **Tu ressembles à ta mère. Moi, je ressemble à mon père. Je viens des États-Unis. Je suis de Dallas.**

Situated in the Loire Valley, Tours is the capital of the Touraine region of France. The area around Tours has many beautiful castles, such as

Enquête culturelle

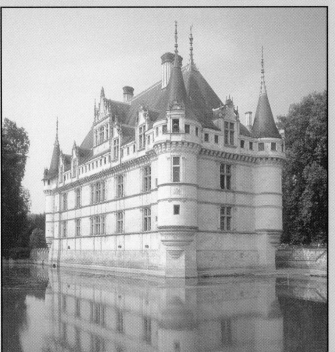

Azay-le-Rideau, like the other Renaissance castles, was built in the 16th century.

Chenonceaux and Chambord. The city's cultural and intellectual life centers around its university, which attracts students from all over the world. Many American teachers and students study in Tours.

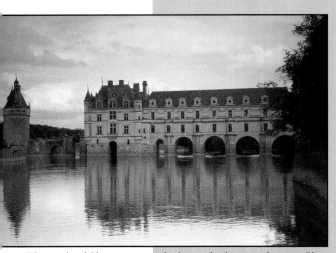

The castle of Chenonceaux is built on a bridge over the river Cher.

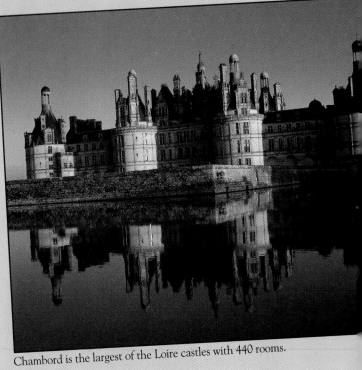

Chambord is the largest of the Loire castles with 440 rooms.

European teenagers have many opportunities to travel to other countries. Because of the relatively small size of the European continent, it doesn't take long by car or train to arrive in another country. Europeans often vacation in neighboring countries. Rather than simply visiting famous monuments, people in Europe often like to explore quaint villages, camp in quiet parks or get to know other people. Therefore, Europeans find

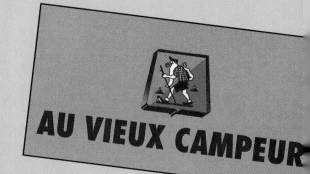

AU VIEUX CAMPEUR

an immediate use for speaking a second language, and international study programs are very popular.

Complétez les phrases avec la lettre du mot convenable d'après le dialogue.
(Complete the sentences with the letter of the appropriate word according to the dialogue.)

1. José vient du....
2. José et son père sont....
3. La... de José est japonaise.
4. Petra est....
5. Petra vient d'....
6. Petra ressemble à sa....
7. Sandy ressemble à son....
8. Sandy vient des....

a. États-Unis
b. allemande
c. mère
d. Mexique
e. belle-mère
f. père
g. mexicains
h. Allemagne

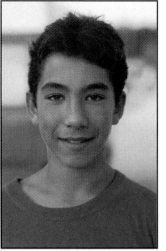

Manuel vient d'Espagne. Il est espagnol.

Azteca   MEXICAIN
7, rue Sauval Paris 1er, tél : 42 36 11 16.
Ce charmant restaurant propose une agréable cuisine mexicaine. Musiciens et chanteurs le soir. *A nice restaurant serving a good Mexican cuisine.*
■ Menus déj. / *Luncheon menus :* 58 & 89 FF.

Match the letter of the sentence that describes each person's nationality with the sentence that tells the country he or she comes from.

1. Rolf vient d'Allemagne.
2. Gina vient d'Italie.
3. Tim vient des États-Unis.
4. Francisco vient d'Espagne.
5. Diana vient d'Angleterre.
6. Liu vient de Chine.
7. Sei vient du Japon.
8. Yolanda vient du Mexique.

a. Il est espagnol.
b. Elle est mexicaine.
c. Elle est anglaise.
d. Elle est japonaise.
e. Elle est italienne.
f. Il est allemand.
g. Il est chinois.
h. Il est américain.

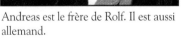

Andreas est le frère de Rolf. Il est aussi allemand.

LA BOCCA

RESTAURANT ITALIEN - BAR
59, rue Montmartre 75002 Paris
Tel: 42 36 71 88
Fermé le dimanche

CHEZ NGO

 Haute gastronomie chinoise et thaïlandaise. Spécialités de poissons frais et crustacés vivants, préparées par 2 chefs, l'un chinois l'autre thaïlandais.

3 *C'est à toi!*

1. Tu viens d'où?
2. Tes parents, ils viennent d'où?
3. Tu ressembles à un membre de ta famille?
4. Tu étudies le français, l'espagnol ou l'allemand?
5. Ton professeur d'anglais, il/elle est américain(e)?

Structure

Present tense of the irregular verb *venir*

The verb **venir** (*to come*) is irregular.

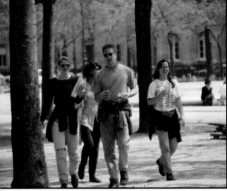

Qui vient? (Paris)

venir			
je	**viens**	Je **viens** d'Allemagne.	*I come from Germany.*
tu	**viens**	Tu **viens** d'où?	*Where are you from?*
il/elle/on	**vient**	Juan **vient** du Mexique.	*Juan comes from Mexico.*
nous	**venons**	Nous **venons** ensemble.	*We're coming together.*
vous	**venez**	Vous ne **venez** pas demain?	*Aren't you coming tomorrow?*
ils/elles	**viennent**	Ils **viennent** chez moi.	*They're coming to my house.*

Tout vient à point
à qui sait attendre demain
vendredi 13.

Pratique

4 Some of your friends are meeting at a café after school. Tell who's coming with whom.

Thérèse vient avec Dominique.

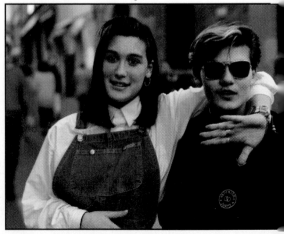

1. je/avec Charles
2. David et Renée/ ensemble
3. Sandrine/avec Latifa
4. Charles et moi, nous/ ensemble
5. tu/avec Delphine
6. Bruno/avec Louis
7. Françoise et Cécile/ ensemble
8. Delphine et toi, vous/ ensemble

Modèle:

Théo et Stéphanie/ensemble
Théo et Stéphanie viennent ensemble.

With a partner, take turns asking and telling who's coming to the school dance. Follow the models.

1. Margarette/non
2. tu/oui
3. Daniel et toi, vous/oui
4. Abdou/non
5. Anne-Marie et Benjamin/non
6. Nathalie et moi, nous/oui
7. Béatrice et Karine/oui
8. le prof de français/non

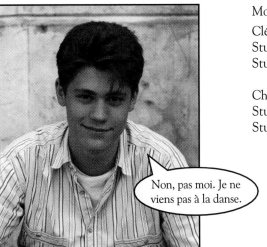

Non, pas moi. Je ne viens pas à la danse.

Modèles:

Clément/oui
Student A: Clément vient?
Student B: Oui, il vient.

Chloé et Alain/non
Student B: Chloé et Alain viennent?
Student A: Non, ils ne viennent pas.

De + definite articles

The preposition **de** (*of, from*) does not change before the definite articles **la** and **l'**.

C'est l'ordinateur de la fille.   *It's the girl's computer.*
Où est le cahier de l'élève?   *Where is the student's notebook?*

Before the definite articles **le** and **les**, however, **de** changes form. **De** combines with **le** and **les** as follows:

de + le = du	*from (the), of (the)*
de + les = des	*from (the), of (the)*

Je viens des États-Unis.   *I'm from the United States.*
José vient du Mexique.   *José is from Mexico.*

To say that someone is from a country with a masculine name, use a form of **venir de** with the definite article: **Je viens du Canada. Elle vient des États-Unis.** To say that someone is from a country with a feminine name, do not use the definite article after **de** or **d'**: **Il vient de Chine. Elles viennent d'Angleterre.** (To say that someone is from a certain city or town, use a form of **être de**: **Je suis de Chicago.**)

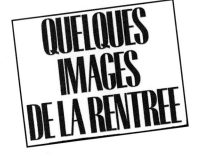

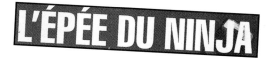

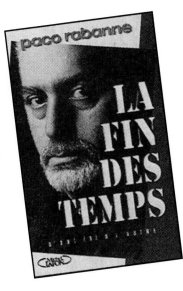

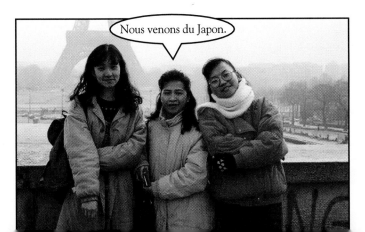

Nous venons du Japon.

Pratique

Modèle:

Minou
C'est le chat de la mère.

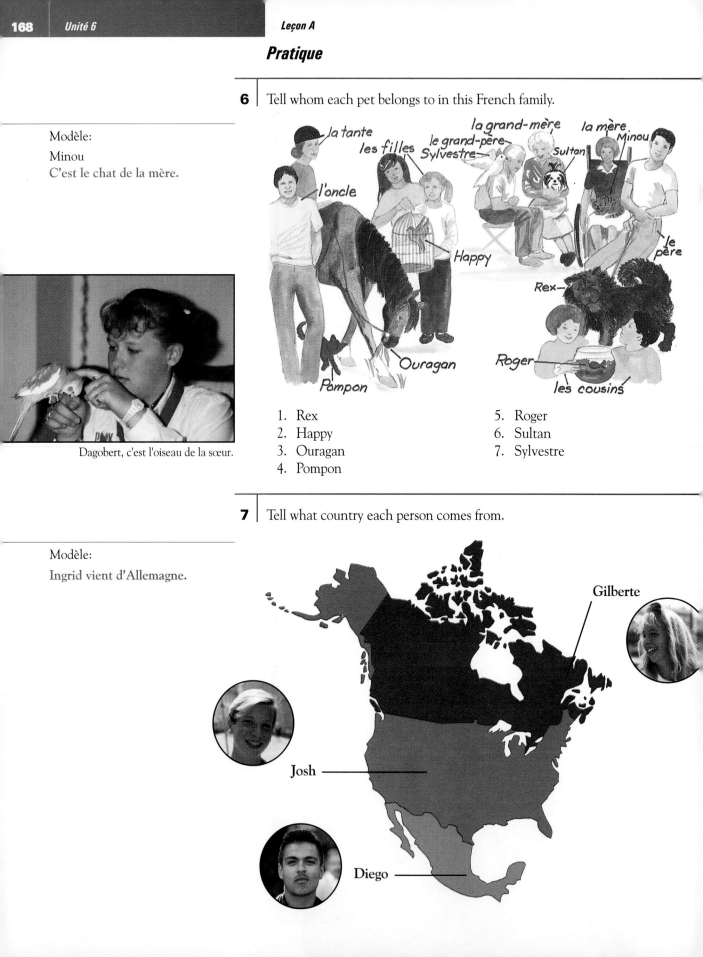

Dagobert, c'est l'oiseau de la sœur.

6 | Tell whom each pet belongs to in this French family.

1. Rex
2. Happy
3. Ouragan
4. Pompon
5. Roger
6. Sultan
7. Sylvestre

7 | Tell what country each person comes from.

Modèle:

Ingrid vient d'Allemagne.

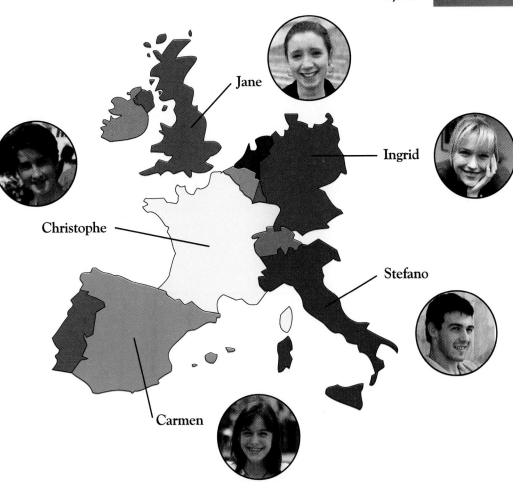

Forming questions

Questions can be divided into two groups:

1. questions that can be answered by "yes" or "no"
    Is it raining?
2. questions that ask for information
    What time is it?

In spoken French there are three basic ways to ask a question that can be answered by "yes" or "no":

1. Make your tone of voice rise at the end of a sentence.
    (It rises at the end of all "yes" or "no" questions.)

    C'est ta famille sur la photo? *Is this your family in the photo?*

2. Put the expression **est-ce que** right before the subject of the sentence. **Est-ce que** has no meaning by itself; it serves only to change a statement into a question. Before a word beginning with a vowel sound, **est-ce que** becomes **est-ce qu'**.

    Est-ce que Normand   *Is Normand Canadian?*
    est canadien?
    Est-ce qu'il est de Montréal? *Is he from Montreal?*

Vous venez des États-Unis, n'est-ce pas?

3. Add the expression **n'est-ce pas** to the end of a sentence. **N'est-ce pas** basically means "isn't that so" and may be interpreted in various ways, depending on context.

C'est ta sœur, **n'est-ce pas?** *She's your sister, isn't she?*
Vous venez du Mexique, *You're from Mexico, aren't you?*
n'est-ce pas?

In spoken French you form a question that asks for information by using a specific question word followed by **est-ce que**, a subject and a verb. Some question words you have already seen are **comment**, **qui**, **pourquoi**, **combien** and **où**.

Où est-ce que tu vas? *Where are you going?*
Avec **qui est-ce que** tu *With whom are you playing tennis?*
joues au tennis?

Pratique

8 | You are going to conduct a survey about what teenagers do in their free time. Prepare some questions for your survey.

Modèle:

skier
Est-ce que tu skies?

1. jouer au basket
2. nager
3. danser
4. aller au cinéma
5. manger au fast-food
6. regarder la télé
7. étudier
8. téléphoner

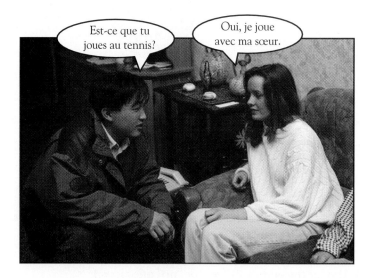

Est-ce que tu joues au tennis?

Oui, je joue avec ma sœur.

9 | Now prepare some follow-up survey questions to ask the participants if they answer "yes" to any of your original questions.

Modèle:

skier (pourquoi)
Pourquoi est-ce que tu skies?

1. jouer au basket (avec qui)
2. nager (comment)
3. danser (comment)
4. aller au cinéma (avec qui)
5. manger au fast-food (pourquoi)
6. regarder la télé (à quelle heure)
7. étudier (où)
8. téléphoner (à qui)

Communication

A group of French-speaking international exchange students is going to visit your French class. You volunteered to make name tags for the visitors and to introduce them to your classmates. To practice your introductions, look at each name tag you made and then give the appropriate information.

Modèle:

> Bonjour! Je m'appelle
>
> *Renée Tremblay*
> *canadienne*
> *Montréal*

Voilà Renée Tremblay. Elle vient du Canada. Elle est de Montréal.

> Bonjour! Je m'appelle
>
> *Jacques Delorme*
> *français*
> *Paris*

> Bonjour! Je m'appelle
>
> *Margaret Tate*
> *anglaise*
> *Northampton*

> Bonjour! Je m'appelle
>
> *Paola Malpezzi*
> *italienne*
> *Milan*

> Bonjour! Je m'appelle
>
> *Jun An*
> *chinoise*
> *Bei-jing*

> Bonjour! Je m'appelle
>
> *Karl Kohl*
> *allemand*
> *Bonn*

> Bonjour! Je m'appelle
>
> *María Herrera*
> *mexicaine*
> *Veracruz*

> Bonjour! Je m'appelle
>
> *Diego Botero*
> *espagnol*
> *Madrid*

> Bonjour! Je m'appelle
>
> *Akio Kusumoto*
> *japonais*
> *Tokyo*

> Bonjour! Je m'appelle
>
> *Loan Cao*
> *vietnamienne*
> *Hô Chi Minh-Ville*

11 Some of the international exchange students that are visiting your class have brought family pictures along with them. With a partner, look at these pictures and then take turns discussing some of the family resemblances you notice. Also see if you can remember where each student is from. Follow the model.

Modèle:

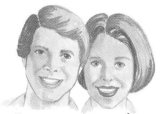

Jacques et sa mère

Student A: Tiens, Jacques ressemble à sa mère!
Student B: Oui, il a ses cheveux blonds.
Student A: Il vient d'où?
Student B: Il vient de France.

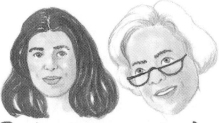

Paola et sa grand-mère

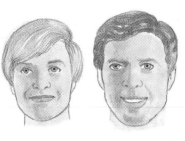

Karl et son père

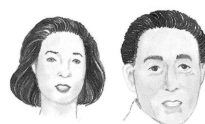

Loan et son père

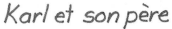

Margaret et sa sœur

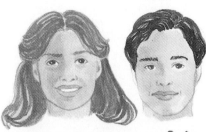

María et son frère

You and your friend Melissa Montoya are applying for a homestay program in Paris. At the end of the application form you are asked to write a short composition in French about yourself. Melissa has already finished her composition, but you haven't started yours. Take a look at Melissa's composition for ideas. Then write your own paragraph.

Je m'appelle Melissa Montoya. Je suis américaine. J'ai 15 ans. Mes parents sont Eduardo et Kay Montoya. J'ai un frère, Andy, et deux sœurs, Katie et Ana. Nous avons un chat qui s'appelle Harley. Mon professeur de français s'appelle Madame Darber. J'ai six cours: français, anglais, histoire, biologie, maths, musique. J'aime faire du footing et du vélo. J'aime aussi lire, aller au cinéma, regarder la télé et écouter de la musique. Je voudrais aller à Paris parce que j'aime la France et le français.

Intonation

Prononciation

In spoken French the voice rises slightly after each group of related words. The voice then falls back to the beginning pitch to start the next phrase. Finally, at the end of the statement, the voice falls to the lowest point. This rising and falling of the voice is called intonation. The lines above the sentence show how the voice rises and falls. Say each of these sentences.

Clarisse ressemble à sa mère.

Elle a ses yeux bleus et ses cheveux bruns.

Mon père et moi, nous sommes américains, et ma belle-mère est japonaise.

In French there are basically two intonation patterns for questions. Questions requiring a "yes" or "no" answer have a rising intonation pattern. Say each of these questions:

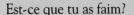

On y va?

Est-ce que tu as faim?

Information-seeking questions have a falling intonation pattern. Say each of these questions:

Où est le cahier?

Qui aime étudier?

Leçon B

In this lesson you will be able to:

➤ identify professions

➤ ask for information

➤ give information

➤ explain something

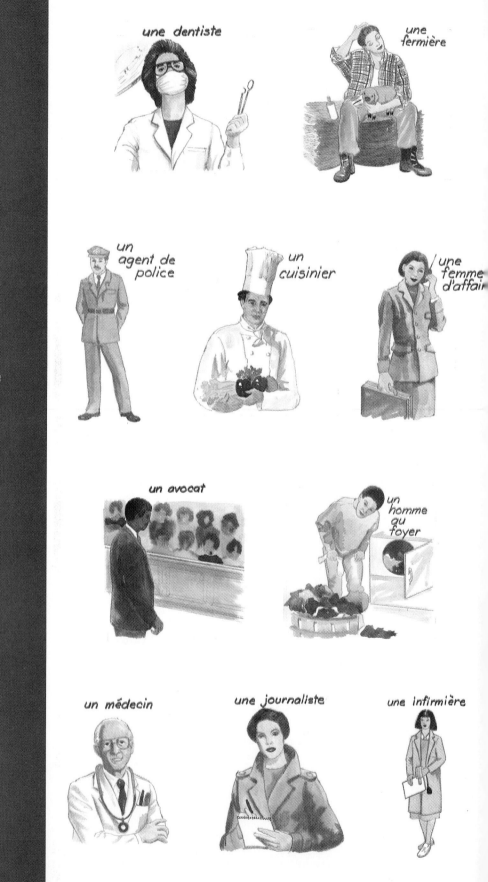

une dentiste

une fermière

un agent de police

un cuisinier

une femme d'affai

un avocat

un homme au foyer

un médecin

une journaliste

une infirmière

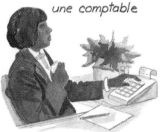
une comptable

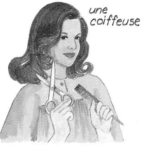
une coiffeuse

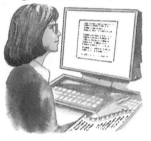
une informaticienne

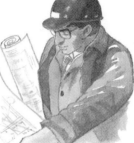
un ingénieur

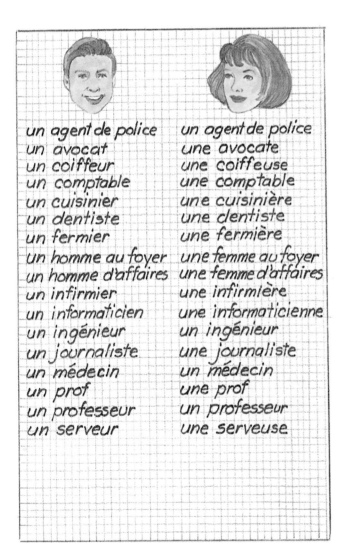

un agent de police	un agent de police
un avocat	une avocate
un coiffeur	une coiffeuse
un comptable	une comptable
un cuisinier	une cuisinière
un dentiste	une dentiste
un fermier	une fermière
un homme au foyer	une femme au foyer
un homme d'affaires	une femme d'affaires
un infirmier	une infirmière
un informaticien	une informaticienne
un ingénieur	un ingénieur
un journaliste	une journaliste
un médecin	un médecin
un prof	une prof
un professeur	un professeur
un serveur	une serveuse

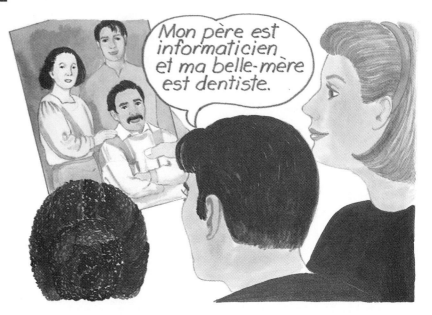

Petra, Sandy and José continue to exchange information about their families.

Petra: **Mon père, il est homme d'affaires. Il voyage beaucoup. Ma mère travaille beaucoup aussi. Elle est femme au foyer. Et tes parents, José?**

José: **Mon père est informaticien et ma belle-mère est dentiste. Sandy, quelle est la profession de tes parents?**

Sandy: **Je n'ai pas de mère. Mon père est prof de français.**

Petra: **Tiens, c'est pourquoi tu parles si bien le français!**

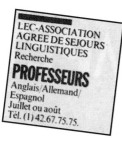

LEC-ASSOCIATION
AGREE DE SEJOURS
LINGUISTIQUES
Recherche

PROFESSEURS

Anglais/Allemand/
Espagnol
Juillet ou août
Tél. (1) 42.67.75.75.

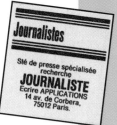 Enquête culturelle

Students over the age of 14 may work during their school vacations. Since school is required until the age of 16, people younger than 16 do not work full-time. The official work week in France is 39 hours, but naturally the actual number of hours spent working depends on the specific job and worker. In offices and stores, the work day typically begins around 8:00 A.M. or 9:00 A.M. and finishes between 5:00 P.M. and 7:00 P.M. All people who are salaried for 12 months are given six weeks of vacation. Many people take up to four weeks of vacation in the summer; the

Journalistes

Sté de presse spécialisée
recherche
JOURNALISTE
Ecrire APPLICATIONS
14 av. de Corbera,
75012 Paris.

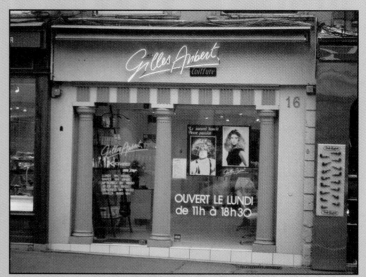

How many hours is this hairdresser open on Monday?

other weeks must be taken at a different time of the year. In addition, employers must pay salaried employees for 11 holidays each year. Another benefit that French workers receive is the opportunity to take continuing education courses. By law, French firms must offer these courses to their employees, who may, for example, perfect their professional knowledge or learn a foreign language.

Répondez par "vrai" ou "faux" d'après le dialogue.
(Answer "true" or "false" according to the dialogue.)

1. Le père de Petra est informaticien.
2. La mère de Petra voyage beaucoup.
3. La belle-mère de José n'est pas femme au foyer.
4. Le père de José est dentiste.
5. Le père de Sandy est professeur de français.
6. Sandy ne parle pas très bien le français.

Match the picture and the description to answer the question **Quelle est sa profession?**

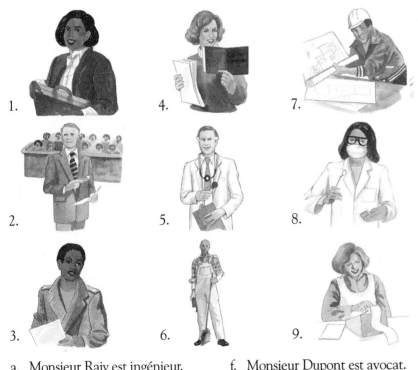

1.
2.
3.
4.
5.
6.
7.
8.
9.

a. Monsieur Rajy est ingénieur.
b. Mademoiselle Sorlot est dentiste.
c. Monsieur Géraud est médecin.
d. Monsieur Odier est fermier.
e. Madame Toussaint est femme d'affaires.
f. Monsieur Dupont est avocat.
g. Madame Pinot est comptable.
h. Mademoiselle Blot est journaliste.
i. Madame Vasconi est professeur.

3 | *C'est à toi!*

1. Quelle est la profession de tes parents?
2. Est-ce que tu préfères être journaliste ou comptable?
3. Est-ce que tu préfères être agent de police ou médecin?
4. Est-ce que tu voyages beaucoup?
5. Dans la salle de classe, qui parle bien le français?

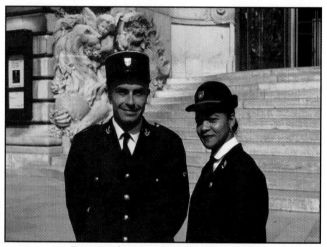

Est-ce qu'ils sont agents de police ou médecins? (Paris)

Structure

Indefinite articles in negative sentences

The indefinite articles **un**, **une** and **des** become **de** or **d'** (*a, an, any*) in a negative sentence.

Tu as **un** frère?	Non, je n'ai pas **de** frère.
Est-ce que Marcel a **une** tante?	Non, il n'a pas **de** tante.
M. Rondeau a **des** enfants?	Non, il n'a pas **d'**enfants.

However, **un**, **une** and **des** do not change after a form of the verb **être** in a negative sentence.

Ce sont des photos de mes parents; ce ne sont pas **des** photos de mes profs.

These are pictures of my parents; they're not pictures of my teachers.

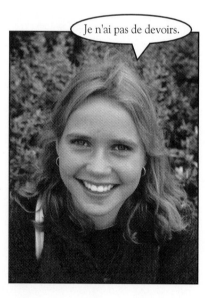

Je n'ai pas de devoirs.

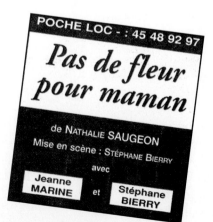

POCHE LOC - : 45 48 92 97

Pas de fleur pour maman

de Nathalie SAUGEON
Mise en scène : Stéphane Bierry

avec

Jeanne **MARINE** et Stéphane **BIERRY**

Pratique

Because of a mix-up in the school cafeteria, many students are missing a part of their lunch. Tell what each person doesn't have.

Modèle:

Mélanie

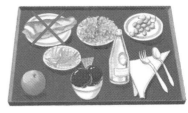

Mélanie n'a pas de sandwich.

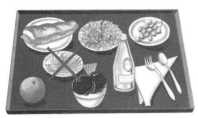

1. Jérôme

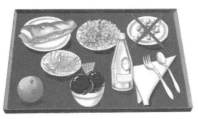

4. Suzanne

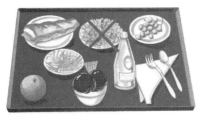

2. Anne-Marie

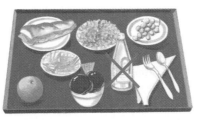

5. Assane

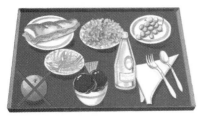

3. je

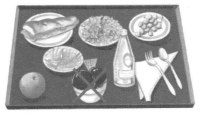

6. tu

With a partner, take turns asking and telling whether or not you have the following relatives and pets. Follow the model.

1. une sœur
2. un oiseau
3. un chat
4. des oncles
5. un cheval
6. des poissons rouges
7. une cousine
8. un chien

Modèle:

un frère

Student A: Est-ce que tu as un frère?
Student B: Oui, j'ai un frère. Et toi, est-ce que tu as un frère?
Student A: Non, je n'ai pas de frère.

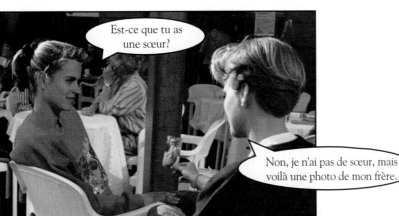

The interrogative adjective *quel*

The adjective **quel** means "which" or "what" and is used to ask questions. **Quel** comes before the noun it describes.

	Masculine	Feminine
Singular	quel	quelle
Plural	quels	quelles

Tu préfères **quel** coiffeur?	*Which hairdresser do you prefer?*
Quelle femme d'affaires voyage beaucoup?	*Which businesswoman travels a lot?*

The forms of **quel** may also come directly before the verb **être**. In this case **quel** agrees with the noun after **être**.

Quelle est la profession de tes parents?	*What are your parents' occupations?*

Pratique

6 Bruno is trying to tell you who's talking to whom, but he isn't being very clear. Ask him to be more specific.

Modèle:

Véronique parle avec un professeur.
Quel professeur?

1. Adja parle avec un coiffeur.
2. Ariane et Alain parlent avec une journaliste.
3. Paul parle avec des agents de police.
4. Monique parle avec une prof.
5. Mme Manet et son fils parlent avec un médecin.
6. Le prof de français parle avec des hommes d'affaires.
7. M. Lafitte parle avec des avocates.
8. Jean parle avec des informaticiennes.

C'est vs. *il/elle est*

Both **c'est** and **il/elle est** mean "he is" or "she is" as well as "it is."

Use **c'est** when the noun that follows is modified by an article, an adjective or both. In a negative sentence, **c'est** becomes **ce n'est pas**.

C'est ma dentiste; c'est une Italienne.	*She's my dentist; she's Italian.*
C'est un bon infirmier; ce n'est pas un médecin.	*He's a good nurse; he's not a doctor.*

Use **il/elle est** when the following word is an adjective or a noun that functions as an adjective (for example, the name of a nationality or an occupation).

Elle est italienne.	*She's Italian.*
Elle est dentiste.	*She's a dentist.*
Il est bavard.	*He's talkative.*

The corresponding plural forms are **ce sont** and **ils/elles sont**.

Ce sont des avocats.	*They are lawyers.*
Ils sont américains.	*They are American.*

Note that a noun of nationality is capitalized but an adjective of nationality is not.

C'est un **J**aponais.	
Il est **j**aponais.	*He's Japanese.*

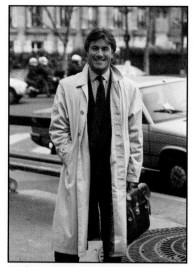

Voilà M. Lussac. Il est avocat.

Pratique

With a partner, talk about the occupations of various people. Student A asks questions and Student B answers them. Follow the model.

1. Mme Robert (prof de français/prof d'anglais)
2. Mlle Chartrier (coiffeuse/infirmière)
3. Jean-Michel (cuisinier/serveur)
4. M. et Mme Tremblay (médecins/dentistes)
5. M. Godot (ingénieur/comptable)
6. Mme Peyrot et Mme Renault (femmes au foyer/femmes d'affaires)
7. Mlle Olivari (informaticienne/journaliste)

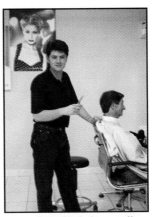
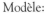

Jean-Michel est coiffeur.

Modèle:

M. Nataf (avocat/agent de police)
Student A: **Voilà Monsieur Nataf. Il est avocat?**
Student B: **Non, il est agent de police.**

Complete Béatrice's descriptions of the following people. Follow the model.

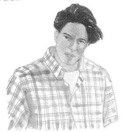

1. C'est Max. ... un bon élève. ... très beau! Max est de Montréal. ... canadien. ... un garçon timide. ... bavard.

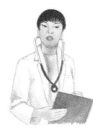

2. C'est Madame Tran. ... une infirmière. ... médecin. ... une femme très intelligente. ... vietnamienne. ... la femme de mon prof de maths.

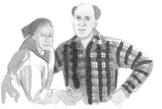

3. Ce sont mes parents. ... des fermiers. ... très diligents. Ma mère vient d'Espagne. ... espagnole. Mais mon père, ... un Français. ... des parents super!

4. Ce sont Clémence et Magali. ... mes cousines. ... étudiantes, mais elles travaillent aussi. Clémence travaille dans un café. ... serveuse. Magali travaille aussi dans un café, mais ... serveuse. ... une cuisinière.

Modèle:

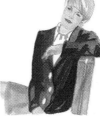

C'est Madame Gagner. **C'est** la mère de David, un garçon dans mon cours d'anglais. **Elle est** française. **Ce n'est pas** une femme au foyer. **C'est** une femme d'affaires. **Elle est** très sympa.

Communication

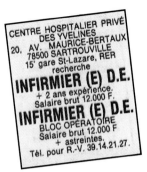

9 You are starting to think seriously about possible careers. Look at this list of ten occupations and on a separate sheet of paper rank them from one to ten in order of your preference.

dentiste	infirmier, infirmière
avocat, avocate	informaticien, informaticienne
fermier, fermière	comptable
professeur	journaliste
cuisinier, cuisinière	coiffeur, coiffeuse

10 For each of your top five career choices in Activity 9, determine what three classes in high school you might need to take in order to enter this profession.

11 Your assignment for current events day in social studies class is to find a newspaper article about jobs. To give your assignment a global perspective, you found an article in a French newspaper that reports the results of a survey taken in France. Two hundred students were surveyed about their parents' occupations. Read the article that follows and then, in order to share the results with students in your social studies class, make two bar graphs on a separate sheet of paper that show how many people are in each profession. In the first one, graph the occupations of the men; in the second one, graph the occupations of the women.

Bourges, le 23 septembre

Deux cents élèves ont participé à un sondage hier pour indiquer les professions et les métiers de leurs parents. Cent élèves de lycée technique, 50 élèves de collège et 50 élèves d'école primaire ont rempli ce sondage. Voilà les résultats.

Les Hommes

Il y a beaucoup de médecins et d'informaticiens parmi les hommes. Il y a 34 informaticiens et 28 médecins. Vingt de ces hommes sont dentistes, 10 sont avocats, six sont professeurs et cinq sont ingénieurs. Dans ce groupe il y a neuf journalistes, trois infirmiers, sept agents de police et 14 comptables. Quinze hommes travaillent comme cuisiniers et huit sont fermiers. Cinq travaillent à la maison comme hommes au foyer et 13 ne travaillent pas.

Les Femmes

Les femmes ont aussi beaucoup de professions différentes. Les professions les plus populaires pour les femmes sont médecin, professeur et ingénieur. Vingt-deux de ces femmes sont médecins, 21 sont professeurs et 20 sont ingénieurs. Dans ce groupe il y a 12 infirmières, 12 dentistes et sept journalistes. Il y a aussi 13 coiffeuses, 15 serveuses, sept comptables, deux fermières et neuf cuisinières. Dix-sept sont femmes au foyer et 16 ne travaillent pas.

2 Here are some employment ads from a newspaper in Nice. Study them and then answer the questions that follow by giving the letter of the appropriate ad.

a.
> Clinique Nice cherche infirmier, service chirurgie, temps plein, poste à pourvoir à partir du 26 août. Tél. 93.13.65.20 de 9 à 16 heures.

b.
> Cherche serveuse. Se présenter RESTAURANT DE PARIS, 28 rue d'Angleterre, Nice, ce jour à partir de 18h.

c.
> Hôtel 4 étoiles recherche secrétaire réception, expérience, anglais courant, libre de suite pour saison, tél. 93.50.02.02. Vence.

d.
> Cherche apprenti(e) coiffeur(euse). 1ère année et 3ème année. Tél. 93.31.12.65.

e.
> CNRS pour laboratoire de recherche Sophia-Antipolis recrute sur concours, un assistant ingénieur en Biologie, ayant bonnes connaissances en biologie moléculaire, culture de cellules, biologie et physiologie cellulaires (DUT ou équivalence). 93.95.77.05.

f.
> INTERNATIONAL HOUSE, 90 écoles de langues dans 20 pays, recrute en septembre pour son centre de Nice, secrétaire commerciale bilingue confirmée. Ecrire 22 boulevard Dubouchage, Nice.

g.
> Restaurant poissons Cagnes-Sur-Mer, cherche cuisinier ou commis de cuisine qualifié, de langue maternelle française, pour saison, libre de suite, bien rémunéré. Tél. pour rendez-vous, au 93.07.36.59 le matin avant 12h00.

h.
> Clinique Nice cherche un infirmier psychiatrique ou DE, jour, temps complet. Tél. 93.13.65.00.

i.
> Restaurant cherche jeune cuisinier, connaissances pâtisserie, sérieuses références contrôlables. Tél. 93.67.14.06.

1. Which ads are for cooking positions?
2. Which ads are for secretarial positions?
3. Which ad is for an apprentice hair stylist?
4. Which ad is for an organization looking for a biological engineer?
5. Which ad is for a waitressing job?
6. Which ad is for a surgical nurse?
7. Which other ad is for a nurse?
8. Which ads are for jobs that require a knowledge of English?

Mise au point sur... la France et ses voisins

Rugged coastlines, sunlit beaches, snowcapped mountains and fields of lavender: this is the landscape of France. In the shape of a hexagon, France is bordered on three sides by water and on three sides by land. This diverse country, slightly smaller than the state of Texas, contains a variety of picturesque scenery.

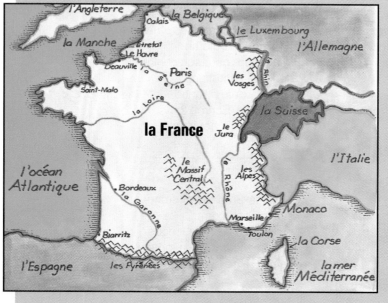

To the north of France lies the English Channel, called **la Manche** by the French because it narrows from the Atlantic Ocean to the North Sea much like a shirt sleeve. Here the beaches blur under a frequent foggy haze and the coastline is rocky. Nevertheless, the cities of Saint-Malo, Étretat and Deauville attract thousands of tourists each year. A 31-mile-long tunnel under the English Channel now joins Folkestone, England, with Calais, France. The French wanted an easy way to cross the Channel for hundreds of years, but it was only recently that the English agreed to be joined "by land" to the continent. The sleek Eurostar bullet train makes the trip between London and Paris in just under four hours.

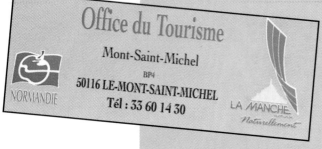

Office du Tourisme
Mont-Saint-Michel
BP4
50116 LE-MONT-SAINT-MICHEL
Tél : 33 60 14 30
NORMANDIE
LA MANCHE
Naturellement

During the Hundred Years War (1337-1453), the English were going to destroy the city of Calais, but six men volunteered to be killed to save it. Th Queen later intervened on their behalf and they were never killed. Rodin's life-size statue, *les Bourgeois de Calais*, honors their memory. (Calais)

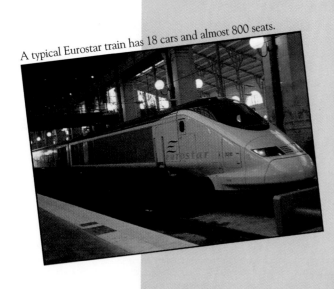

A typical Eurostar train has 18 cars and almost 800 seats.

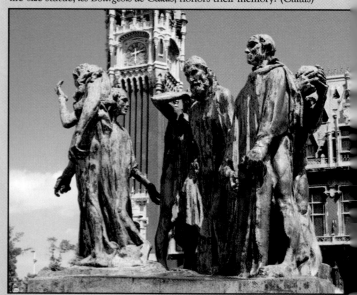

England, France and many of their neighbors have joined to form the European Union, an organization which promotes the economic growth of its members. Most of the barriers to the movement of money, goods, people and services among EU members have been removed, forming the largest single market in the world. Citizens of the 15 EU countries may travel to other member nations without passports, may work in other EU countries and are not required to pay import or export taxes on products purchased in other member countries.

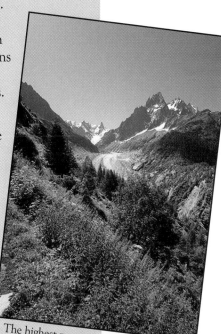

Belgium, Luxembourg, Germany, Switzerland and Italy border France on the east. French is spoken in France, Belgium, Luxembourg and Switzerland. Three mountain ranges, **les Vosges** (between France and Germany), **le Jura** (between France and Switzerland) and **les Alpes** (between France and Italy) form natural boundaries between France and its neighbors. Skiing and mountain climbing are popular hobbies in these regions.

The highest mountains in western Europe, the Alps extend from France into Switzerland, Italy and Austria.

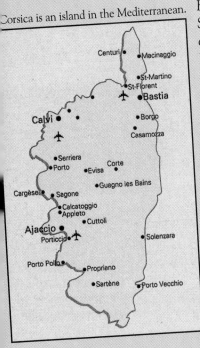

Corsica is an island in the Mediterranean.

To the south of France lie the Mediterranean Sea, the tiny principality of Monaco and the island of Corsica. The beaches of the French Riviera, stretching from near the city of Toulon to the Italian border, appeal to vacationers from all over the world.

Colors seem brighter in the south of France and even the food, spiced with olive oil, garlic and tomatoes, has a unique flavor. Monaco is an independent country where citizens speak French. Napoléon Bonaparte was born in Corsica, a department of France.

Monaco, ruled by Prince Rainier, covers less than one square mile.

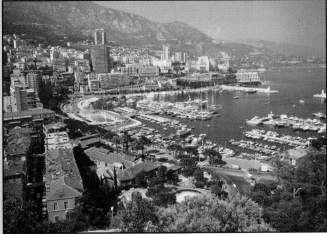

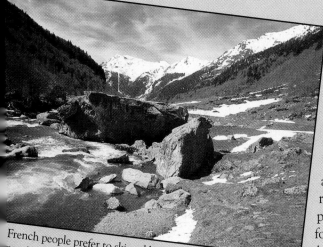

French people prefer to ski and hike in *les Pyrénées* because it's ~~pensive~~ than in *les Alpes*. (Col du Pourtalet)

The mountains called **les Pyrénées** form a natural boundary between France and Spain on the west. The resort city of Biarritz and the port city of Bordeaux, famous for its vineyards, are on the Atlantic Ocean.

There are several important rivers in France. **La Seine** divides the capital city of Paris in half before it meanders north to the city of Le Havre on the English Channel. Along the tranquil banks of **la Loire**, the longest river in France, kings had beautiful châteaux built during the Renaissance. **Le Rhône** empties into the Mediterranean Sea near the city of Marseille, the largest French port. Two other important rivers in France are **la Garonne**, near Bordeaux, and **le Rhin**, which forms a border between France and Germany.

The Gulf Stream from the Atlantic Ocean keeps the climate of France quite mild throughout the year. However, **le mistral**, a powerful wind, blows dry air through the mountains of **le Massif Central** in central France during the spring and summer.

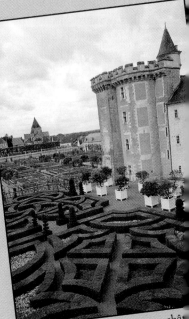

Villandry, another 16th century châ is less remarkable for its castle than gardens, laid out as three terraces.

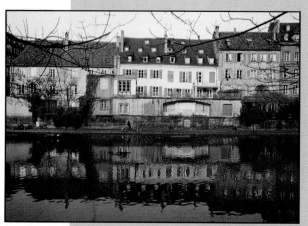

Strasbourg, in the province of Alsace, reflects both French and German heritage.

France used to be divided into provinces; people still maintain pride in the food, wine, architecture, art, dialects and traditional costumes associated with these provinces. Several of the more well-known French provinces are Brittany and Normandy to the north, Provence to the south, Aquitaine to the west, and Alsace and Lorraine to the east. Alsace and Lorraine have belonged to either Germany or France at various times throughout history; many of the people in these provinces speak both German and French, as well as local dialects.

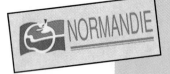

Today France is divided into smaller **départements** for governmental purposes. You can tell what department people are from by the last two numbers of their license plates and also by the first two numbers of their zip codes.

A combination of the traditional and the contemporary, beautiful countryside and bustling cities, France, the largest country in western Europe, is rightly called **la Belle France**.

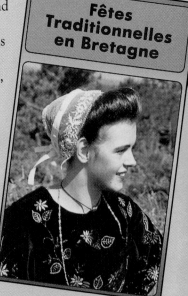

Fêtes Traditionnelles en Bretagne

3   Answer the following questions.

1. France is in the shape of what geometrical figure?
2. Why do the French call the English Channel **la Manche**?
3. What is the purpose of the European Union?
4. What are three European countries, other than France, where citizens speak French?
5. What three mountain ranges are located in the eastern part of France?
6. What is the name of the small principality located in the southern part of France?
7. How is the food in the southern part of France unique?
8. What river divides the city of Paris in half?
9. What two cities are important French ports?
10. What is responsible for France's moderate climate?
11. Why are the French proud to be associated with the former provinces?
12. How is France divided for governmental purposes today?
13. What is France often called?

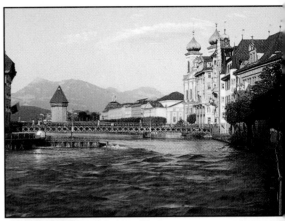

Knowing French would make it easier to visit Lucerne, Switzerland.

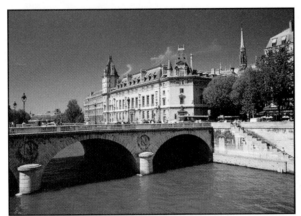

The "N" on this bridge, one of 33 that cross the Seine in Paris, stands for Napoléon.

4   Here is France's weather report for October 30. Answer the questions that follow.

1. All temperatures in this weather report are given in Celsius degrees (°C). What five French cities had temperatures of 10°C?
2. With the exception of Bastia on the island of Corsica, which city had the warmest temperature?
3. What was the temperature in Biarritz?
4. For soccer players was the weather better in Rennes or Bordeaux?
5. It was 9°C in Dijon. What else can you say about the weather there?
6. What city is located on the Rhône River between Lyon and Marseille? What was the temperature in this city?
7. What city is located near the border between France and Belgium? What was the weather like there?
8. In what two mountain ranges did it snow?
9. The accompanying chart shows cities from 12 of the countries that belong to the European Union and their temperatures from October 29. At what time were these temperatures recorded?
10. In what city was the temperature 22°C?
11. Was it warmer in Greece or Spain?

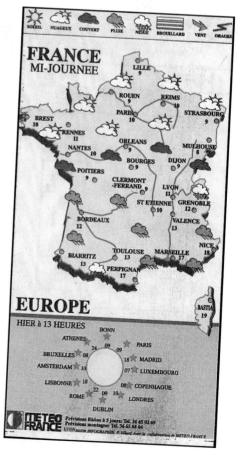

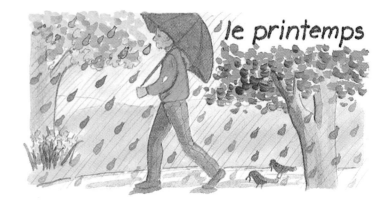

le printemps

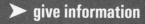

Leçon C

In this lesson you will be able to:

➤ give information

➤ invite

➤ express emotions

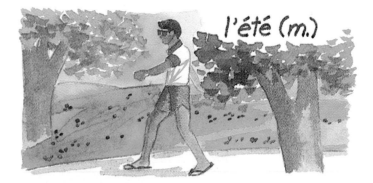

l'été (m.)

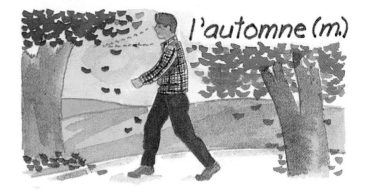

l'automne (m.)

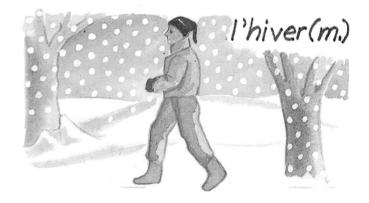

l'hiver (m.)

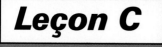

Quel temps fait-il?

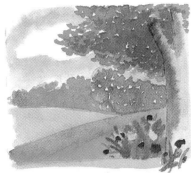 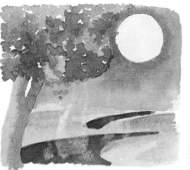 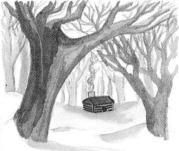

Il fait beau.   Il fait chaud.   Il fait froid.

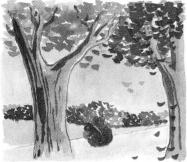 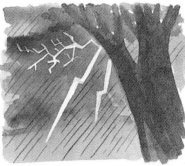 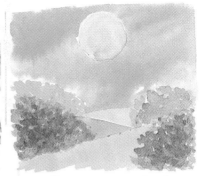

Il fait frais.   Il fait mauvais.   Il fait du soleil.

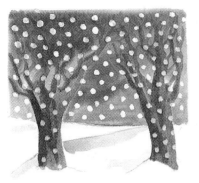 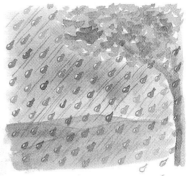 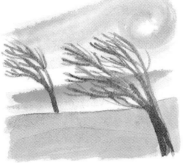

Il neige.   Il fait du vent.   Il pleut.

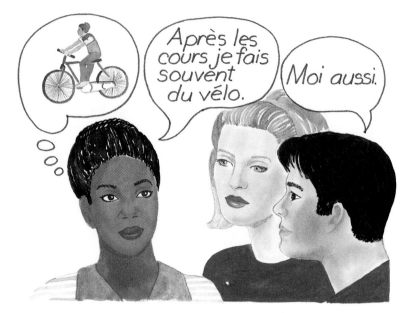

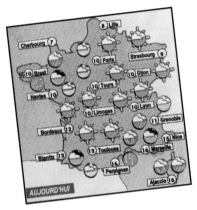

Petra, Sandy and José are talking about how they spend their free time.

Sandy: **Il fait beau à Tours en automne. Après les cours je fais souvent du vélo.**

José: **Moi aussi. Et quand il fait mauvais, je joue aux jeux vidéo.**

Petra: **J'aime aussi faire du vélo. Mais je n'ai pas de vélo ici.**

José: **Ma famille a un autre vélo.**

Sandy: **Alors, on fait un tour ensemble aujourd'hui?**

Petra: **D'accord. Quelle chance! J'ai déjà deux amis à Tours.**

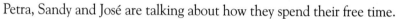

👁️ *Enquête culturelle*

Temperatures (**les températures**) in all French-speaking countries and most other countries in the world are calculated on the basis of the Celsius scale. Like all scales in the metric system, invented by the French, the Celsius scale is based on a division of measurements into hundredths or thousandths. Water freezes at 0° Celsius and boils at 100° Celsius. (It freezes at 32° Fahrenheit and boils at 212° Fahrenheit.)

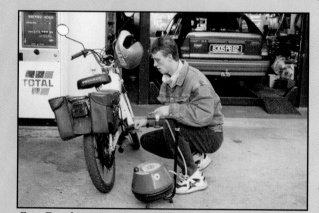

Many people ride bicycles in France both for pleasure and as a means of transportation. Mopeds (**les mobylettes**) are another popular way to get around. **Les mobs,** as they are often called, get through traffic easily and relatively quickly. Teenagers find **les mobs** to be economical, easy to park and simple to operate. People over the age of 14 may operate **une mobylette** without a driver's license as long as they drive under 45 kilometers per hour and wear a helmet.

For a French teenager a moped offers freedom and independence.

1 | Answer the following questions.

1. At what temperature (Celsius) does water boil?
2. What are two advantages of driving a **mobylette**?
3. How old must a person be to drive a **mobylette**?
4. Do you need a driver's license to drive a **mobylette**?
5. If you are over the age of 14 but don't have a driver's license, what is the speed limit you must observe when driving a **mobylette**?

2 | *Répondez en français.*

1. Sandy, José et Petra, ils sont où?
2. Quel temps fait-il à Tours en automne?
3. Est-ce que Sandy fait souvent du vélo?
4. Qui joue aux jeux vidéo quand il fait mauvais?
5. Qui n'a pas de vélo à Tours?
6. Quand est-ce qu'on fait un tour ensemble?
7. Qui sont les deux amis de Petra à Tours?

3 | *Quel temps fait-il? Répondez en français.*

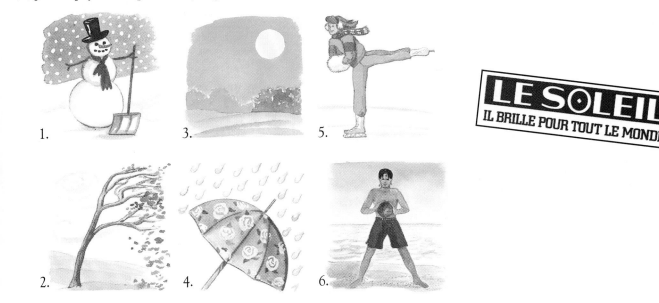

1.

2.

3.

4.

5.

6.

LE SOLEIL
IL BRILLE POUR TOUT LE MONDE!

4 | *Complétez le dialogue suivant.*

Fred: Tu... d'où?

Maria: Je viens... ..... Je suis.... Et toi?

Fred: Je viens... ..... Je suis....

Maria: Quel temps fait-il chez toi en...?

Fred: Il fait.... Moi, j'aime.... Qu'est-ce que tu aimes faire en...?

Maria: Moi, j'aime... en....

5 | *C'est à toi!*

1. Est-ce que tu préfères l'automne ou le printemps? Pourquoi?
2. Qu'est-ce que tu aimes faire en été?
3. Qu'est-ce que tu aimes faire en hiver?
4. Tu as un vélo?
5. Est-ce que tu aimes jouer aux jeux vidéo?
6. Est-ce que tu travailles après les cours?

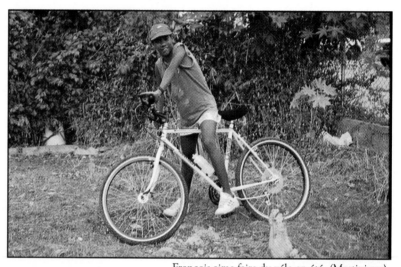

François aime faire du vélo en été. (Martinique)

Structure

Present tense of the irregular verb *faire*

The basic meaning of the irregular verb **faire** is "to do" or "to make," but it has other meanings as well.

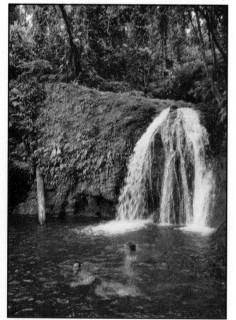

Il fait très chaud en Guadeloupe.
(Cascade Écrevisses)

faire			
je	**fais**	Je **fais** du vélo.	*I'm going biking.*
tu	**fais**	Qu'est-ce que tu **fais?**	*What are you doing?*
il/elle/on	**fait**	Quel temps **fait**-il?	*What's the weather like?*
nous	**faisons**	Nous **faisons** des omelettes.	*We're making omelettes.*
vous	**faites**	Vous ne **faites** pas de sport?	*You don't play (any) sports?*
ils/elles	**font**	Ils **font** un tour.	*They're going for a ride.*

Like the irregular verbs **aller** and **avoir**, **faire** is used in many expressions where a different verb is used in English. You have already seen expressions with **faire** when talking about participating in various activities, prices and what the weather's like.

Tu **fais** du footing?	*Are you going running?*
Ça **fait** combien?	*How much is it/that?*
Il **fait** chaud.	*It's (The weather's) hot/warm.*

Pratique

6 It's noon. Tell what the following people are making for lunch.

1. Jean-Michel

2. je

3. Ahmed et Aïcha

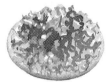

4. nous

5. tu

6. vous

7. Benjamin et Olivier

Modèle:

Christine

Christine fait un hamburger.

---

7 It's Saturday afternoon. Tell what various people are doing by combining each subject in column A with the appropriate form of one of the expressions in column B.

A	B
Grégoire	faire du vélo
tu	faire les devoirs
nous	faire du shopping
Karine et Denise	faire du roller
vous	faire un tour
je	faire du sport
ils	faire du footing

Modèle:

Grégoire fait du roller.

---

8 With a partner, take turns asking and telling what you normally do in certain types of weather. Follow the model.

1. Il fait chaud.
2. Il fait froid.
3. Il pleut.
4. Il fait beau.
5. Il fait mauvais.

Modèle:

Il neige.

Student A: Qu'est-ce que tu fais quand il neige?

Student B: Je skie. Et toi?

Student A: Je joue aux jeux vidéo.

Forming questions with inversion

A more formal way to ask a question in French, especially in written French, is to invert, or reverse, the order of the verb and its subject pronoun. With simple inversion the order is:

> **verb + subject pronoun**

Quelle heure est-il? [t]	*What time is it?*
Avez-vous faim?	*Are you hungry?*
Mangeons-nous au fast-food?	*Shall we eat at the fast-food restaurant?*

Note that a hyphen connects the verb and its subject pronoun.

Inverting the pronoun **je** and its verb is not common. Form **je** questions either by making your tone of voice rise at the end or by using **est-ce que**.

When the **il**, **elle** or **on** form of the verb ends with a vowel, a **t** is added between the verb and its subject pronoun. This **t** is pronounced.

Ressemble-t-il à son père? [t]	*Does he look like his father?*
A-t-il les cheveux blonds? [t]	*Does he have blond hair?*

If the subject of the sentence is a noun, inversion is formed by adding the appropriate subject pronoun after the verb. This pronoun agrees with the subject noun in gender and in number.

Les filles font-**elles** du sport?	*Do the girls play sports?*
Valérie joue-t-**elle** au basket?	*Is Valérie playing basketball?*

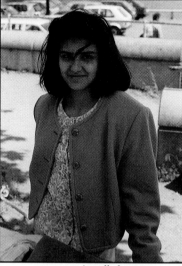

A-t-elle les yeux noirs?

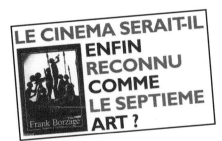

LE CINEMA SERAIT-IL ENFIN RECONNU COMME LE SEPTIEME ART ?

Frank Borzage

Pratique

9 | Find out if your friends are doing what you think they're doing by forming questions using inversion.

Modèle:

Anne/étudier la biologie
Anne étudie-t-elle la biologie?

1. Valérie/finir les devoirs
2. Christophe/parler avec le prof
3. Fatima/travailler
4. Marc et Fabrice/jouer au foot
5. Cécile et Patricia/faire un tour
6. Laurent/écouter de la musique
7. Stéphanie et Nadia/venir au café
8. Chloé et Daniel/manger des frites

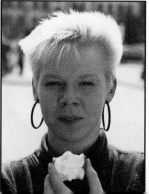

Sophie mange-t-elle une pomme?

10 You're talking to your French pen pal on the phone. Unfortunately, you have a bad connection. Rephrase each question you ask using inversion.

1. —Est-ce que tu danses bien?
   —Pardon?
2. —Tes amis et toi, vous allez souvent en boîte?
   —Pardon?
3. —Tu fais du sport?
   —Pardon?
4. —Tu étudies beaucoup?
   —Pardon?
5. —Tes professeurs sont sympa?
   —Pardon?
6. —Est-ce que tu ressembles à ton frère?
   —Pardon?
7. —Est-ce que ton frère est méchant?
   —Pardon?
8. —Ton frère et toi, vous avez un chien?
   —Pardon?
9. —Est-ce que ta famille voyage beaucoup?
   —Pardon?
10. —Tu viens ici?
    —Pardon?

Modèle:
—Tu aimes le rock?
—Pardon?
—Aimes-tu le rock?

11 Get to know your partner better by asking and answering questions. Student A asks questions using inversion. Student B asks questions using **est-ce que**. Follow the model.

1. avec qui/aller au cinéma
2. quand/étudier
3. quels professeurs/aimer bien
4. à qui/ressembler
5. où/aller en vacances

Modèle:
quels sports/faire
Student A: Quels sports fais-tu?
Student B: Je fais du footing et du roller. Quels sports est-ce que tu fais?
Student A: Je joue au tennis.

Communication

12 With two partners, play the roles of an American student and two French-speaking exchange students. It's the last class of the day. The American student asks what the two exchange students are doing after class. After they respond, the American student suggests an activity for all of them to do together. The exchange students either agree or disagree, depending on the weather. If someone disagrees, that person suggests another activity. Finally, all three students decide what they are going to do after class.

Modèle:
Student A: Salut, Cédric! Qu'est-ce que tu fais après les cours aujourd'hui?
Student B: Moi, j'ai besoin de faire les devoirs.
Student A: Et toi, Farid?
Student C: Je regarde la télé.
Student A: Moi, je joue au foot. On joue ensemble?
Student B: Ah zut! Il pleut.
Student C: Pas possible! Alors, on va au fast-food?
Student A: Super! J'ai faim.
Student B: Moi aussi. Allons-y ensemble!

13 You want to know your classmates' favorite seasons. Write the names of the four seasons. Then poll as many of your classmates as you can in five minutes to find out their favorite season. For example, **Est-ce que tu préfères l'été, l'hiver, le printemps ou l'automne? Je préfère l'été.** As each classmate answers your question, make a check by the appropriate response. After you have finished asking questions, count how many people like each season and be ready to share your findings with the rest of the class.

14 Your new pen pal from Guadeloupe is curious to find out if the seasons change where you live and what the weather is like. In a note to your pen pal, tell what the weather is like during the four seasons in your area. Give a typical temperature for each season using the Celsius scale. (**Il fait... degré(s) Celsius.**) Also mention what your favorite indoor and outdoor activities are during the various seasons.

Sur la bonne piste

Reading is made up of at least three speeds: skimming, scanning and digesting. Skimming—reading very quickly—is a high-speed technique used to figure out context. (For most readings, skimming should be the first technique you use.) Scanning—hunting for a precise idea or word—is a medium-speed technique used to search for specific information. (Scanning helps you answer questions about a reading.) Digesting—reading very thoroughly to accomplish a task—is a low-speed technique. Digesting requires a lot of time and should not be the first or the only reading technique you use. If you approach a reading with the intent of digesting all the details, you waste both time and thinking energy. Instead, first skim the reading and make use of a very helpful skill: predicting. Reading becomes easier and much more interesting when you try to guess what comes next!

The following reading is a dialogue that takes place at a party. As you skim the dialogue, stop after each person's portion of the conversation. Then look at who will speak next and predict what that person will say. Finally, continue reading to find out if your prediction was correct.

La Soirée de Papa

Chez les Piedbois. Paul Piedbois, le père d'Olivier, ouvre la porte.

M. Piedbois:	Bonsoir, Charles!
M. Théron:	Salut, Paul!
M. Piedbois:	Entre! Tu préfères un coca, une limonade ou un café?
M. Théron:	Une limonade, s'il te plaît. Tiens, qui est ce beau garçon, Paul?
M. Piedbois:	C'est mon fils.
Olivier:	Bonsoir, Monsieur. Je m'appelle Olivier. Et vous?
M. Théron:	Je m'appelle Charles Théron.
M. Piedbois:	Monsieur Théron est musicien professionnel.
Olivier:	Musicien? C'est super génial! Papa, tu peux me présenter aux autres invités?
M. Piedbois:	D'accord. Ah, Martin! Je te présente mon fils, Olivier. Il s'intéresse beaucoup aux professions de mes amis.
M. Nanteuil:	Martin Nanteuil. Enchanté de faire ta connaissance, Olivier. Je suis dentiste.
Olivier:	Enchanté!
M. Piedbois:	Et voilà Fernando Ortiz. Il est ingénieur.
Olivier:	Il est français?
M. Piedbois:	Non, mexicain. Tu vois la fille brune?

Olivier:	Oui.
M. Piedbois:	C'est Danielle Graedel. On l'appelle "Dana." Elle vient de Suisse.
Olivier:	Quelle est sa profession?
M. Piedbois:	C'est une interprète. Elle parle français, italien, allemand, japonais et russe. Et là-bas, l'homme aux yeux noirs, c'est Marco Casati. Il est de Florence. Il assiste à une conférence de pharmaciens demain. Voilà Cathy Collins, une Anglaise. Mademoiselle Collins désire être prof de français à Londres, mais pour le moment elle est serveuse.
Olivier:	Et la femme blonde?
M. Piedbois:	C'est Astrid Schiller, une copine de Cathy. C'est une cuisinière.
Olivier:	Elle est anglaise aussi?
M. Piedbois:	Non, elle est allemande. Et voilà Hisatake Tanaka. Il vient du Japon. C'est un pilote pour Air France. À côté il y a Mercedes Pizano, une Espagnole. Elle est comptable.
Olivier:	C'est une soirée internationale, papa! Tu as des copains intéressants!

15   Scan the reading to find answers to the following questions.

1. Where is Fernando Ortiz from? Where is Cathy Collins from?
2. Who has a nickname?
3. What is Danielle Graedel's profession? Which guests could she talk to in their native language?
4. Who is Italian? Who is Swiss? Who is Japanese?
5. Cathy Collins and Astrid Schiller are friends. How do you suppose they know each other?
6. Why does Olivier like his father's party?
7. What do you think Paul Piedbois does for a living?

Nathalie et Raoul

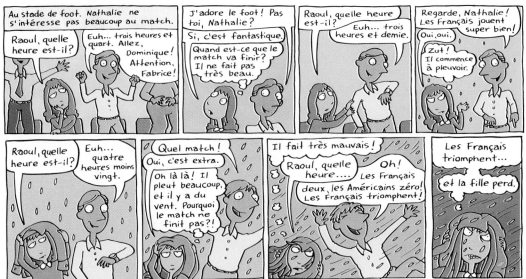

C'est à moi!

Now that you have completed this unit, take a look at what you should be able to do in French. Can you do all of these tasks?

➤ I can tell someone's nationality.

➤ I can ask and tell what country and what city someone is from.

➤ I can identify someone's profession.

➤ I can ask for and give information about various topics, including the weather.

➤ I can explain why.

➤ I can invite someone to do something.

➤ I can express emotions.

Here is a brief checkup to see how much you understand about French culture. Decide if each statement is **vrai** or **faux**.

Juanita María est mexicaine.

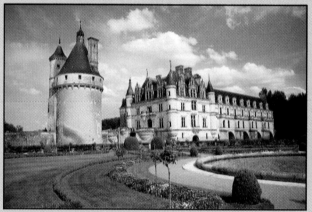

Which Loire castle spans a river?

1. Chenonceaux and Chambord are two of the many beautiful castles located in the Loire Valley.
2. Teenagers in Europe frequently vacation in neighboring countries and therefore find it practical to speak a second language.
3. All people who receive a salary for 12 months are entitled to six weeks of vacation each year.
4. France is bordered on three sides by water: the English Channel, the Atlantic Ocean and the Mediterranean Sea.

The Seine River empties into the English Channel at Le Havre.

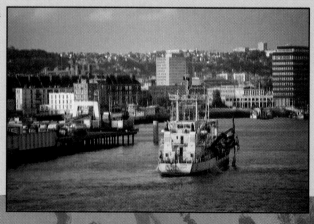

5. The European Union is a new underwater tunnel that connects France and England.
6. French is spoken in four European countries: France, Belgium, Luxembourg and Switzerland.
7. The three mountain ranges in France are **les Vosges, le Jura** and **le Rhône**.
8. Today France is divided into provinces for governmental purposes.
9. Temperatures are measured in degrees Fahrenheit in most European countries.
10. You must be at least 16 years old to operate a **mobylette** in France.

Communication orale

Businesspeople from foreign countries often visit the United States to learn more about our institutions and way of life. In addition to business establishments, they occasionally visit schools. To be prepared for an upcoming visit to your school from businesspeople representing various countries, have a conversation with your partner about these guests. Here is a list of guests and the countries they are from.

M. Jouffret - France

Mlle Castillo - Mexico

Mlle DiPiazza - Italy

M. Kraft - Germany

Mme Paquette - Canada

M. Cortés - Spain

Mme Chatton - France

M. Alonso - Mexico

Mlle Ounsworth - England

Mme Liu - China

M. Pagnucci - Italy

Mlle Peltier - Canada

Take turns naming at least eight different visitors. Tell their names, what countries and cities they are from, their professions, the languages they speak and the family members, if any, who are coming along with them. Follow the model.

Modèle:

Student A: M. Jouffret vient de France. Il est de Marseille. Il parle français et anglais. Il vient ici avec sa femme et son fils.

Student B: Quelle est sa profession?

Student A: M. Jouffret est informaticien.

Communication écrite

Unfortunately, your French teacher was absent on the day the school administrator met with the staff to go over all the details about the prospective visit from international businesspeople to your school. Write a note to your teacher telling him or her who all these visitors are, what cities and countries they are from, what languages they speak, what their professions are and what family members, if any, are coming with them. Also tell your teacher which businessperson you would like to speak with.

Communication active

To identify someone's nationality, use:

Il est français.
C'est un Français. } *He is French.*

Elle est japonaise.
C'est une Japonaise. } *She is Japanese.*

To ask where someone is from, use:
Tu viens/Vous venez d'où? *Where are you from?*

To tell where someone is from, use:
Il/Elle est de New York. *He/She is from New York.*
Il/Elle vient du Canada. *He/She is from Canada.*

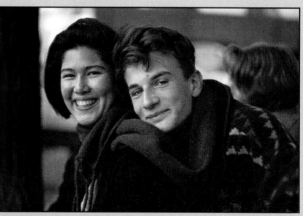

Lien vient de Chine, et Mark vient du Canada.

Il/Elle vient de Chine. *He/She is from China.*
Il/Elle vient d'Angleterre. *He/She is from England.*
Il/Elle vient des États-Unis. *He/She is from the United States.*

To identify someone's profession, use:

Il est avocat.
C'est un avocat. } *He's a lawyer.*

Elle est journaliste.
C'est une journaliste. } *She's a journalist.*

To ask for information, use:

C'est qui?   *Who is it?*

Quelle est la profession de   *What is Mr. Desmarais' occupation?*
Monsieur Desmarais?

Il fait beau, **n'est-ce pas?**   *It's nice, isn't it?*

Est-ce que tu es allemande?   *Are you German?*

Quand viens-tu?   *When are you coming?*

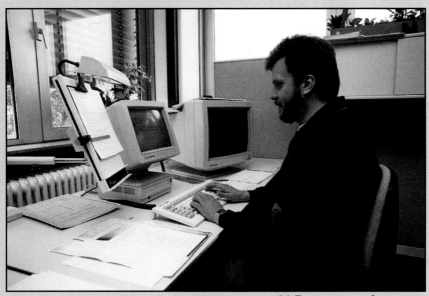

M. Desmarais est informaticien.

To give information, use:

Il voyage beaucoup.   *He travels a lot.*

Elle travaille beaucoup.   *She works a lot.*

Je n'ai pas de mère.   *I don't have a mother.*

Il fait beau en automne.   *It's nice in autumn.*

Il fait mauvais en hiver.   *The weather's bad in the winter.*

To explain something, use:

C'est pourquoi tu parles si bien   *That's why you speak French so well!*
le français!

To invite someone to do something, use:

On fait un tour **ensemble?**   *Do you want to take a trip together?*

To express emotions, use:

Quelle chance**!**   *What luck!*

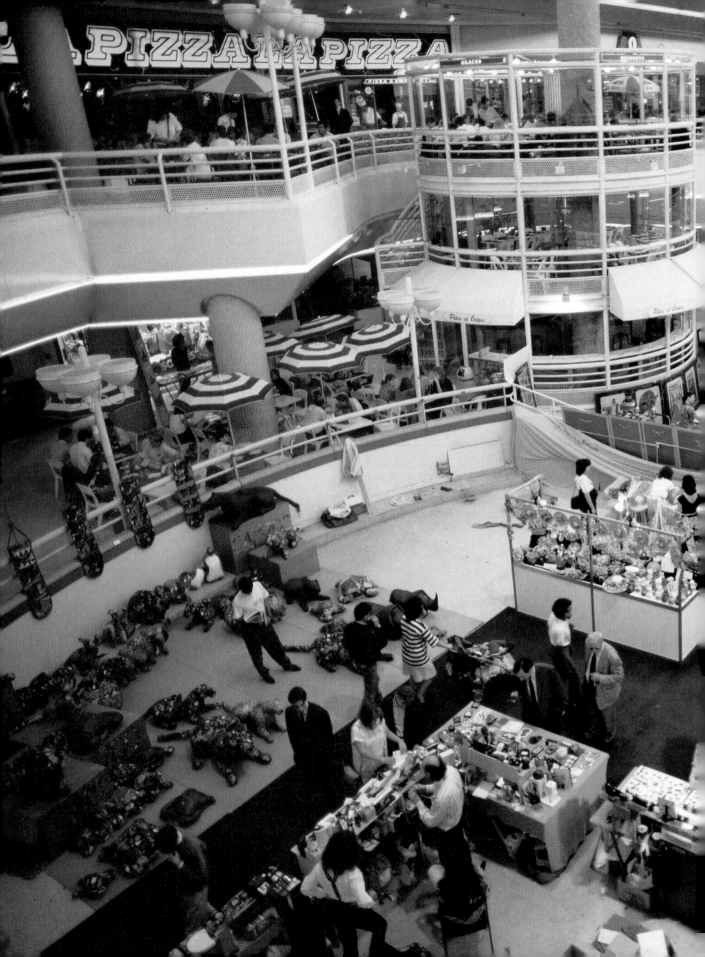

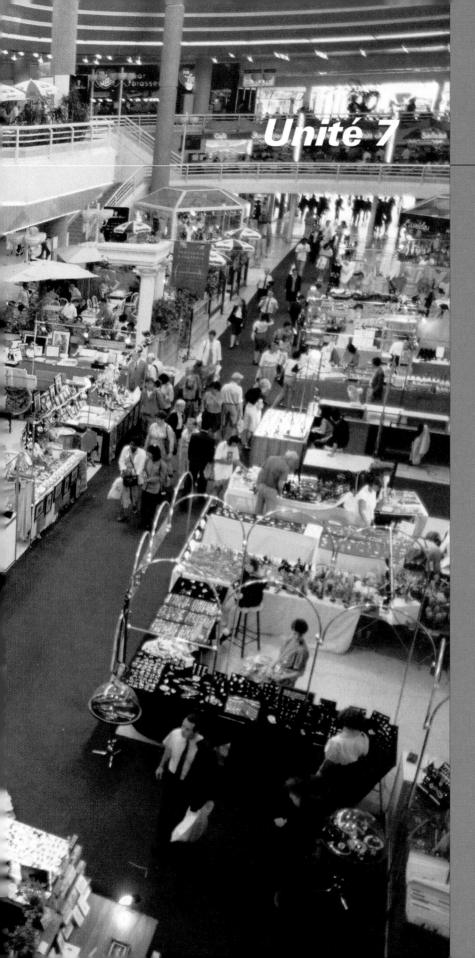

Unité 7

On fait les magasins.

In this unit you will be able to:

➤ express likes and dislikes

➤ agree and disagree

➤ express need

➤ express intentions

➤ invite

➤ inquire about and compare prices

➤ ask for information

➤ give information

➤ ask someone to repeat

➤ choose and purchase items

Leçon A

In this lesson you will be able to:

➤ **express intentions**

➤ **express need**

➤ **invite**

➤ **express likes and dislikes**

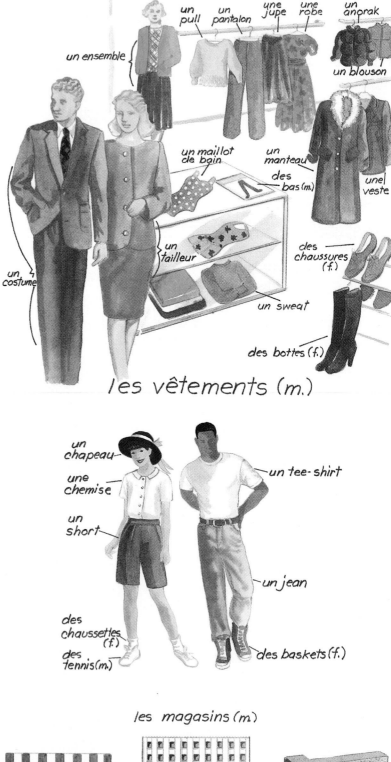

un ensemble

un pull   un pantalon   une jupe   une robe   un anorak

un blouson

un maillot de bain   un manteau   des bas (m.)   une veste

un tailleur

un costume

des chaussures (f.)

un sweat

des bottes (f.)

les vêtements (m.)

un chapeau

une chemise   un tee-shirt

un short

un jean

des chaussettes (f.)

des tennis (m.)   des baskets (f.)

les magasins (m.)

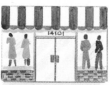

une boutique

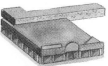

un grand magasin

un centre commercial

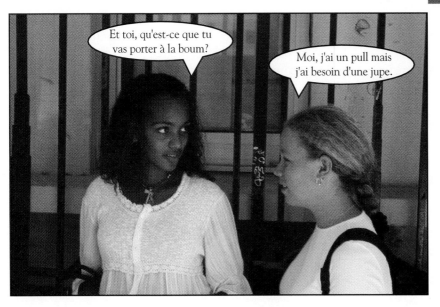

Lamine and Ariane are talking about what they're going to wear to a party.

Lamine: **Je vais aller au centre commercial pour chercher un jean et un tee-shirt pour samedi soir. Et toi, qu'est-ce que tu vas porter à la boum?**

Ariane: **Moi, j'ai un pull mais j'ai besoin d'une jupe.**

Lamine: **Allons ensemble au grand magasin! On va peut-être trouver quelque chose là-bas.**

Ariane: **D'accord. J'aime bien faire les magasins!**

Enquête culturelle

There are huge shopping malls in France but fewer than in the United States. However, small specialized stores still do a brisk business. Just as in the United States, you can go to **le pressing** or **la teinturerie** (*dry cleaner's*) to have your clothes dry-cleaned, **le tailleur** (*tailor*) to have your clothes altered and **la cordonnerie** (*shoe repair shop*) to have your shoes repaired.

OPERA PRESSING

OPERA PRESSING

CONFIEZ VOS VETEMENTS A UN MAITRE-TEINTURIER A VOTRE SERVICE DU LUNDI AU VENDREDI

14 rue St Anne
75001 Paris — — — — (1) 42 96 07 81

CORDONNERIE NEUCHATELOISE
G. Jeanneret Fondée en 1918
Maître-cordonnier
La Tradition dans le Beau Travail
Toutes Réparations, Ville et Montagne
Ressemelage entier
Chaussures médicales
Bottes - Bottillons, Chaussons agneau
Produit et accessoires
pour articles de cuir
5, r. Gubernatis
06000 NICE   **93 80 46 74**

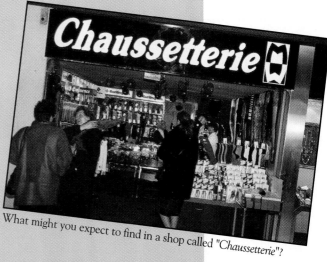

What might you expect to find in a shop called "*Chaussetterie*"?

Like other teenagers around the world, French teens follow fashion trends closely. They like to dress up for special occasions. In general, the French place more importance on having quality clothing that is the latest style than on having many different outfits.

Certain areas of larger French cities attract teenagers and young adults. For example, **le Quartier latin**, near the University of Paris, is an area where students often find clothes, international restaurants and entertainment which appeal to their contemporary tastes.

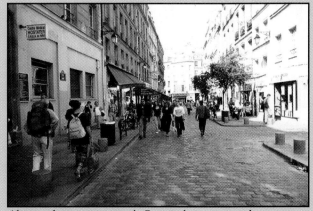

Along pedestrian streets in *le Quartier latin*, you can shop, go to movies and eat in international restaurants. (Paris)

Open-air markets, featuring fresh fruits and vegetables as well as seafood and meat, are located in most French-speaking cities. In large cities, neighborhood markets may be open every day except Monday. In smaller towns, markets may be open only one day a week. At **le marché aux puces** (*flea market*) you can purchase a variety of

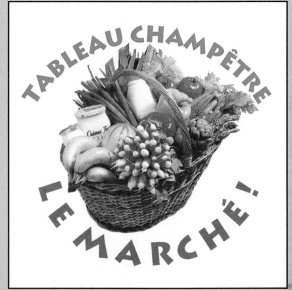

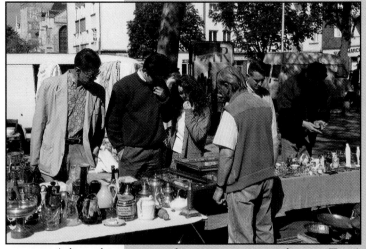

At *le marché aux puces* vendors expect customers to bargain. (Tours)

items ranging from antique lamps to secondhand clothing. At such outdoor markets buyers often try bargaining with vendors to get a reduced price. These lively markets attract many tourists and shoppers who have figured out a way to stretch their income.

1   *Répondez en français.*

1. Qui va faire les magasins?
2. Qu'est-ce que Lamine va porter à la boum?
3. La boum, c'est quand?
4. Qu'est-ce qu'Ariane a déjà pour la boum?
5. De quoi Ariane a-t-elle besoin?
6. Ariane et Lamine, est-ce qu'elles vont au grand magasin ou à la boutique?

2   Identify each numbered item you see in the illustration.

Modèle:

Ce sont des bas.

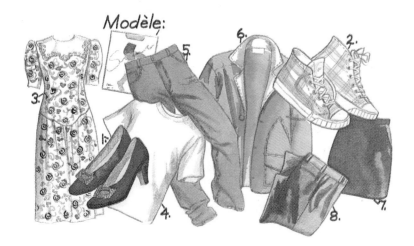

Modèle:

3   Choose the letter of the item of clothing that each person must be wearing.

1. Sabrina skie. Elle porte....
   a. une jupe   b. un anorak   c. une robe

2. Mamadou nage. Il porte....
   a. une veste   b. des baskets   c. un maillot de bain

3. Michèle joue au volley. Elle porte....
   a. un blouson   b. des bas   c. un short

4. Nadia porte des tennis. Elle porte aussi....
   a. des chaussettes   b. des bottes   c. des bas

5. Il fait froid. Catherine porte une robe et aussi....
   a. un ensemble   b. un sweat   c. un manteau

6. Sylvie porte une jupe et aussi....
   a. un pull   b. un pantalon   c. un costume

7. Diana voyage beaucoup. Elle porte un ensemble: des chaussures, un tailleur et....
   a. des tennis   b. un chapeau   c. un tee-shirt

8. Édouard va au café avec ses parents. Il porte un pantalon et....
   a. une chemise   b. un jean   c. un tailleur

4 | *C'est à toi!*

1. Est-ce que tu aimes faire
   les magasins?
2. Où est-ce que tu préfères faire les
   magasins, au centre commercial, au
   grand magasin ou à une boutique?
3. Qu'est-ce que tu portes aujourd'hui?
4. Qu'est-ce que ton ami(e) porte
   aujourd'hui?
5. Qu'est-ce que tu portes quand tu vas
   à une boum?
6. Qu'est-ce que tu portes en été?

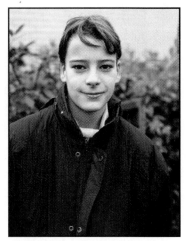

Qu'est-ce que Christian porte
aujourd'hui?

Structure

Aller + infinitive

One way to express what you are going to do in the near future is to
use the present tense form of **aller** that agrees with the subject plus
an infinitive.

Je **vais faire** les magasins.	*I'm going to go shopping.*
Qu'est-ce que tu **vas chercher**?	*What are you going to look for?*

To make a negative sentence, put **ne (n')** before the form of **aller** and
pas after it.

André **ne** va **pas** porter	*André's not going to wear*
son costume noir.	*his black suit.*

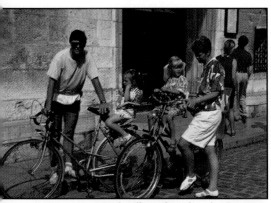

La famille va faire du vélo. (Beaune)

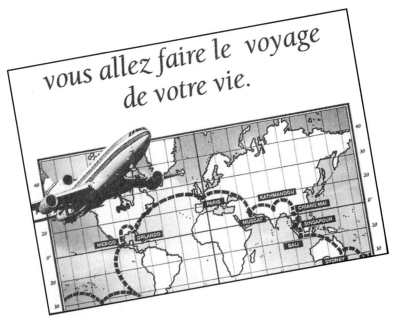

vous allez faire le voyage
de votre vie.

Pratique

5 Tell what the following people are going to do this weekend.

Modèle:

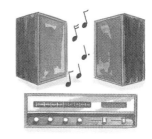

Véro
Véro va écouter de la musique.

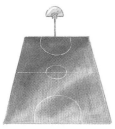

1. nous

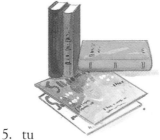

5. tu

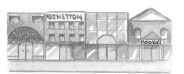

2. je

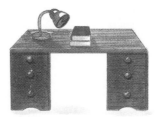

6. Vincent

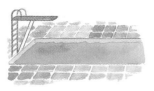

3. Nadine et Jeanne

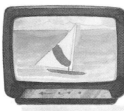

7. vous

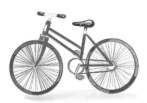

4. Normand et Gilbert

6 Forecasters have predicted that the storm of the decade will hit your area tomorrow. Knowing that everyone will be stranded at home, tell whether or not the following people are going to do what they had planned.

1. Antonine et Marie/téléphoner à leurs amis
2. nous/étudier
3. vous/skier
4. Mme Delacroix/dormir
5. je/faire des crêpes
6. Étienne/sortir avec Sara
7. Emmanuel et Fabrice/manger au café
8. tu/aller à la boum de Monique

Modèles:

M. Martin/écouter de la musique
Monsieur Martin va écouter de la musique.

les filles/faire les magasins
Les filles ne vont pas faire les magasins.

7 With a partner, take turns asking and telling whether or not you're going to do certain things during your next vacation.

Modèle:

nager

Student A: Est-ce que tu vas nager?

Student B: Oui, je vais nager. Et toi, est-ce que tu vas nager?

Student A: Non, je ne vais pas nager.

1. skier
2. aller au centre commercial
3. voyager
4. jouer au foot
5. faire les devoirs
6. regarder la télé
7. travailler

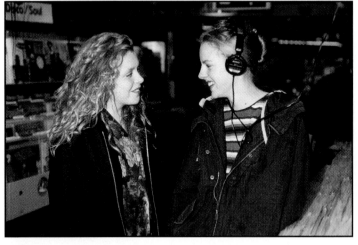

Thérèse et Marianne vont faire du shopping.

À + definite articles

The preposition **à** (*to, at, in*) does not change before the definite articles **la** and **l'**.

Allons ensemble à la boutique!	*Let's go to the boutique together!*
Pas possible. Je finis mes devoirs à l'école.	*Not possible. I'm finishing my homework at school.*

Before the definite articles **le** and **les**, however, **à** changes form. **À** combines with **le** and **les** as follows:

à + le = au	*to (the), at (the), in (the)*
à + les = aux	*to (the), at (the), in (the)*

Qui va **au** centre commercial?	*Who is going to the mall?*
Jean et moi, nous allons **aux** grands magasins.	*Jean and I are going to the department stores.*

Au and **aux** are used before countries with masculine names.

Tu vas **aux** États-Unis ou **au** Canada?	*Are you going to the United States or to Canada?*

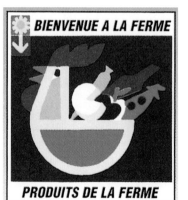
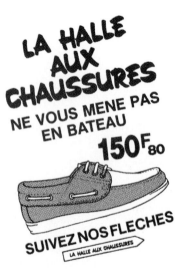

Pratique

Tell where some of your friends are going, choosing from the locations in the following list.

la boum de Marc	la boutique	le cinéma	l'école
le Mexique	le fast-food	les États-Unis	

Modèle:

Ariane va parler espagnol.
Elle va au Mexique.

1. Béatrice et Éric vont danser samedi soir.
2. Catherine et Florence ont faim.
3. Salim va parler anglais.
4. Yasmine a besoin de chercher un jean et un tee-shirt.
5. Magali et Patrick désirent regarder un film de Spielberg.
6. Thomas a besoin de parler avec le prof d'informatique.

You are in charge of giving away items left over from the school's rummage sale. Tell which items you're going to give to the following people.

Modèle:

le frère de Stéphanie
Je vais donner le blouson au frère de Stéphanie.

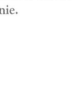

1. les profs de français
2. la prof de musique
3. le fils de la prof de biologie
4. l'informaticien de l'école
5. le prof de géographie
6. la sœur de David

Communication

Your French pen pal has sent you a message by E-mail to find out what American students wear when they do certain things. Make a list of four items of clothing that you normally wear, according to each situation.

jouer au basket
aller à l'école
aller à une boum
aller au café avec les parents

Quand Jean-Claude fait du vélo, il porte un tee-shirt, un short, des chaussettes et des tennis. (Montréal)

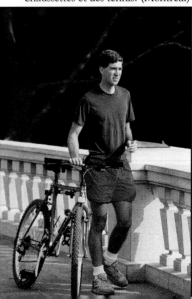

11 Imagine that you work at a travel agency. Clients ask you what they should pack when planning a trip to certain French-speaking vacation spots during the winter and spring travel seasons. According to the weather report you receive from each city's tourist bureau, select at least three clothing items for male travelers and three clothing items for female travelers to take to each destination.

1. À Québec, au Canada, il fait très froid et il neige beaucoup en hiver. Il fait -15° C.
2. À Fort-de-France, à la Martinique, il fait du soleil et il fait très chaud en hiver. Il fait 28° C.
3. À la Nouvelle-Orléans, aux États-Unis, il fait beau et il fait chaud au printemps. Il fait 24° C.
4. À Paris, en France, il fait frais et il pleut au printemps. Il fait 12° C.

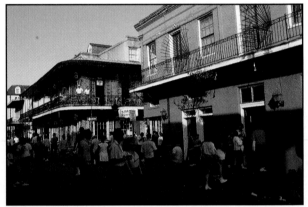

Il fait chaud à la Nouvelle-Orléans au printemps.

12 With a partner, have a phone conversation about going shopping. Student A needs to go to the mall to buy some clothes and calls Student B to see if he or she would like to go along. Student B also needs to buy something and agrees to go with Student A. Decide on a time and tell each other good-bye.

Prononciation

The sound [ɔ]

The sound [ɔ], or "open o," is just one of the sounds corresponding to the letter **o** in French. It is called "open **o**" because your mouth must be more open than closed to form it. Say each of these words:

robe   anorak   short   costume   botte   porter

The sound [õ]

The sound [õ] is an open nasal sound. It is represented by the letters **on** and **om**. In either case, the **n** or **m** is not pronounced and the sound [õ] comes out through your nose. Say each of these words:

pantal**on**   all**ons**   blous**on**   Jap**on**   c**om**bien   c**om**ptable

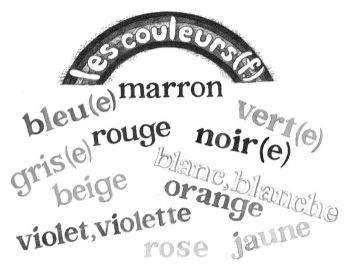

les couleurs (f)

bleu(e) marron vert(e)
gris(e) rouge noir(e)
beige blanc, blanche
violet, violette orange
rose jaune

Leçon B

In this lesson you will be able to:

➤ express likes and dislikes
➤ inquire about and compare prices
➤ agree and disagree

Il est petit.   Il est grand.   Elle est courte. Elle est longue.

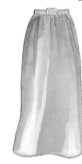

Il est vieux.   Il est nouveau.

Il est bon marché.

Soldes   Il est cher.

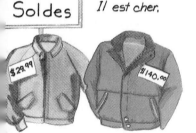

$29.99 $140.00

Elle est moche.   Elle est belle. Elle est jolie.

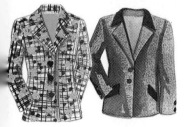

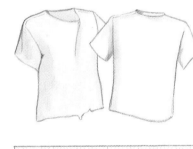

petit	petite
grand	grande
joli	jolie
beau	belle
moche	moche
nouveau	nouvelle
vieux	vieille
court	courte
long	longue
cher	chère
bon marché	bon marché

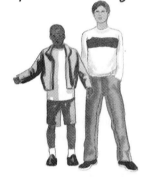

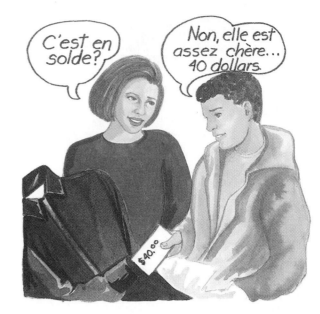

Madame Desrosiers is shopping with her son Jean at a boutique in Montreal.

Madame Desrosiers:	**J'adore la chemise bleue! Et elle est bon marché. Elle coûte 18 dollars.**
Jean:	**Beurk! Je ne vais pas acheter ça! Elle est moche. Mais j'ai besoin d'une nouvelle chemise.**
Madame Desrosiers:	**Il y a beaucoup de belles chemises ici - noires, blanches, vertes....**
Jean:	**C'est vrai. Tiens, j'aime la grande chemise noire.**
Madame Desrosiers:	**C'est combien? C'est en solde?**
Jean:	**Non, elle est assez chère... 40 dollars.**

Enquête culturelle

There are many opportunities for shopping in Montreal, the second largest French-speaking city in the world. Beneath Montreal's busy streets in the midtown area, and literally carved from the rock that supports them, lies the world's largest subterranean city. Shopping, strolling, eating, doing business and finding entertainment are easy at any time of the day or night, with no worries about the cold Canadian winters. Department stores, hotels, restaurants, movie theaters and many businesses are located in and around large

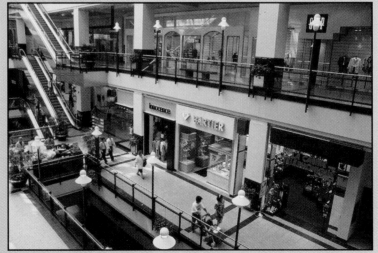

Underground Montreal is essentially one large shopping mall.

squares, such as the **Place Ville-Marie** and the **Place Bonaventure**. The four-line **métro** (*subway*) system and a series of walkways, stairways and elevators connect this underground complex. Decorations, such as stained glass windows, murals and ceramic artworks, beautify the modern **métro**

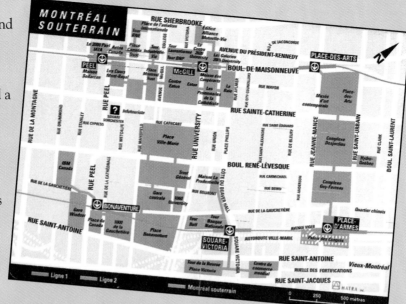

stations, each designed by a different architect. Aboveground, concrete and glass skyscrapers top the subterranean complex. The idea of an underground structure separating road traffic from pedestrian traffic is not new. Five centuries ago, the Italian artist Leonardo da Vinci envisioned a two-level city.

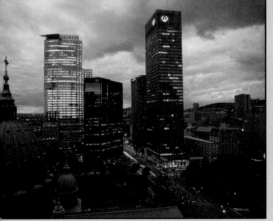

Montreal has immense skyscrapers aboveground; underground lies another complete city.

When items are **en solde** (*on sale*) in French shops, they are sometimes displayed on the sidewalk in front of the store marked with the sign **Soldes** to attract customers.

What word tells you that this shop is having a sale?

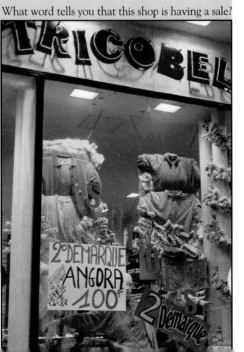

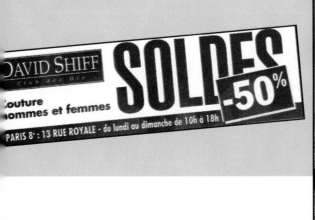

1 | *Répondez en français.*

1. Qui fait les magasins?
2. Qui aime la chemise bleue?
3. La chemise bleue, est-elle chère ou bon marché?
4. Est-ce que Jean aime la chemise bleue?
5. Pourquoi est-ce que Jean ne va pas acheter la chemise bleue?
6. La chemise noire, est-elle grande ou petite?
7. Combien coûte la chemise noire?

2 | Write the name of the person that fits each description.

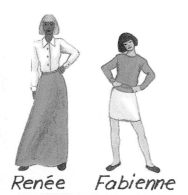
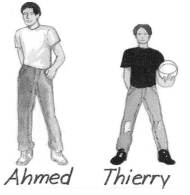

Renée   *Fabienne*   *Ahmed*   *Thierry*

1. Son pull est bleu.
2. Il porte des baskets noires.
3. Elle est petite.
4. Son tee-shirt est blanc.

5. Il porte un vieux jean.
6. Sa jupe est longue.
7. Il est grand.
8. Sa jupe est courte.

3 | *C'est à toi!*

1. Avec qui fais-tu souvent les magasins?
2. Où vas-tu pour acheter des vêtements?
3. Est-ce que tu aimes acheter des vêtements en solde?
4. Qui porte un tee-shirt aujourd'hui?
5. Qui porte un jean aujourd'hui? Est-il nouveau ou vieux?
6. Qu'est-ce que tu portes aujourd'hui?

Claire fait souvent les magasins avec son amie Catherine.

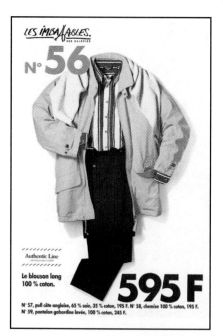

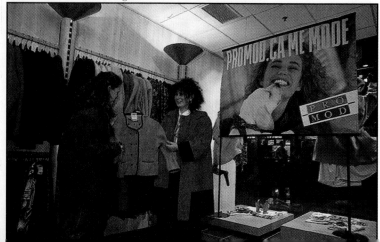

Structure

Irregular adjectives

You already know that most feminine adjectives are formed by adding an **e** to masculine adjectives.

gris	gri**se**
bleu	bleu**e**

You also know that if a masculine adjective ends in **-e**, the feminine adjective is identical.

rouge	rouge
moche	moche

Some irregular adjectives never change form, even in the plural.

orange	orange
marron	marron
super	super
sympa	sympa
bon marché	bon marché

Some feminine adjectives are formed by doubling the final consonant of a masculine adjective and adding an **e.**

bon	bon**ne**
quel	quel**le**
violet	violet**te**
italien	italien**ne**

To form a feminine adjective from a masculine adjective that ends in **-er,** change the ending to **-ère.**

cher	ch**ère**
premier	premi**ère**

Some other masculine adjectives also have irregular feminine forms.

blanc	**blanche**
frais	**fraîche**
long	**longue**

The adjectives **nouveau** and **vieux,** like the adjective **beau,** have irregular feminine forms as well as irregular forms before a masculine noun beginning with a vowel sound.

<table>
<tr><td>Masculine Singular
before a Consonant
Sound</td><td>Masculine Singular
before a Vowel
Sound</td><td>Feminine
Singular</td></tr>
<tr><td>un **beau** magasin</td><td>un **bel** homme</td><td>une **belle** affiche</td></tr>
<tr><td>un **nouveau** pantalon</td><td>un **nouvel** ami</td><td>une **nouvelle** robe</td></tr>
<tr><td>un **vieux** costume</td><td>un **vieil** anorak</td><td>une **vieille** photo</td></tr>
</table>

The irregular masculine plural forms of these adjectives are **beaux,** **nouveaux** and **vieux.**

les beaux vêtements   les nouveaux élèves   les vieux pulls
[z]

Le Vieux Bistro

14, rue du Cloître Notre-Dame Paris 4ème
Tél : 43 54 18 95, M° Cité.

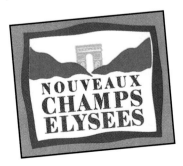

Pratique

4 | Sophie and Jérémy are going out tonight. Tell what they are going to wear.

Modèle:

Sophie va porter un pull noir....

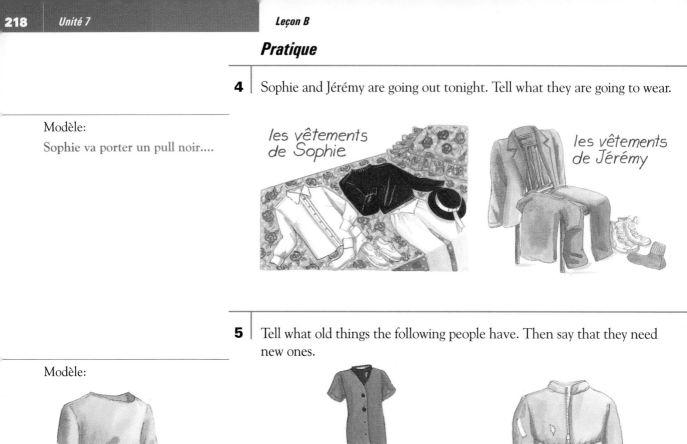

5 | Tell what old things the following people have. Then say that they need new ones.

Modèle:

Bruno
Bruno a un vieux sweat. Il a besoin d'un nouveau sweat.

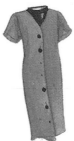

1. Mme Duval

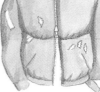

4. Sabrina

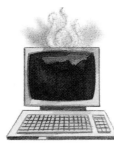

2. M. Bureau

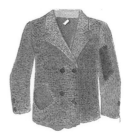

5. M. Piedbœuf

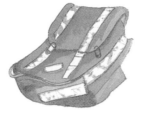

3. Anne

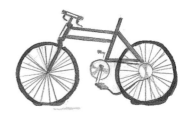

6. Dikembe

With a partner, take turns asking and telling what you think about the items of clothing you see in the store window. When answering each question, use the appropriate form of one of the following adjectives.

| beau | moche | cher | bon marché | long | court |

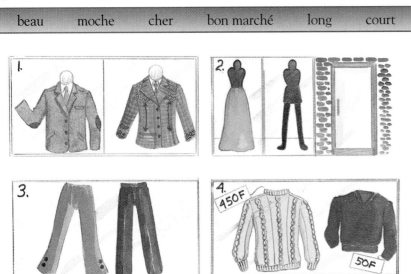

1. 2.

3. 4. 450F 50F

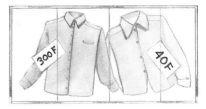

Student A: Comment est-ce que tu trouves la chemise beige?
Student B: Elle est très chère. Comment est-ce que tu trouves la chemise jaune?
Student A: Elle est bon marché.

Position of adjectives

In French, adjectives usually follow the nouns they describe.

> Donnez-moi une boisson **chaude**.
> Je voudrais un café **noir**.
> Mario est un serveur **italien**.

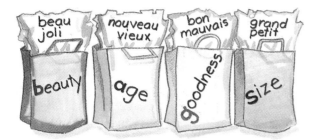

Some frequently used adjectives precede the nouns they describe. These adjectives often express *beauty*, *age*, *goodness* and *size*. (You can remember these categories easily by associating them with the word "bags.") Some of these adjectives are **beau, joli, nouveau, vieux, bon, mauvais, grand** and **petit**.

> Ma **petite** sœur va faire les magasins.
> Elle cherche un **nouveau** jean.
> Elle trouve un **beau** pull rose.
> Quelles **bonnes** soldes!

> *My little sister is going to go shopping.*
> *She's looking for new jeans.*
> *She finds a beautiful pink sweater.*
> *What good sales!*

LA PETITE VALISE POUR UN GRAND TOUR DU MONDE

Pratique

7 | Agree with what the French exchange student says about some of the people in your school. Use the indicated noun in each of your sentences.

Modèle:

Lisa est intelligente. (une élève)
Oui, c'est une élève intelligente!

1. Matt est timide. (un garçon)
2. Mrs. Johnson est bavarde. (une prof)
3. Amy est méchante. (une fille)
4. Mr. Ross est diligent. (un homme)
5. Paul est paresseux. (un élève)
6. Mr. Gray est super. (un professeur)
7. Ms. Lell est généreuse. (une femme)
8. Ryan est sympa. (un ami)

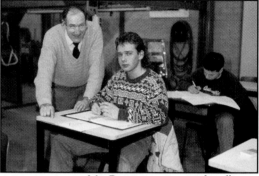

Mr. Gray est aussi un prof intelligent.

8 | Tell what each child has for show-and-tell, using the appropriate form of the indicated adjective.

Modèle:

Joséphine/une photo (vieux)
Joséphine a une vieille photo.

1. Pauline/un chat (joli)
2. Alice/une affiche (nouveau)
3. André/un sac à dos (grand)
4. Manu/un chien (petit)
5. Alexandre/une cassette (bon)
6. Jamila/un oiseau (beau)

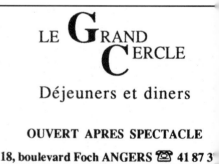
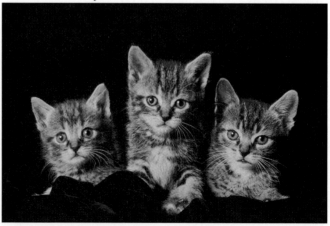

– Chouette, une petite valise! Chouette, une petite valise! Chouette, une petite valise!

Aïcha a trois beaux petits chats.

Describe the items you find in the school's lost-and-found department as you look for your missing sweater. Use two adjectives from the list that follows in each of your descriptions. Make sure the adjectives agree with the nouns they describe.

vieux	jaune	joli	blanc	grand	bleu	nouveau	vert
bon	noir	beau	mauvais	rouge	moche	petit	marron

Modèle:

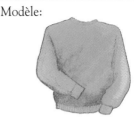

Il y a un grand sweat vert.

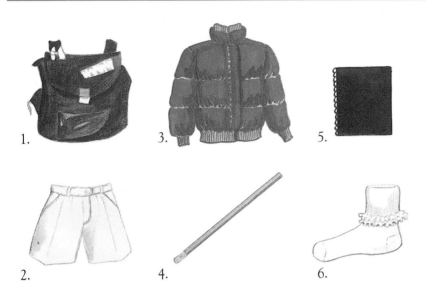

1.

2.

3.

4.

5.

6.

Present tense of the verbs *acheter* and *préférer*

The endings of the verbs **acheter** (*to buy*) and **préférer** (*to prefer*) are regular, but there is an **accent grave** over the final **e** (**è**) in the stem of the **je, tu, il/elle/on** and **ils/elles** forms.

Tu préfères le bleu ou le vert?   *Do you prefer the blue (one) or the green (one)?*

Je n'achète pas ça!   *I'm not buying that!*

Céline achète un nouveau jean.

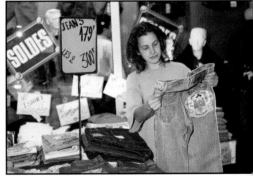

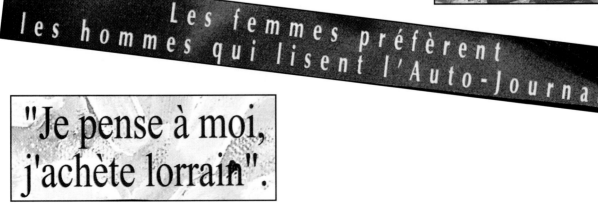

Les femmes préfèrent les hommes qui lisent l'Auto-Journal...

"Je pense à moi, j'achète lorrain".

Pratique

10 Say that although the following people prefer the items on the left, they're buying the items on the right.

Modèle:

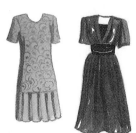

Valérie
Valérie préfère la robe bleue, mais elle achète la robe rouge.

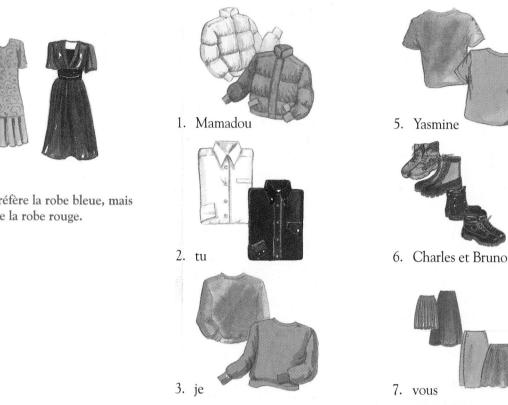

1. Mamadou

5. Yasmine

2. tu

6. Charles et Bruno

3. je

7. vous

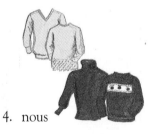

4. nous

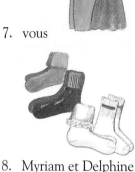

8. Myriam et Delphine

Communication

11 To find out what your classmates' favorite colors are, take a sheet of paper and list as many colors as you can think of in French. Then poll as many of your classmates as you can. In your survey:

1. Ask each classmate what color he or she prefers.
2. As each person answers your question, make a check on your paper by the appropriate color.
3. After you have finished asking questions, count how many people like each color and be ready to share your findings with the rest of the class.

Modèle:

Chantal: Quelle couleur préfères-tu?

Marc: Moi, je préfère le vert.

. . . .

Chantal: Trois élèves préfèrent le vert, quatre élèves préfèrent le noir....

2 It's near the end of your trip to France. You decide to do some comparative clothes shopping before you spend the 650 French francs you saved to buy clothes with. Your two favorite stores are a big department store and a small boutique. Compare the items that you see at each store. Then, on a separate sheet of paper, make a list of what you are going to buy at each one. In the column **Au grand magasin**, write each item along with its color and price. Do the same in the column **À la boutique**. Finally, total each column and make sure the combined amount doesn't exceed 650 francs.

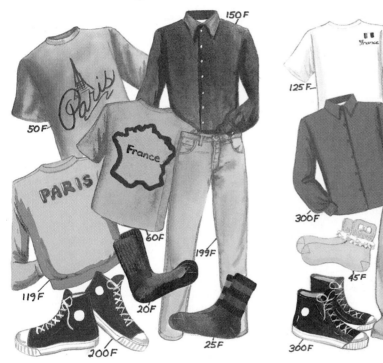

Grand magasin

Boutique

3 With a partner, discuss what you decided to purchase in Activity 12. From the lists you made, read each item you are going to buy to your partner and get his or her opinion.

Modèle:

Student A: Je vais acheter le tee-shirt bleu au grand magasin.

Student B: J'adore le tee-shirt bleu, et il est bon marché.

Mise au point sur... les vêtements

Whether they are digging through racks of secondhand clothes at the **marché aux puces** on the outskirts of Paris or window-shopping (**faire du lèche-vitrines**) at the **haute couture** (*high fashion*) shops along the **rue du Faubourg Saint-Honoré** in the heart of the city, French teenagers follow fashion trends (**la mode**) and strive to achieve their individual "look" (**le look**).

La mode c'est une question d'idées pas une question de prix.

LAURENE M

COUNTRY FOR KIDS

new look CREATION

Marc Anthony

miss HELEN

Bout'Chou

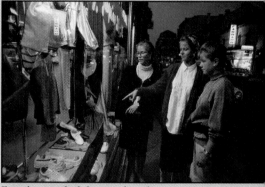

French teens find that window-shopping is a great way to catch up on the latest styles.

French teens, like their American counterparts, spend quite a bit of their free time and money on clothes. In larger

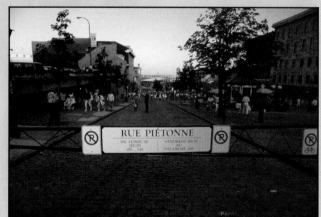

RUE PIÉTONNE
DU LUNDI AU JEUDI VENDREDI 16h30 AU DIMANCHE 24h

The *rues piétonnes* usually have a wide selection of shops and restaurants without the interference of traffic and parked cars. (Montréal)

cities, they go to the **centre commercial** to shop. In smaller towns, they often browse along the **rues piétonnes** (*streets reserved only for pedestrians*), looking in department stores or boutiques for a unique outfit at an affordable price.

Different stores cater to people with a wide variety of tastes. You can find anything from a discarded designer dress to old army boots at the open-air markets. Small boutiques offer personalized service and specialized lines of clothing. Here customers may shop in a more relaxed setting as salespeople hand them clothing from racks and shelves to try on or purchase.

Les grands magasins, such as the Galeries Lafayette, Printemps, and the Samaritaine, have branches all over France and sell a large variety of goods. The oldest department store in the world, Au Bon Marché in Paris, opened in 1852

GALERIES Lafayette

PRINTEMPS

OU TROUVER CE QUE VOUS CHERCHEZ ?

64, Boulevard Haussmann - 75009 PARIS
Ouvert de 9h35 à 19h - du Lundi au Samedi
Nocturne le Jeudi jusqu'à 22h
Métro : Havre-Caumartin - RER : Auber

and is famous for its extensive **épicerie** (*food market*) that sells everything from **escargots** (*snails*) to champagne. When you shop in a **grand magasin**, a salesclerk helps you select the item you want to buy, then brings it to a cashier. Usually stores also wrap the purchase free of charge when you say that it's for a gift. This comes in handy if you have been invited to a French home for a meal and want to bring something to your hosts, as is the custom. **Les grandes surfaces** (*large supermarket and discount stores*), also called **hypermarchés**, offer customers moderate prices along with a wide selection of merchandise.

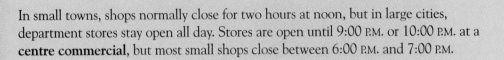

In small towns, shops normally close for two hours at noon, but in large cities, department stores stay open all day. Stores are open until 9:00 P.M. or 10:00 P.M. at a **centre commercial**, but most small shops close between 6:00 P.M. and 7:00 P.M.

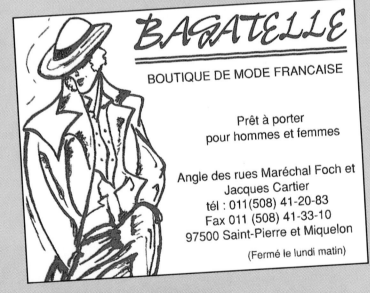

The entire world looks to French fashion houses, such as Cardin, Dior, Lacroix, Chanel, Saint Laurent and Nina Ricci, for the latest styles. Fashion shows twice a year in Paris attract buyers from all around the globe to see the **défilés** (*showings*). Most designers also create **prêt-à-porter** (*ready-to-wear*) clothing which is more affordable for the average customer. If you can't get a ticket to a fashion show, you can always go to Angelina. In the spring and fall, you can get a seat near the window of this tea salon on the **rue de Rivoli** and watch models and designers rushing off to exhibit the latest collections.

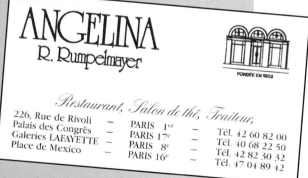

But French teenagers are interested in more than high fashion. For school, casual clothing is the usual attire; many students wear jeans to class. On weekends and for parties, students have a chance to show off their own personal style. Some prefer an upscale, conservative look called **B.C.B.G.** Others favor a more radical style. For French teenagers, tastes in **fringues** (slang for *clothes*) vary just as they do in the rest of the world.

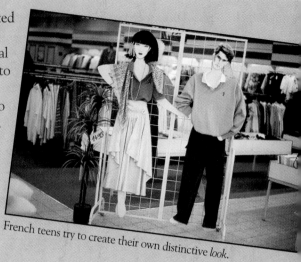

French teens try to create their own distinctive look.

14 Answer the following questions.

1. Where do teenagers often go in Paris to find secondhand clothing?
2. Along what street in Paris are the boutiques of the leading fashion designers located?
3. What is the French term for streets reserved only for pedestrians?
4. Why do some people prefer to shop in a small boutique?
5. In a small boutique is it the customer or the salesperson who takes clothing from racks and shelves?
6. What are the names of two French department stores?
7. In what country did the concept of a department store originate?
8. If you are invited to eat at a French person's home, what is it customary to bring?
9. What are the names of two famous French designers?
10. What are the initials used to describe a rather expensive, conservative style of clothing?

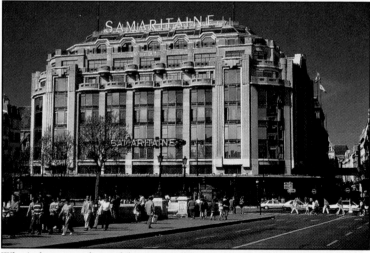

What's the name of one of the more well-known French department stores? (Paris)

5 **Au Vieux Campeur** is a sporting goods chain with stores located throughout Paris. Each individual store specializes in certain areas. Match the people with the address of the store they should visit, based on what they want or need.

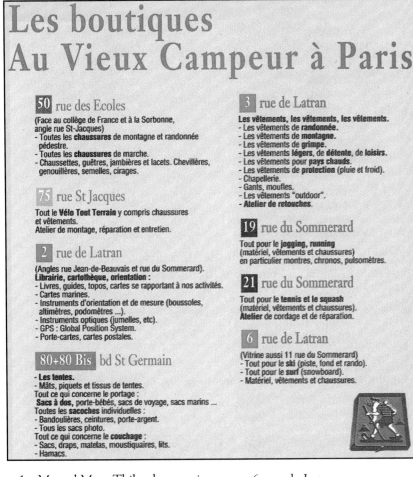

Les boutiques
Au Vieux Campeur à Paris

50 rue des Écoles

(Face au collège de France et à la Sorbonne, angle rue St-Jacques)
- Toutes les **chaussures** de montagne et randonnée pédestre.
- Toutes les **chaussures** de marche.
- Chaussettes, guêtres, jambières et lacets. Chevillères, genouillères, semelles, cirages.

75 rue St Jacques

Tout le **Vélo Tout Terrain** y compris chaussures et vêtements.
Atelier de montage, réparation et entretien.

2 rue de Latran

(Angles rue Jean-de-Beauvais et rue du Sommerard).
Librairie, cartothèque, orientation :
- Livres, guides, topos, cartes se rapportant à nos activités.
- Cartes marines.
- Instruments d'orientation et de mesure (boussoles, altimètres, podomètres ...).
- Instruments optiques (jumelles, etc).
- GPS : Global Position System.
- Porte-cartes, cartes postales.

80+80 Bis bd St Germain

- **Les tentes.**
- Mâts, piquets et tissus de tentes.
Tout ce qui concerne le portage :
Sacs à dos, porte-bébés, sacs de voyage, sacs marins ...
Toutes les **sacoches** individuelles :
- Bandoulières, ceintures, porte-argent.
- Tous les sacs photo.
Tout ce qui concerne le **couchage** :
- Sacs, draps, matelas, moustiquaires, lits.
- Hamacs.

3 rue de Latran

Les vêtements, les vêtements, les vêtements.
- Les vêtements de **randonnée.**
- Les vêtements de **montagne.**
- Les vêtements de **grimpe.**
- Les vêtements **légers,** de **détente,** de **loisirs.**
- Les vêtements pour **pays chauds.**
- Les vêtements de **protection** (pluie et froid).
- Chapellerie.
- Gants, moufles.
- Les vêtements "outdoor".
- **Atelier de retouches.**

19 rue du Sommerard

Tout pour le **jogging, running**
(matériel, vêtements et chaussures)
en particulier montres, chronos, pulsomètres.

21 rue du Sommerard

Tout pour le **tennis et le squash**
(matériel, vêtements et chaussures).
Atelier de cordage et de réparation.

6 rue de Latran

(Vitrine aussi 11 rue du Sommerard)
- Tout pour le **ski** (piste, fond et rando).
- Tout pour le **surf** (snowboard).
- Matériel, vêtements et chaussures.

1. M. and Mme Thibault are going camping and need to buy a tent and two backpacks.
2. Issa needs to have her mountain bike repaired.
3. Mlle Bernier needs to have her tennis racket restrung.
4. Fabrice wants to buy some new ski poles.
5. M. Martin wants to buy some running shoes and a windbreaker.
6. The Dubois family is planning a trip to Normandy and wants to find some guidebooks and maps of the region.
7. Jean-Philippe is spending the month of January in Montreal and needs to buy some new winter clothing, including a coat and some gloves.
8. Martine is going hiking and needs to buy some thick socks.

a. 6, rue de Latran
b. 3, rue de Latran
c. 50, rue des Écoles
d. 19, rue du Sommerard
e. 80 + 80 bis, boulevard Saint-Germain
f. 2, rue de Latran
g. 21, rue du Sommerard
h. 75, rue Saint-Jacques

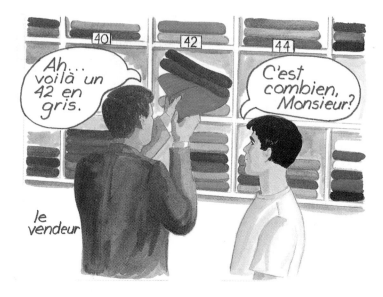

Leçon C

In this lesson you will be able to:

➤ choose and purchase items

➤ ask someone to repeat

➤ ask for information

➤ give information

A salesclerk in a small boutique offers to help Théo.

Le vendeur: **Oui, Monsieur?**
Théo: **Je cherche un pantalon gris. Je fais du 42.**
Le vendeur: **Voici les pantalons. Excusez-moi, quelle taille?**
Théo: **42, s'il vous plaît.**
Le vendeur: **Ah... voilà un 42 en gris.**
Théo: **C'est combien, Monsieur?**
Le vendeur: **219 francs.**
Théo: **D'accord. Est-ce que vous vendez aussi des chaussures?**
Le vendeur: **Non, nous ne vendons pas de chaussures ici.**

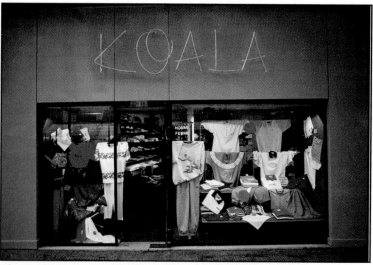

Théo va dans une petite boutique pour chercher un pantalon.

If you haven't heard what someone has said, you may ask the person to repeat by saying **Pardon?** or **Excusez-moi?** You may also say **Comment?**, or in less formal situations, **Quoi?** or **Hein?**

To ask a salesclerk the size of an item of clothing, you say **C'est quelle taille?** To ask the size of a pair of shoes, you say **C'est quelle pointure?** The accompanying chart compares sizes in the United States with those in France and Great Britain.

Size comparison
Table de comparaison de tailles

Women's dresses, knitwear and blouses. Robes, chemisiers et tricots femmes.

F	36	38	40	42	44	46	48
GB	10	12	14	16	18	20	22
USA	8	10	12	14	16	18	20

Women's stockings. Bas et collants femmes.

F	1	2	3	4	5
USA	8½	9	9½	10	10½

Women's shoes. Chaussures femmes.

F	35½	36	36½	37	37½	38	39
GB	3	3½	4	4½	5	5½	6
USA	4	4½	5	5½	6	6½	7½

Men's shoes. Chaussures hommes.

F	39	40	41	42	43	44	45
GB	5½	6½	7	8	8½	9½	10½
USA	6	7	7½	8½	9	10	11

Men's suits. Costumes hommes.

F	36	38	40	42	44	46	48
GB	35	36	37	38	39	40	42
USA	35	36	37	38	39	40	42

Men's shirts. Chemises hommes.

F	36	37	38	39	40	41	42
USA	14	14½	15	15½	16	16½	17

Men's sweaters. Tricots hommes.

F	36	38	40	42	44	46
GB	46	48	51	54	55	59
USA	46	48	51	54	56	59

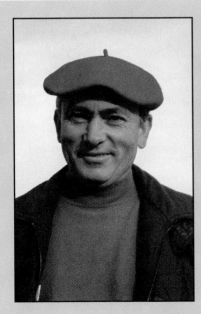

Many English words related to clothing originally came from French. For example, we use the word **chic** for "stylish," **boutique** for a "shop" and **béret** for the small round cap that was first worn in **les Pyrénées**. The French also gave us the word for "jeans." French tailors created denim pants, called **gênes**, which were named after the city of Genoa, Italy. They were first worn there by sailors during the Middle Ages. Later the word was modified to "jeans." The fabric that is used to make jeans was originally called **serge de Nîmes** after the town in France where it was loomed. This was eventually shortened to "denim."

Bérets, traditionally worn by older men, are becoming more and more fashionable among younger women. (Saint-Jean-de-Luz)

1 | Answer the following questions.

1. What would you say if you didn't hear what your teacher said the first time?
2. What would you say if you didn't hear what your friend said the first time?
3. What is the French word for "size" if you are referring to an article of clothing?
4. If a woman wears a size 38 shoe in France, what size does she wear in the United States?
5. If a man wears a size 15 shirt in the United States, what size does he wear in France?
6. If a woman wears a size 38 dress in France, what size does she wear in the United States?
7. If a man wears a size 9 shoe in the United States, what size does he wear in France?
8. What are several French words related to clothing that are commonly used in English?
9. What two French words were combined to give us the word "denim"?

2 | *Choisissez la bonne réponse.*

1. Qui cherche un pantalon?
2. Qui parle à Théo?
3. De quelle couleur est le pantalon?
4. Théo, quelle taille fait-il?
5. Combien coûte le pantalon?
6. Qu'est-ce que Théo cherche aussi?

a. gris
b. 219 francs
c. le vendeur
d. des chaussures
e. Théo
f. du 42

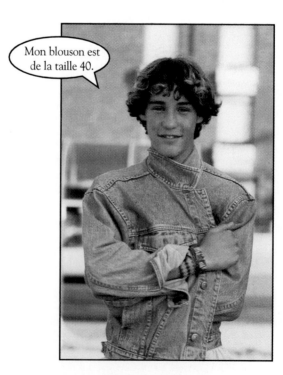

Mon blouson est de la taille 40.

What would you say in French in the following situations?

1. You suggest to a friend that you go shopping together at the mall.
2. You tell a salesclerk that you're looking for some black jeans.
3. You didn't hear what a salesclerk said and ask him or her to repeat.
4. You ask a salesclerk the size of a shirt.
5. You ask a salesclerk how much a sweater costs.
6. You tell a salesclerk that you are going to buy the yellow ski jacket.
7. You ask a salesclerk if he or she also sells socks.

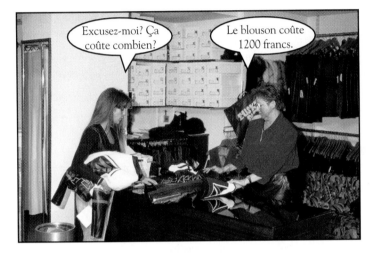

C'est à toi!

1. Est-ce que tu travailles dans une boutique, un magasin ou un grand magasin?
2. Est-ce que tu aimes acheter des vêtements?
3. Qu'est-ce que tu cherches quand tu vas dans une petite boutique?
4. Le pantalon coûte 219 francs. Est-ce qu'il est cher ou bon marché?
5. Qu'est-ce que tu préfères porter à l'école, un ensemble ou un jean et un sweat?
6. Est-ce que tu préfères porter un vieux jean ou un nouveau jean?

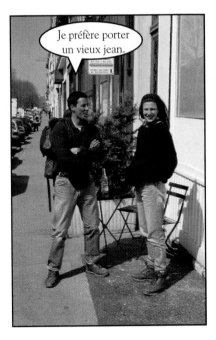

Structure

Present tense of regular verbs ending in -re

The infinitives of many French verbs end in **-re**. Most of these verbs, such as **vendre** (*to sell*), are regular. To form the present tense of a regular **-re** verb, first find the stem of the verb by removing the **-re** ending of the infinitive.

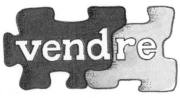

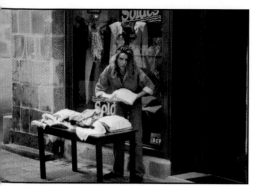

Joanne vend des fringues. (Brive-la-Gaillarde)

Now add the endings (**-s, -s, —, -ons, -ez, -ent**) to the stem of the verb depending on the corresponding subject pronouns. Note that no ending is added to the stem in the **il/elle/on** form.

vendre			
je	**vends**	Je **vends** des vêtements.	*I sell clothes.*
tu	**vends**	Qu'est-ce que tu **vends**?	*What are you selling?*
il/elle/on	**vend**	On **vend** des baskets ici?	*Do they sell hightops here?*
nous	**vendons**	Oui, nous **vendons** des chaussures.	*Yes, we sell shoes.*
vous	**vendez**	Vous ne **vendez** pas de pulls?	*Don't you sell sweaters?*
ils/elles	**vendent**	Ils **vendent** des jeans.	*They sell jeans.*

Pratique

5 Tell what the following people sell, based on where they work.

Modèle:

Sophie travaille à Bananas. Alors, elle vend des maillots de bain.

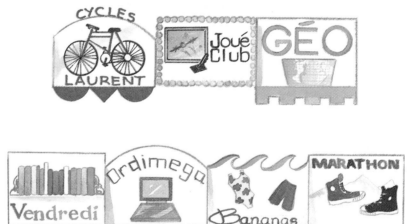

1. Christine et Jean-Michel travaillent à Joué Club.
2. Mme Picard travaille à Vendredi.
3. Thierry travaille à Marathon.
4. Béatrice et sa sœur travaillent à Géo.
5. Abdoul et Khadim travaillent à Cycles Laurent.
6. Mlle Lambert travaille à Ordimega.

The French Club at your school is sponsoring a **marché aux puces** to raise money for a trip to France. Tell what the club members are selling.

Modèle:

Jean-Paul
Jean-Paul vend des cahiers.

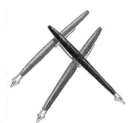

1. Margarette

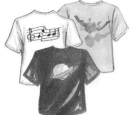

5. tu

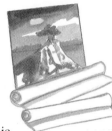

2. nous

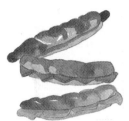

6. Guillaume

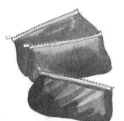

3. je

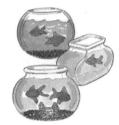

7. vous

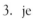

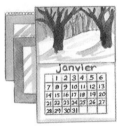

4. Pierre et Amine

8. Delphine et Françoise

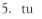

Communication

With a partner, play the roles of an American student who is shopping at a ski resort in the French Alps and the salesclerk at the resort's boutique. The customer's brother wants a nice French ski jacket and has given the customer enough money to buy it. During the course of the conversation, the customer and the salesclerk should talk about what size ski jacket the customer's brother wears, what color he prefers and the prices of various jackets. Finally, the customer decides on a jacket and purchases it.

8 | *Trouvez une personne qui....* Interview your classmates to find out about their shopping habits and tastes in clothes. On a separate sheet of paper, number from 1 to 14. Circulate around the classroom asking your classmates one at a time the questions that follow. When someone answers a question affirmatively, have that person write his or her name next to the number of the appropriate question. Continue asking questions, trying to find a different person who answers each question affirmatively.

Est-ce que tu...

1. aimes les shorts très grands?
2. portes souvent un tee-shirt noir?
3. préfères porter un sweat?
4. vas faire du shopping aujourd'hui?
5. aimes le jaune?
6. as un pull rouge?
7. as un pantalon beige?
8. aimes les manteaux longs?
9. as un chapeau?
10. as un anorak bleu?
11. vas souvent au centre commercial?
12. aimes faire les magasins?
13. as des baskets?
14. aimes acheter les vêtements en solde?

Modèle:

Jacques: **Tu aimes les shorts très grands?**

Christiane: **Oui, j'aime les shorts très grands.** (Writes her name beside number 1.)

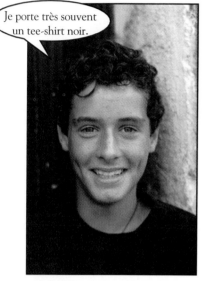

Je porte très souvent un tee-shirt noir.

Est-ce qu'Estelle et Lydie ont un anorak bleu?

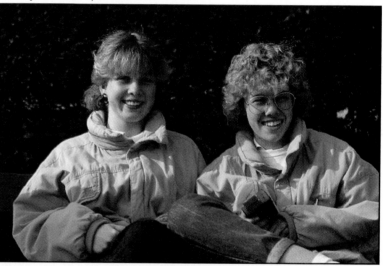

Sur la bonne piste

One of the major keys to understanding a reading is being able to evaluate it. Asking yourself whether you agree or disagree with the information in the reading will give you a reason to look at it in more depth. For instance, if a store advertisement claims that a shirt is stylish and guarantees popularity, you, the reader, need to evaluate this statement. Do you like the style of the shirt? Some readers may not. Can a shirt really make you popular? Most readers would doubt this. Evaluating information as you read it is called critical reading. Critical reading helps you separate fact from opinion. When you no longer simply accept what you read and begin to form your own opinions about it, you are using more advanced reading and thinking skills (especially if what you are reading is written in another language!).

The reading that follows is part of an article from a back-to-school issue of a French magazine. Read critically the three clothing descriptions.

Dans la mode c'est déjà la rentrée!

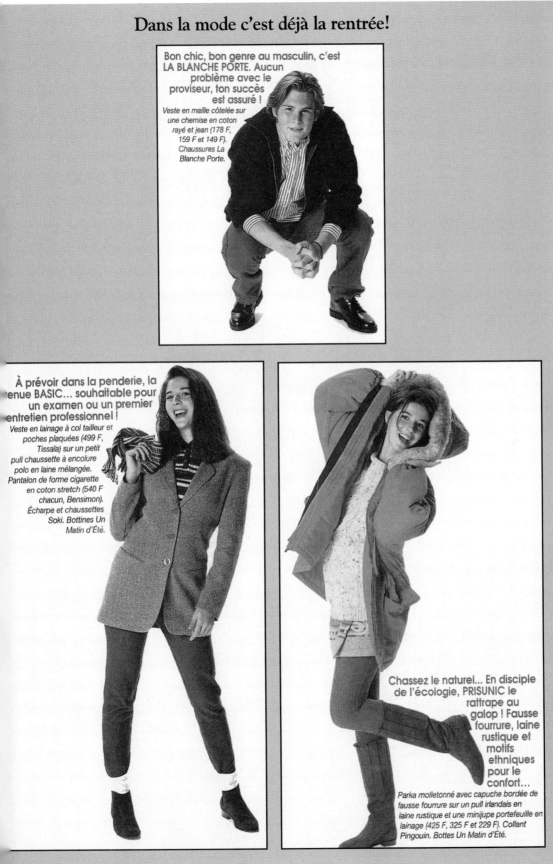

Bon chic, bon genre au masculin, c'est LA BLANCHE PORTE. Aucun problème avec le proviseur, ton succès est assuré !
Veste en maille côtelée sur une chemise en coton rayé et jean (178 F, 159 F et 149 F). Chaussures La Blanche Porte.

À prévoir dans la penderie, la tenue BASIC... souhaitable pour un examen ou un premier entretien professionnel !
Veste en lainage à col tailleur et poches plaquées (499 F, Tissaïa) sur un petit pull chaussette à encolure polo en laine mélangée. Pantalon de forme cigarette en coton stretch (540 F chacun, Bensimon). Écharpe et chaussettes Soki. Bottines Un Matin d'Été.

Chassez le naturel... En disciple de l'écologie, PRISUNIC le rattrape au galop ! Fausse fourrure, laine rustique et motifs ethniques pour le confort...
Parka molletonné avec capuche bordée de fausse fourrure sur un pull irlandais en laine rustique et une minijupe portefeuille en lainage (425 F, 325 F et 229 F). Collant Pingouin. Bottes Un Matin d'Été.

9 | Answer the following questions.

1. You know that the French word for "boot" is **botte**. What is the French word for "short boot"?

2. Which of the three outfits is the most expensive? Which is the least expensive?

3. Is the fur on the parka from Prisunic real or fake? Is this outfit ecologically correct?

4. According to the article, wearing the outfit from La Blanche Porte guarantees that you won't have any problems with your school principal. What assumption is this claim based on?

5. Which outfits, if any, are appropriate to wear...
   a. to school?
   b. to a job interview?
   c. to a party?
   d. at home while watching television?

6. Does one of these outfits reflect your own personal style? Why or why not?

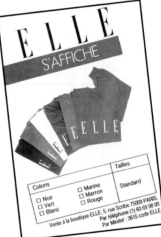

Nathalie et Raoul

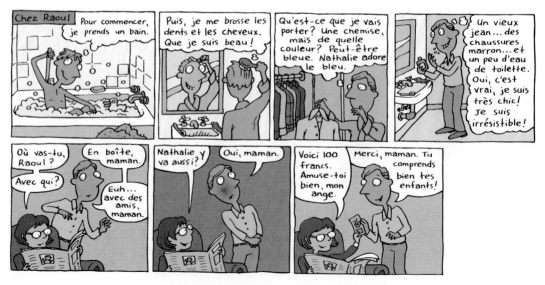

C'est à moi!

Now that you have completed this unit, take a look at what you should be able to do in French. Can you do all of these tasks?

➤ I can tell what I like and what I dislike.

➤ I can agree with someone.

➤ I can say what I need.

➤ I can say what someone is going to do.

➤ I can invite someone to do something.

➤ I can inquire about and compare prices.

➤ I can ask for and give information about various topics, including colors and sizes of clothing.

➤ I can ask someone to repeat.

➤ I can choose and purchase clothing.

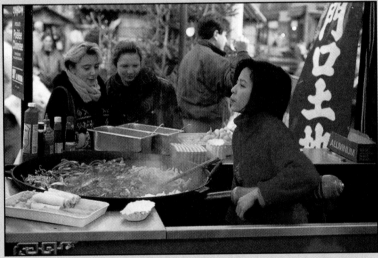

Brigitte et Véro vont manger chinois.

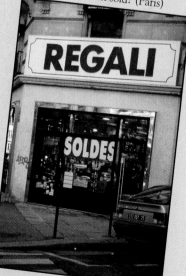

Does the sign in the window mean this store has been sold? (Paris)

Here is a brief checkup to see how much you understand about French culture. Decide if each statement is **vrai** or **faux**.

1. Small specialized stores still flourish in France even though there are giant shopping malls.
2. Generally the French prefer having stylish clothing of good quality rather than simply having a lot of different outfits.
3. At **le marché aux puces** customers are expected to bargain with vendors.
4. Montreal is the largest French-speaking city in the world.
5. Living and shopping in Montreal can be done entirely underground if you choose to remain in the subterranean part of the city.
6. If you see the sign **Soldes** on items displayed on the sidewalk in front of a French store, it means that someone else has already purchased them.

7. At Parisian department stores, such as the Galeries Lafayette and Printemps, you can find men's and women's fashions.
8. Department stores in large French cities close for two hours at noon.
9. Shoe sizes are the same in both France and the United States.
10. The French gave us the word for "jeans."

Communication orale

Imagine that you and your partner live in Montreal and are planning to go to the **Place Ville-Marie** on a big shopping spree tomorrow. Have a conversation in which each of you talks about several items of clothing you have that are old. Also give some other information about these items, for example, their color. Then say that you need new ones. Suggest that you go shopping together tomorrow. Next name several stores that you are going to shop at and tell what they sell. Finally, set a time to meet tomorrow.

Communication écrite

No one is at home when you and your partner decide to go to the **Place Ville-Marie** on your shopping spree tomorrow. Write a note in French to the rest of your family in which you tell them what you are going to do and why. Begin by saying at what time and where you and your friend are going shopping. Then mention what clothes you have that are old and say that you need new ones. Next tell the cost of each item you are going to buy. Finally, name several stores where you are going to shop and say what they sell.

Communication active

To say what you like, use:

J'aime bien faire les magasins.	*I really like to go shopping.*
J'adore la chemise bleue.	*I love the blue shirt.*

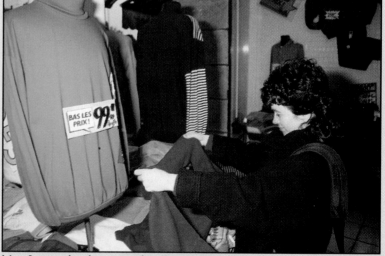

Mme Legras adore le sweat violet. (Bayonne)

To say what you dislike, use:
Beurk! *Yuk!*

To agree with someone, use:
C'est vrai. *This is/It's/That's true.*

To say you need something, use:
J'ai besoin d'un pull. *I need a sweater.*
J'ai besoin d'une chemise. *I need a shirt.*

To express intentions, use:
Je vais aller au centre
commercial. *I'm going to go to the mall.*

To invite someone to do something, use:
Allons ensemble au *Let's go to the department store*
grand magasin! *together!*

To inquire about prices, use:
C'est combien? *How much is it?*
C'est en solde? *Is it on sale?*

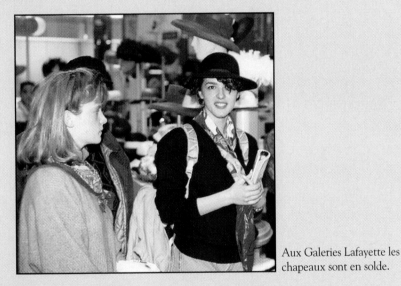

Aux Galeries Lafayette les
chapeaux sont en solde.

To compare prices, use:
Il/Elle est assez cher/chère. *It's rather expensive.*
Il/Elle est bon marché. *It's cheap.*

To ask for information, use:
Quelle taille? *What size?*
Est-ce que **vous vendez** aussi *Do you also sell shoes?*
des chaussures?

To give information, use:
Je fais du 42. *I wear size 42.*

To ask someone to repeat, use:
Excusez-moi? *Excuse me?*

To choose and purchase an item, use:
Je cherche un pantalon gris. *I'm looking for gray pants.*

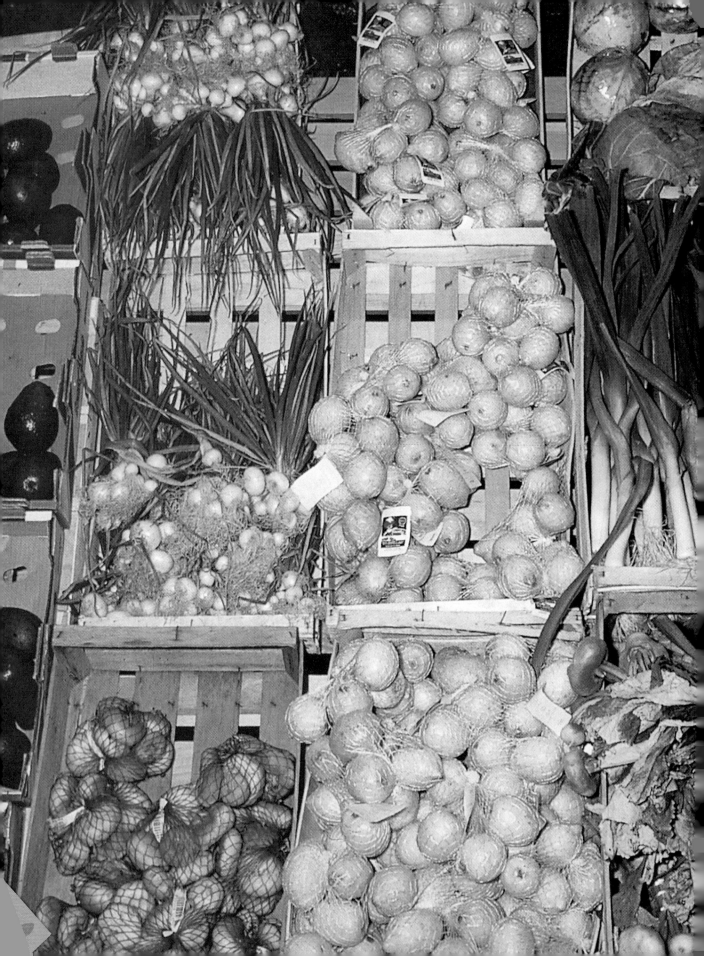

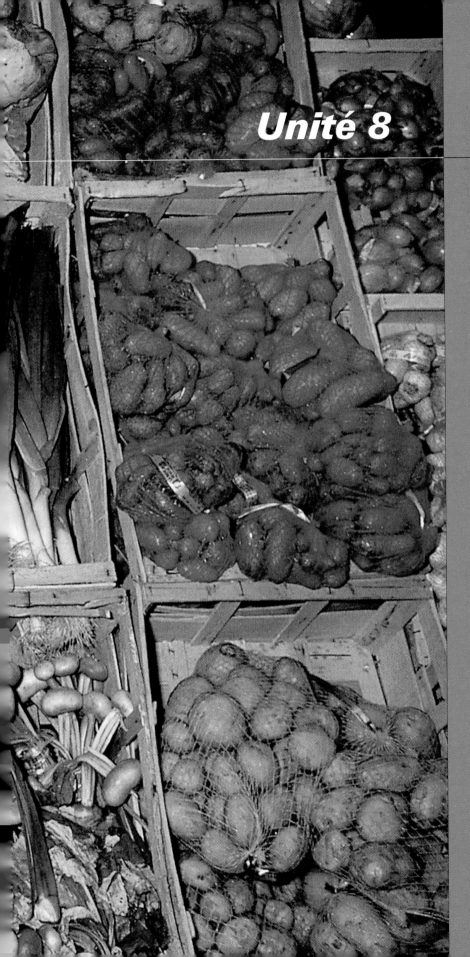

Unité 8

On fait les courses.

In this unit you will be able to:

➤ ask for information
➤ give information
➤ express likes and dislikes
➤ agree and disagree
➤ identify objects
➤ ask for permission
➤ ask for a price
➤ state prices
➤ inquire about and compare prices
➤ make a complaint
➤ insist
➤ negotiate
➤ choose and purchase items

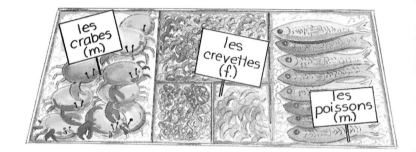

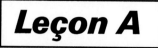

Leçon A

In this lesson you will be able to:

➤ ask for information

➤ give information

➤ agree and disagree

➤ identify objects

➤ ask for permission

les légumes (m.)

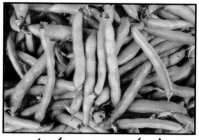

les haricots verts (m.)

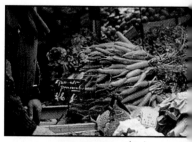

les carottes (f.)

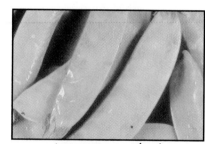

les petits pois (m.)

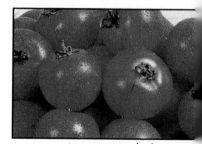

les tomates (f.)

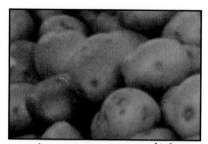

les pommes de terre (f.)

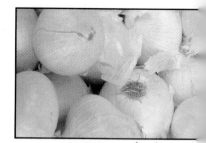

les oignons (m.)

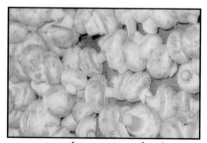

les champignons (m.)

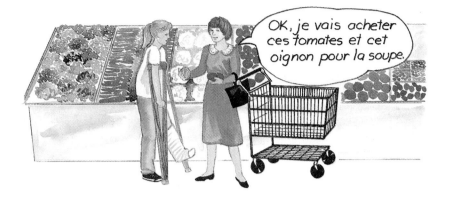

Madame Laurier and her daughter Madeleine are at the supermarket in Marseille.

Mme Laurier: **Qu'est-ce que tu veux manger ce soir?**

Madeleine: **Euh... tu peux faire une bouillabaisse?**

Mme Laurier: **OK, je vais acheter ces tomates et cet oignon pour la soupe. Maintenant on va chercher les crabes et les poissons.**

Madeleine: **Nous pouvons acheter des oranges aussi?**

Mme Laurier: **Oui, ton père veut toujours un fruit après le repas.**

Enquête culturelle

Marseille is France's largest seaport and oldest city. Tourists often visit **le Vieux Port**, a small port near the center of the city filled with recreational and fishing boats, and **la Canebière**, the main commercial street lined with many shops. Ships from all over the world dock at the modern, international port nearby. One of the well-known churches of the city, **Notre-Dame-de-la-Garde**, has a golden statue of the Virgin Mary on its steeple. This statue still guides sailors safely to the port, since it can be seen far out into the Mediterranean Sea. The French national anthem, the "Marseillaise," received its name from the city of Marseille.

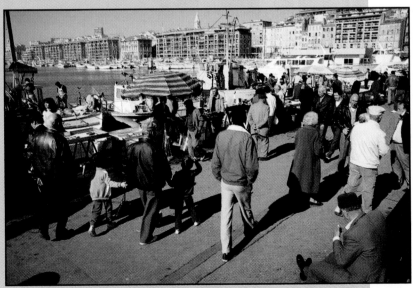

Early in the morning people head to *le Vieux Port* to buy fresh fish. (Marseille)

Regional specialties from all over the country may be found in French food stores as well as in restaurants. **Bouillabaisse**, a fish soup, is a specialty of Marseille. **Pâté de foie gras**, a pork and goose liver pâté, comes from the

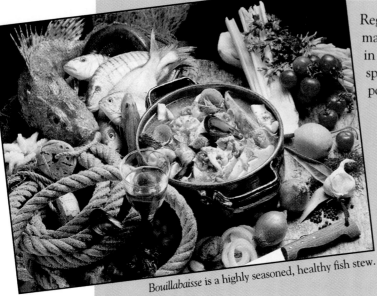

Bouillabaisse is a highly seasoned, healthy fish stew.

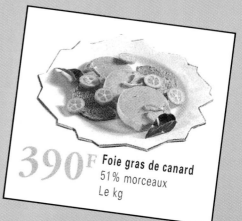

390^F **Foie gras de canard**
51% morceaux
Le kg

Choumieux

SPECIALITE DE CASSOULET
et CONFIT DE CANARD
Tous les jours jusqu'à minuit Tél. (1) 47.05.49.75
79, rue Saint-Dominique (7ᵉ)

---

city of Strasbourg. **Cassoulet**, from the southwestern part of France, is a stew made from duck, goose or sausage and white beans. **Quiche lorraine**, a quiche containing bacon, onions and cheese, was created in the province of Lorraine. **Bœuf bourguignon**, a meat stew cooked in red wine, originated in the Burgundy region.

There are different types of *quiche* depending on the region and ingredients used. (Bayonne)

Pains spéciaux au blé complet

Ingrédients: Farine complète de blé (67%), farine de blé, matière grasse végétale, sucre, levure et sel.

Valeur nutritive par 100 g:
Protéines	12 g
Matières grasses	7 g
Hydrates de carbone	75 g
dont fibres	7 g
1640 kJ (390 kcal)	

A conserver dans un endroit sec.

A consommer de préférence avant fin: voir la face principale du paquet.

e **225 g**

Healthy ingredients are often emphasized on food packages in France, just as they are in the United States. Labels in grocery stores highlight expressions such as **pas d'additifs** (*no additives*), **1% de matière grasse** (*1% fat content*) and **fort en vitamines** (*high in vitamins*).

Il y a des poissons dans une bouillabaisse. (Lyon)

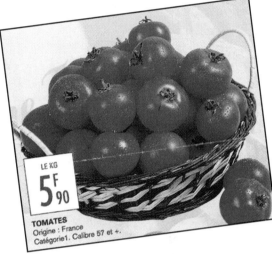

1 | *Répondez en français.*

    1. Qu'est-ce que Mme Laurier va faire ce soir?

    2. La bouillabaisse, c'est un dessert?

    3. Quels légumes est-ce qu'il y a dans une bouillabaisse?

    4. Qu'est-ce qu'il y a aussi dans une bouillabaisse?

    5. Quel fruit est-ce que Mme Laurier et Madeleine vont acheter?

    6. Qu'est-ce que les Français mangent souvent après le repas?

2 | *Choisissez la bonne réponse.*

    1. Les... sont des légumes longs.   a. tomates

    2. Les... sont des fruits.   b. oignon

    3. Les... sont des légumes orange.   c. haricots verts

    4. L'... est un légume blanc.   d. crabes

    5. Les... sont des légumes blancs.   e. carottes

    6. Les... sont des légumes rouges.   f. oranges

    7. Les frites sont des....   g. champignons

    8. On trouve les... dans   h. pommes de terre
       la Méditerranée.

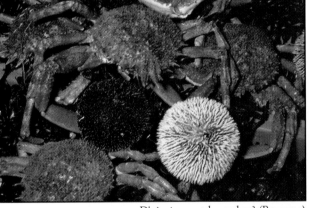

D'où viennent les crabes? (Bayonne)

TOMATES
Origine : France
Catégorie1. Calibre 57 et +.

3 | Say how much you like each of the following foods, using **J'aime
beaucoup, J'aime un peu** or **Je n'aime pas.**

Qui n'aime pas les crevettes? (Bayonne)

    1. les petits pois

    2. les crevettes

    3. les légumes

    4. les champignons

    5. les poissons

    6. les oignons

    7. les fruits

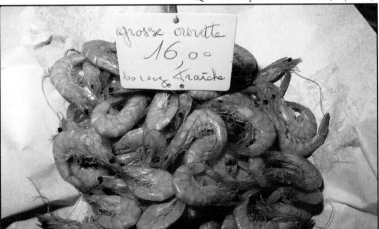

4 | *C'est à toi!*

1. Est-ce que tu manges beaucoup de légumes?
2. Quels légumes aimes-tu?
3. Est-ce que tu préfères le poisson ou le steak?
4. Quand est-ce que tu aimes manger de la soupe, en été ou en hiver?
5. Dans ta famille, qui aime les oranges?
6. Qu'est-ce que tu vas manger ce soir?

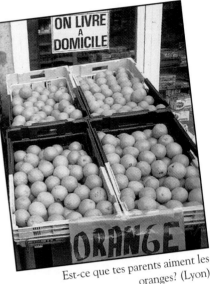

Est-ce que tes parents aiment les oranges? (Lyon)

Structure

Present tense of the irregular verb *vouloir*

The verb **vouloir** (*to want*) is irregular.

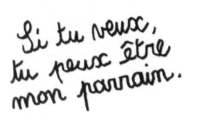

vouloir			
je	**veux**	Je **veux** un sandwich.	*I want a sandwich.*
tu	**veux**	Qu'est-ce que tu **veux**?	*What do you want?*
il/elle/on	**veut**	Ton père **veut** un fruit.	*Your father wants (a piece of) fruit.*
nous	**voulons**	Nous ne **voulons** pas ces tomates.	*We don't want these tomatoes.*
vous	**voulez**	Où **voulez**-vous manger?	*Where do you want to eat?*
ils/elles	**veulent**	Ils **veulent** faire une quiche.	*They want to make a quiche.*

You already know one form of the verb **vouloir** that you use when you ask for something: **Je voudrais....** (*I would like . . . .*) The French often use this form, which is more polite than **je veux**.

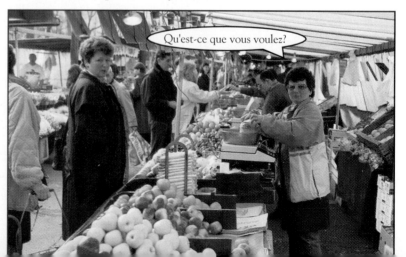

Qu'est-ce que vous voulez?

Pratique

You and your friends are trying to decide where to have lunch. Tell who wants to eat at a café and who wants to eat at a fast-food restaurant.

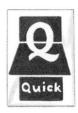

Clément
Clément veut manger au fast-food.

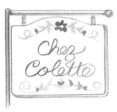

Luc et Marie-Alix
Luc et Marie-Alix veulent manger au café.

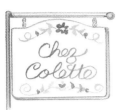

1. Christine

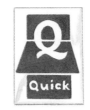

5. David

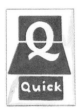

2. nous

6. je

3. Jamila et Latifa

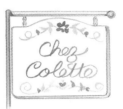

7. Laurent et Philippe

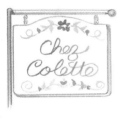

4. tu

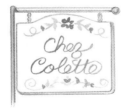

8. vous

Tell what the following people want, depending on whether they are hungry or thirsty.

1. Édouard a soif. (une eau minérale/une crêpe)
2. J'ai soif. (une orange/un café)
3. Mme Pinetti et son fils ont faim. (des jus d'orange/des légumes)
4. Tu as faim. (des crevettes/un jus de pomme)
5. Nous avons soif. (des pommes de terre/des limonades)
6. Vous avez faim. (des fruits/des boissons)

Modèles:

Patricia a soif. (un dessert/un coca)
Elle veut un coca.

M. et Mme Lavigne ont faim.
(des frites/un jus de raisin)
Ils veulent des frites.

Present tense of the irregular verb *pouvoir*

The verb **pouvoir** (*to be able to*) is irregular. In the following examples note the different meanings of **pouvoir** in English.

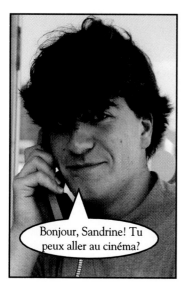

Bonjour, Sandrine! Tu peux aller au cinéma?

	pouvoir		
je	**peux**	Je **peux** sortir?	*May I go out?*
tu	**peux**	Tu **peux** aller au cinéma?	*Can you go to the movies?*
il/elle/on	**peut**	Il ne **peut** pas inviter ses amis.	*He can't invite his friends.*
nous	**pouvons**	Nous **pouvons** acheter des oranges?	*Can we buy some oranges?*
vous	**pouvez**	**Pouvez**-vous venir demain?	*Are you able to come tomorrow?*
ils/elles	**peuvent**	Ils **peuvent** travailler ensemble.	*They can work together.*

Pratique

7 Tell which is the most expensive item the following people can buy, based on how much money they have.

Modèle:

Abdou (cent francs)
Abdou peut acheter le sac à dos.

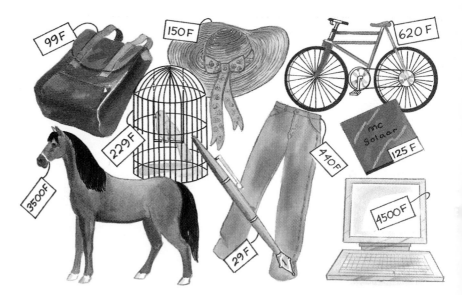

1. M. Prat (cinq mille francs)
2. vous (sept cents francs)
3. Thibault et son frère (cent quarante francs)
4. je (quatre cent soixante francs)
5. Mme Wolff (deux cents francs)
6. les sœurs de Nicolas (deux cent cinquante francs)
7. nous (quatre mille francs)
8. tu (trente francs)

8 The grocery store is closing in five minutes. You and your friends still have to buy some of the things you need to prepare a dinner of fish soup, bread, fruit, cheese and mineral water. Decide who in column A can look for each item in column B.

Modèle:
Gilbert peut chercher les oranges.

A	B
Gilbert	les carottes
Étienne et Diane	les tomates
je	les oignons
Thierry et toi, vous	les crabes
tu	les poissons
Florence	les oranges
Louis et moi, nous	le fromage
Stéphanie et Nadia	l'eau minérale

Demonstrative adjectives

Demonstrative adjectives are used to point out specific people or things. **Ce**, **cet** and **cette** mean "this" or "that"; **ces** means "these" or "those." These adjectives agree with the nouns that follow them.

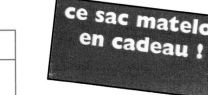
ce sac matelot en cadeau !

	Singular		Plural
Masculine before a Consonant Sound	Masculine before a Vowel Sound	Feminine	
ce chien	cet anorak	cette robe	ces crabes

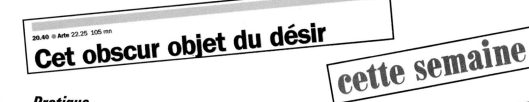
TT
20.40 ● Arte 22.25 105 mn
Cet obscur objet du désir

cette semaine   N° 2510 2 F

Pratique

9 Help your great-grandmother with her grocery shopping by telling her the prices of the food she chooses. Complete each of your sentences with the appropriate demonstrative adjective (**ce**, **cet**, **cette** or **ces**).

1. ... jambon coûte 40F.
2. ... tomate coûte 2F.
3. ... crabe coûte 35F.
4. ... haricots verts coûtent 7F.
5. ... oignon coûte 3F.
6. ... poisson coûte 23F.
7. ... pommes de terre coûtent 11F.
8. ... orange coûte 3F.
9. ... champignons coûtent 8F.

Ces champignons coûtent huit francs. (Montréal)

10 | Find out whether or not you and your partner like the same clothes. Take turns asking and answering questions about the pictured items.

Modèle:

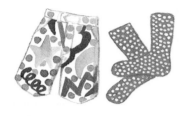

Student A: **Tu aimes ce short?**
Student B: **Oui, j'aime ce short. Tu aimes ces chaussettes?**
Student A: **Non, je n'aime pas ces chaussettes.**

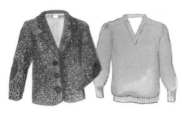

1.

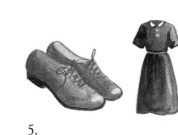

4.

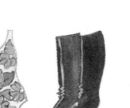

2.

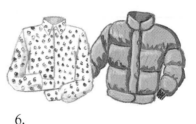

5.

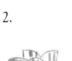

3.

6.

Communication

11 | You are spending the summer with the Garrigues family in the south of France. Mme Garrigues is going to make a fish soup for dinner and asked you to pick up ingredients at the supermarket. Since she was in a hurry this morning, she left you only the recipe (on the left). You've already made a list of what ingredients you have (on the right). Comparing the recipe with what's on hand, write your grocery list.

Modèle:

Nous avons besoin de
15 crevettes....

La Soupe	Nous avons...
20 crevettes	*5 crevettes*
2 crabes	*1 poisson blanc*
3 poissons blancs	*1 oignon*
2 oignons	*2 tomates*
2 tomates	*2 pommes de terre*
2 carottes	
3 pommes de terre	

2 Interview two of your classmates to find out if they like certain foods. Make a grid like the partial one that follows. Write down the names of ten foods. Ask your classmates if they like each of these foods. As they answer each question, write their names in the appropriate column.

Est-ce que vous aimez...		
	oui	non
les crevettes?	*Francis*	*Yasmine*
le fromage?	*Yasmine, Francis*	

Modèles:

Danièle: Est-ce que vous aimez les crevettes?

Francis: Moi, j'aime les crevettes.

Yasmine: Et moi, je n'aime pas les crevettes.

Danièle: Est-ce que vous aimez le fromage?

Yasmine: Moi, j'aime le fromage.

Francis: Et moi aussi, j'aime le fromage.

3 To help you and your partner decide what you are going to do tonight, take turns asking and answering questions. Student A asks if Student B would like to do certain things. Student B either accepts, saying **Oui, je veux bien,** or refuses, saying **Non, je ne peux pas,** depending on the response indicated.

1. aller au centre commercial (J'ai besoin d'un nouveau jean.)
2. venir chez moi (Je travaille à 18 heures.)
3. aller au fast-food (J'ai faim.)
4. étudier avec moi (J'ai une interro demain.)
5. aller en boîte (C'est trop cher.)
6. faire une bouillabaisse (Je vais au café avec la famille.)
7. nager (Je n'ai pas de maillot de bain.)

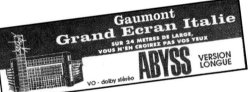

Modèles:

aller au cinéma (On passe un bon film au Gaumont.)

Student A: Tu veux aller au cinéma?

Student B: Oui, je veux bien. On passe un bon film au Gaumont.

faire du vélo (Je n'ai pas de vélo.)

Student A: Tu veux faire du vélo?

Student B: Non, je ne peux pas. Je n'ai pas de vélo.

Prononciation

The sound [ø]

The vowel combination **eu** is pronounced [ø] when it's in the last syllable of a word ending in **-eu, -eut** or **-eux**. Say each of these words:

v**eu**t	chev**eux**
bl**eu**	d**eux**
p**eux**	génér**eux**

The sound [œ]

In most other cases **eu** is pronounced [œ] before a final pronounced consonant other than [z]. The vowel combination **œu** is always pronounced [œ]. Say each of these words:

p**eu**vent	taill**eur**
coul**eur**	vend**eur**
v**eu**lent	s**œur**

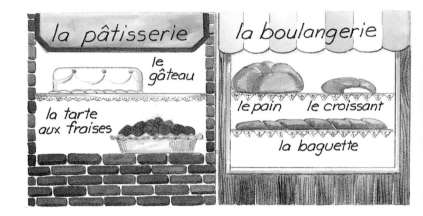

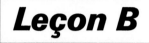

Leçon B

In this lesson you will be able to:

➤ **agree and disagree**

➤ **express likes and dislikes**

➤ **insist**

➤ **give information**

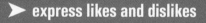

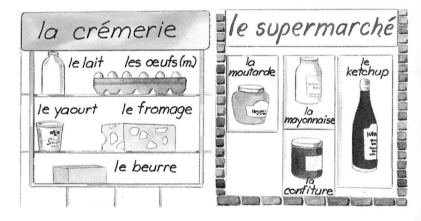

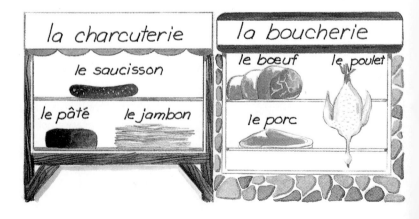

Combien de confiture as-tu?

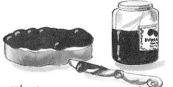

J'ai trop de confiture.

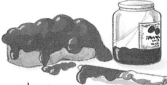

J'ai beaucoup de confiture.

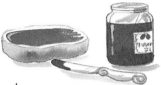

J'ai assez de confiture.

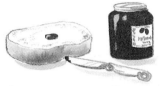

J'ai un peu de confiture.

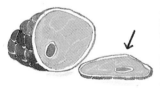

une tranche de
jambon

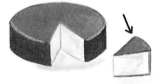

un morceau de
fromage

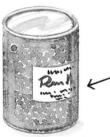

une boîte de
petits pois

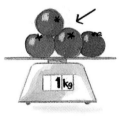

un kilo de
tomates

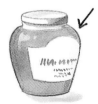

un pot de
moutarde

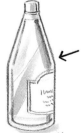

une bouteille d'eau
minérale

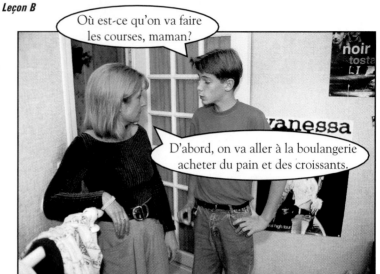

Madame Rousseau and her son Benjamin are talking about going grocery shopping.

Benjamin:	Où est-ce qu'on va faire les courses, maman?
Mme Rousseau:	D'abord, on va aller à la boulangerie acheter du pain et des croissants.
Benjamin:	Ouais! J'aime bien les croissants le matin.
Mme Rousseau:	Puis, on va acheter des yaourts et un peu de fromage, peut-être du camembert, à la crémerie.
Benjamin:	Moi, j'aime aussi le pâté. On ne va pas acheter de pâté?
Mme Rousseau:	Si, si, mais attends! Nous pouvons aussi aller à la charcuterie.

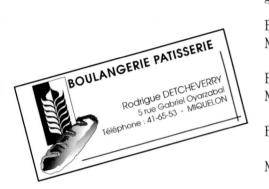

Enquête culturelle

The expression **Repas sans pain, repas de rien** ("A meal without bread is nothing") shows the importance of bread in the French diet. Although French bread comes in many shapes and sizes, the most common

The French buy their *baguettes* fresh every day. (Bayonne)

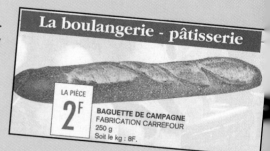

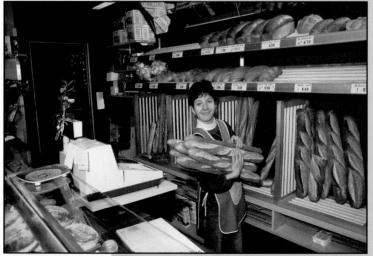

type, the **baguette**, is a long, thin loaf of bread with a crisp crust. This hard crust keeps the bread fresh without being wrapped; people can be seen carrying **baguettes** tucked under their arms or nibbling on the ends of them as they walk home from the **boulangerie**. The bread has such a good taste that the French usually don't butter it, except for breakfast. Other sweeter types of bakery products are just as delicious. A **pain**

You can make your own version of a *pain au chocolat* by baking chocolate chips inside a crescent roll.

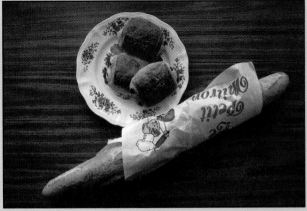

au chocolat tastes like a **croissant** and has a piece of chocolate in the center. Children often eat them for

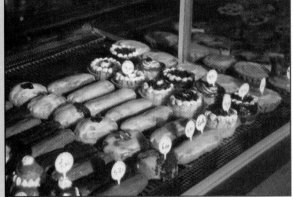

snacks. **Un éclair** is a cream-filled pastry, **un chausson aux pommes** resembles an apple turnover and **une brioche** is a soft, round roll.

Would you choose a chocolate, mocha or vanilla *éclair*? (Angers)

Camembert is a soft cheese with a thin, edible skin.

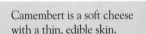

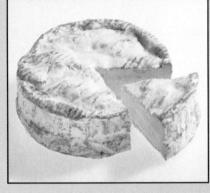

Fruit and cheese, other staples in the French diet, are often served as dessert at the end of a meal. Most regions of France produce their own special cheese, with some 360 different kinds in all to choose from. Camembert, Pont-l'Évêque and Neufchâtel are three of the many famous types of cheese from the northern province of Normandy. Brie, the most famous of all French cheeses, comes from the Parisian area. Roquefort, one of the better-known blue cheeses from the **Massif Central**, is made from sheep's milk.

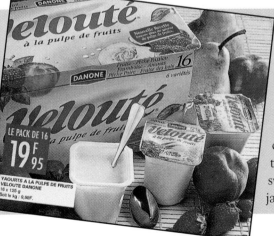

Instead of cheese, the French often eat yogurt for dessert. French yogurt is generally thinner than the custard-type yogurt found in the United States. In general, French teenagers drink less milk than American teens but consume more cheese and yogurt. They generally eat their yogurt plain, but sometimes sweeten it with a little sugar, honey, jam or jelly.

1 | Write a four-sentence paragraph in French that summarizes the conversation between Madame Rousseau and Benjamin. Begin by telling what they are going to do. Then mention what they are going to buy at the bakery and at the dairy store. Also name two foods that Benjamin likes.

2 | You're planning a picnic with some of your friends. Before you go grocery shopping, take turns with your partner asking and telling which foods and beverages each of you prefers.

Modèle:

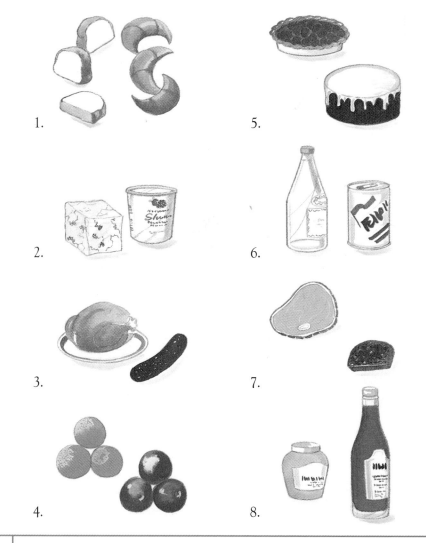

Thomas: Tu préfères le lait ou le jus d'orange?

Amina: Moi, je préfère le jus d'orange.

1.

2.

3.

4.

5.

6.

7.

8.

Combien de tranches de jambon vas-tu acheter? (Bayonne)

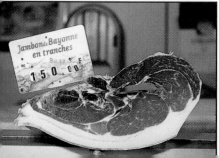

3 | Match the expression of quantity on the left with the appropriate food or beverage on the right.

1. un pot de...   a. eau minérale
2. une tranche de...   b. tomates
3. une boîte de...   c. confiture
4. une bouteille d'...   d. camembert
5. un morceau de...   e. jambon

4 | *C'est à toi!*

1. Dans ta famille, qui fait les courses?
2. Est-ce que tu aimes le fromage français?
3. Est-ce que tu préfères le bœuf, le poulet ou le poisson?
4. Est-ce que tu préfères le ketchup ou la moutarde avec les hamburgers?
5. Est-ce que tu manges beaucoup de pain?
6. Est-ce que tu manges assez de fruits et de légumes?

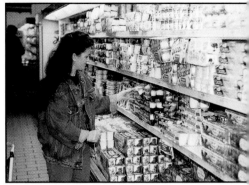

Mme Planchon fait les courses dans sa famille.

Structure

The partitive article

There are some nouns that can't be counted, such as bread, ice cream and water. We often use the words "some" or "any" before these nouns. In French, "some" or "any" is expressed by combining **de** with a singular definite article (**le, la** or **l'**). This forms the partitive article which indicates a part, a quantity or an amount of something.

Masculine before a Consonant Sound	Feminine before a Consonant Sound	Masculine or Feminine before a Vowel Sound
du café	**de la** soupe	**de l'**eau minérale

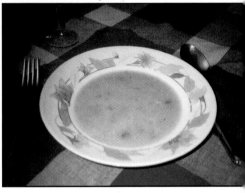

Vous voulez de la soupe?

On va acheter **du** pain.	*We're going to buy (some) bread.*
Vous avez **de la** glace?	*Do you have (any) ice cream?*
Je voudrais **de l'**eau minérale.	*I would like (some) mineral water.*

As you can see in the preceding examples, the partitive article (**du, de la** or **de l'**) is required in French but is often omitted in English.

When talking about things that can be counted, such as potatoes and carrots, "some" or "any" is expressed by **des**, the plural of the indefinite article **un(e)**. Here, too, "some" or "any" is often omitted in English.

Je veux **des** pommes de terre.	*I want (some) potatoes.*

Partitive articles are often used after certain verbs and expressions to indicate quantity: **vouloir, acheter, manger, donner, désirer, avoir, voici, voilà** and **il y a.** Partitive articles are not used after the verbs **aimer, adorer** and **préférer**, which refer to things in general.

Il y a **de la** soupe?	*Is there (any) soup?*
Benjamin adore **la** bouillabaisse.	*Benjamin loves fish soup.*

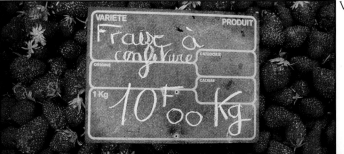

Voici des fraises. (Lyon)

Pratique

5 Your teacher always posts the school lunch menu in French. You're the first one to see this week's menu. Report what's being served in the cafeteria each day. Monday has been done for you.

Modèle:

Lundi il y a du jambon, des carottes et de la glace à la vanille.

lundi	mardi	mercredi	jeudi	vendredi
jambon	porc	hamburgers	poulet	poisson
carottes	haricots verts	frites	petits pois	pommes de terre
glace à la vanille	fromage	glace au chocolat	pain	tarte aux fraises
	raisins		yaourts	

6 You're at a family picnic. Help your young cousin get something to eat and drink by asking him if he wants some of each item on the picnic table.

Modèle:

Tu veux du poulet?

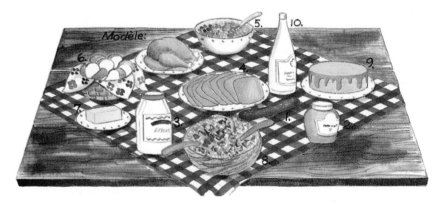

7 You're going to do your weekly grocery shopping at many stores. As you look at each one, say that you're going to buy some of what is indicated.

Modèle:

à la boucherie
Je vais acheter du bœuf.

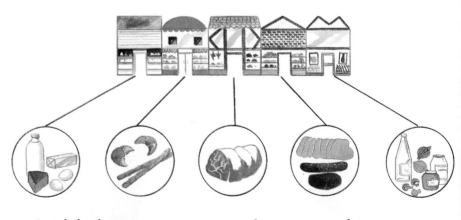

1. à la boulangerie
2. à la crémerie
3. au supermarché
4. à la charcuterie

Complete each short dialogue, using the appropriate articles from the following list.

du	de la	des	le	la	les

1. Karine: Nous pouvons manger... hamburgers ce soir, maman?
   Mme Renard: Oui. Alors, j'ai besoin d'acheter... ketchup et... moutarde au supermarché.

2. Mlle Javert: Avez-vous... tartes aux fraises aujourd'hui?
   M. Arnaud: Non, Mademoiselle, mais voici... tartes aux pommes.

3. Luc: J'adore... quiche.
   Brigitte: Moi, je préfère... omelettes.

4. M. Senghor: Voilà... petits pois.
   Khadim: Je n'aime pas... légumes verts. Il y a... carottes?

5. Amine: Tu veux... soupe?
   Florence: Oui, j'aime bien... bouillabaisse.

6. Serveur: Vous désirez... beurre?
   Mme Carnot: Oui, Monsieur. Donnez-moi aussi... confiture, s'il vous plaît.

7. Mme Vollet: Tu veux... jambon?
   Fred: Non, merci. Je n'aime pas beaucoup... porc.

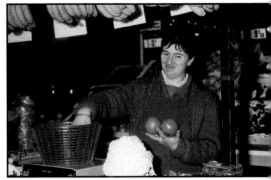
Voulez-vous manger des oranges?

The partitive article in negative sentences

You've already learned that in negative sentences, **des** becomes **de** or **d'**.

Je ne veux pas de pommes de terre.   *I don't want (any) potatoes.*

The partitive articles **du**, **de la** and **de l'** also change to **de** or **d'** in negative sentences.

On ne va pas acheter de fromage.   *We're not going to buy (any) cheese.*

Il n'y a pas d'eau minérale.   *There isn't any mineral water.*

Pratique

Olivier is a vegetarian. Tell whether or not he eats the foods that are indicated.

1. porc
2. steak
3. pâté
4. pain
5. légumes
6. fruits
7. jambon
8. camembert
9. glace
10. bœuf

Modèles:

frites
Il mange des frites.

saucisson
Il ne mange pas de saucisson.

10 With a partner, take turns asking and answering questions about what's in the refrigerator.

Modèle:

salade/beurre

Student A: Il y a de la salade?

Student B: Oui, il y a de la salade. Il y a du beurre?

Student A: Non, il n'y a pas de beurre.

1. moutarde/ketchup
2. lait/jus d'orange
3. fromage/œufs
4. eau/coca
5. pommes de terre/tomates
6. crevettes/poisson
7. pâté/bœuf

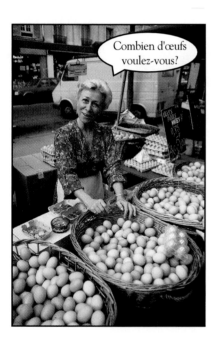

Combien d'œufs voulez-vous?

Expressions of quantity

To ask "how many" or "how much," use the expression **combien de** before a noun.

Combien de croissants est-ce que tu veux?	*How many croissants do you want?*
Il y a **combien d'**œufs dans cette omelette?	*How many eggs are there in this omelette?*

To tell "how many" or "how much," use one of these general expressions of quantity before a noun:

assez de	*enough*
beaucoup de	*a lot of, many*
(un) peu de	*(a) little, few*
trop de	*too much, too many*

Je voudrais **un peu de** fromage.	*I would like a little cheese.*
Non, merci, j'ai **assez d'**eau.	*No thanks, I have enough water.*

Certain nouns express a specific quantity. They are followed by **de** and a noun.

un morceau de	*a piece of*
une tranche de	*a slice of*
un pot de	*a jar of*
une boîte de	*a can of*
une bouteille de	*a bottle of*
un kilo de	*a kilogram of*

Donnez-moi **une tranche de** jambon.	*Give me a slice of ham.*
Je veux acheter **un kilo d'**oranges.	*I want to buy one kilo of oranges.*

Pratique

1 With a partner, take turns asking and telling how much food is left on the buffet table.

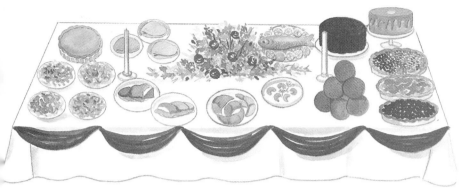

Modèle:

salades/quiches
Student A: Il y a combien
de salades?
Student B: Il y a quatre salades. Il y a combien de quiches?
Student A: Il y a une quiche.

1. omelettes/sandwichs
2. croissants/crevettes
3. poissons/oranges
4. gâteaux/tartes

2 Imagine that you work at a market and are taking inventory. Tell your boss how many of each vegetable or fruit you have using **trop de**, **assez de** or **peu de**.

Modèle:

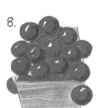

Nous avons peu de haricots verts.

1.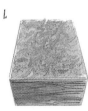

4.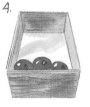

7.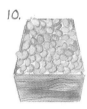

2.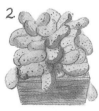

5.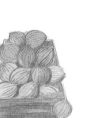

8.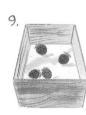

3.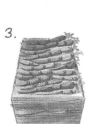

6.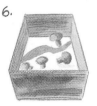

9.

10.

13 Because your neighborhood grocer has rearranged his store, you can't find any of the items you want. Ask him to give you each item you're looking for, using one of the quantities from the following list.

Modèle:

café
Donnez-moi un kilo de café, s'il vous plaît.

un pot de	une tranche de	une boîte de
un kilo de	une bouteille de	

1. pommes de terre
2. jus de pomme
3. mayonnaise
4. jambon

5. confiture
6. petits pois
7. coca
8. pâté

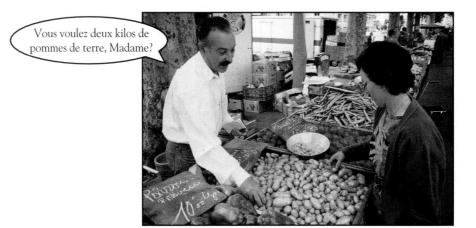

Vous voulez deux kilos de pommes de terre, Madame?

Communication

14 You and the other 20 students that you're traveling through France with have picnic lunches at noon. You are all responsible for planning the daily menus as well as shopping for the food and beverages. You and your partner signed up to plan and shop for tomorrow's picnic lunch, which will consist of a variety of sandwiches, fruits, cheeses, desserts and beverages. With your partner, make the grocery list. Be sure to include the amount of each item you need, for example, **10 tranches de jambon, 7 baguettes, 4 bouteilles de coca**, etc.

On va acheter des fruits au marché. (Paris)

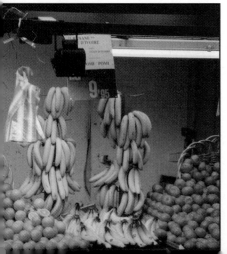

15 With your partner, categorize the food and beverages you chose in Activity 14 according to where you are going to buy them. On a separate sheet of paper, write the headings **crémerie, pâtisserie, boulangerie, charcuterie, marché** and **supermarché.** Then put each food or beverage item under the place where you're going to buy it.

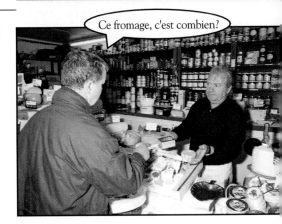

Ce fromage, c'est combien?

6 Before you go shopping for your groceries, you and your partner want to practice a typical conversation between a customer and a shopkeeper or merchant at one of the places you will visit. In the course of your conversation:

1. Greet each other.
2. The customer says that he or she wants a specific quantity of each item he or she wants to buy there.
3. The shopkeeper says that he or she either has or doesn't have each item. If the shopkeeper doesn't have a certain item, the customer should ask for something similar.
4. The customer asks for the total amount.
5. The shopkeeper tells the amount.
6. Say good-bye to each other.

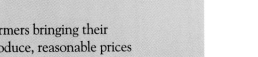

Mise au point sur... les courses

It's easy to find tasty things to eat in France, the country known throughout the world for its good food. However, it may be more difficult deciding where to shop. From open-air markets to specialty food shops, from corner grocery stores to large supermarkets, choices are everywhere.

Open-air markets generally offer the freshest food, with farmers bringing their products directly to the customer. Along with the fresh produce, reasonable prices also attract customers, who sometimes bargain to get an even better buy. Merchants set up stands of regional specialties as well as seasonal fruits, vegetables, meat, seafood and cheese. Few of the products are refrigerated, not even the meat. Often located on a public square, markets open early in the morning. Shoppers arrive with their shopping basket (**un sac à provisions**) in hand, as shopping bags are usually not provided.

Markets in other French-speaking countries reflect the local character. In Senegal, Morocco and Algeria, the smell of exotic spices, the shouts of the merchants tempting customers to their stalls and the bright colors of the merchandise itself all offer a lively shopping experience. Markets on the Caribbean islands of Guadeloupe and Martinique sell tuna, lobster, clams and other products from the sea, as well as bananas, papayas, mangoes, avocados, guavas and yams.

Specialty shops, also popular in French-speaking countries, are often family-owned and operated. Customers appreciate the individualized service they receive at these shops. To buy bakery products, such as bread and rolls, let your nose guide you to **la boulangerie.**

The pungent aroma of spices fills the air in this market in Pointe-à-Pitre. (Guadeloupe)

For special pastries, as well as cakes, pies and cookies, head for **la pâtisserie**. For most meat products, stop in **la boucherie** where the butcher will be happy to advise you on the appropriate cut of meat for a certain recipe and will cut and wrap it for you. **La boucherie chevaline**, a specialized butcher shop, offers only horse meat. For prepared pork products or delicatessen food, including salads and cold meat dishes, go to **la charcuterie**.

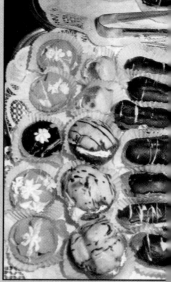

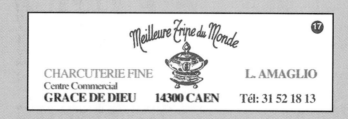

French pastries are like individual works of art.

Convenient corner grocery stores (**les épiceries**) stock many different products. Sidewalk stands in front of these stores sell fruits and vegetables to passersby.

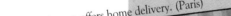

This *épicerie* even offers home delivery. (Paris)

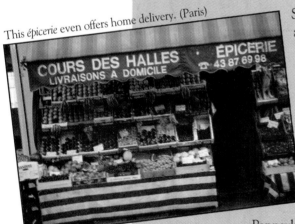

Supermarkets, like Monoprix, Uniprix and Prisunic, sell a variety of merchandise under one roof. Shoppers usually pay a small deposit to rent a shopping cart (**un chariot**) which they fill at different departments before paying at the checkout (**la caisse**). In many ways, French supermarkets resemble those in the United States. In fact, one French supermarket chain, Carrefour, has a store in Pennsylvania. Carrefour stores are so large that some supervisors wear roller skates to move quickly back and forth to help cashiers in the many checkout lines. Yet, in other ways, French supermarkets differ from their counterparts in the United States. For example, the long rows of bottled water, the large cheese section and the limited variety of cold cereal and snack food reflect traditional French shopping habits. Frozen foods (**les produits surgelés**) have become increasingly popular as busy lifestyles limit the time spent on meal preparation.

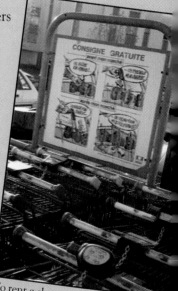

To rent a shopping cart, you insert a ten-franc coin. When you return the cart, you get your money back.

Avec Carrefour je positive! ◀ⓒ

Whether customers pick a place to shop based on fresh products, a large selection, individualized help or convenience, they will find a place to buy good food close to home.

Answer the following questions.

1. Where can a French-speaking shopper bargain for a lower price, at an open-air market, a specialty shop, a corner grocery store or a supermarket?
2. Are products at an open-air market refrigerated?
3. Where are markets often located?
4. Why do shoppers often bring their own **sac à provisions** with them?
5. How would you describe a typical African market?
6. What are three kinds of food that can be found in Caribbean markets?
7. What is the difference between a **boucherie** and a **charcuterie**?
8. What are the names of two supermarket chains in France?
9. Where do you go to pay for your purchases at a supermarket?
10. What section of a French supermarket is larger than its American counterpart? What section is smaller?

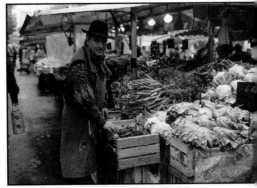

Depending on the quality of their produce, vendors may be willing to bargain at an open-air market.

Here are two grocery store receipts, one from Monoprix and the other from Prisunic. Answer the questions that follow.

```
SOLDES! SOLDES! SOLDES! SOLDES! SOLDES
! SOLDES! SOLDES! SOLDES! SOLDES! SOLD


    EVIAN BTLLE 50        2,95
    PAIN PARISIE          4,00
    CAFE SOLUBLE         21,20
    BABYBEL 200G          9,95
    FRUITERIE             5,40
 ****            TOT     43,50
    ESPECES              45,00
    A RENDRE              1,50
  5.07.98 19:21 0160103 0538 17
*** MERCI D'AVOIR CHOISI MONOPRIX! ***
MONOPRIX 99 FG ST-ANTOINE 75011 PARIS
```

```
 ***     PRISUNIC CAUMARTIN     ***

2x14,50 LAVAZZA EXPRESSO       29,00
        FRUITS ET LEGUMES      11,65
            **** TOTAL         40,65

        ESPECES               100,65

        A RENDRE               60,00

  7.08.98 14:52 1119201 0248 210
 ***    MERCI DE VOTRE VISITE    ***
```

At Monoprix:

1. What brand of mineral water did the customer buy?
2. How much did the bread cost?
3. How many grams did the Babybel cheese weigh?
4. What was the date of the customer's purchase?
5. In what city is this Monoprix?

At Prisunic:

1. How many packages of Lavazza coffee did the customer purchase?
2. How much was the customer's bill?
3. How many francs did the customer give the cashier?
4. How many francs did the customer receive in change?
5. At what time did the customer check out?

Leçon C

In this lesson you will be able to:

➤ ask for a price

➤ state prices

➤ make a complaint

➤ inquire about and compare prices

➤ negotiate

➤ choose and purchase items

les fruits (m.)

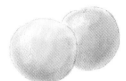

les cerises (f.)   les pêches (f.)

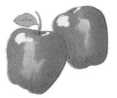

les fraises (f.)   les pommes (f.)

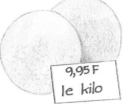
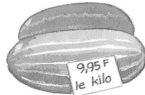

9,95 F le kilo   9,95 F le kilo

les melons (m.)   les pastèques (f.)

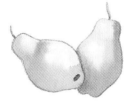
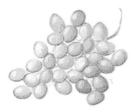

les poires (f.)   les raisins (m.)

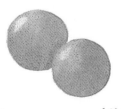
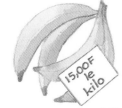

15,00 F le kilo

les oranges (f.)   les bananes (f.)

Les bananes sont plus chères que les pastèques.

Les melons sont aussi chers que les pastèques.

Les melons sont moins chers que les bananes.

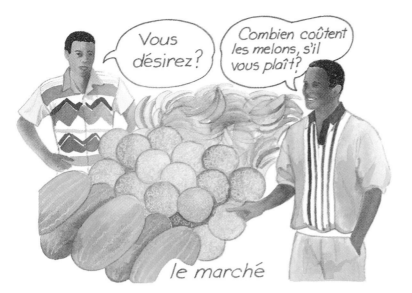

le marché

Monsieur Gagnon is shopping for fruit at an open-air market in Guadeloupe.

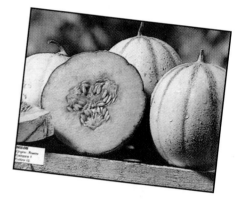

Le marchand:	Bonjour, Monsieur. Vous désirez?
M. Gagnon:	Combien coûtent les melons, s'il vous plaît?
Le marchand:	Les melons... euh... 9,95 francs le kilo.
M. Gagnon:	Mais ils sont déjà mûrs. Je trouve que c'est trop cher. Est-ce que je peux acheter deux kilos pour 15,00 francs?
Le marchand:	D'accord, Monsieur.
M. Gagnon:	Et les bananes, combien coûtent-elles?
Le marchand:	Les bananes sont plus chères que les melons. Elles coûtent 15,00 francs le kilo.
M. Gagnon:	Bon, alors je vais aussi acheter deux kilos de bananes.

The Caribbean island of Guadeloupe, made up of two main islands and some smaller ones, is one of France's overseas departments in the West Indies (**les Antilles**). Its tropical climate encourages the growth of many fruits and vegetables. Some of the island's other exports are cocoa, coffee and sugar cane.

Enquête culturelle

Bananas are one of Guadeloupe's principal fruits.

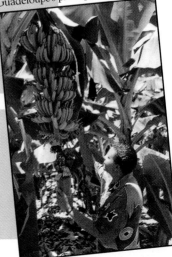

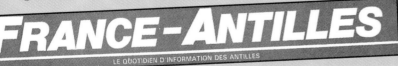
LE QUOTIDIEN D'INFORMATION DES ANTILLES

Since most people in Guadeloupe have fruit trees and gardens near their homes, they need to shop for only some of their fruits and vegetables. When they go shopping at an open-air market, they usually bargain with the merchants. Fruit prices in the Caribbean vary according to the season and the type of fruit. In the metric system, **un kilogramme (un kilo)** equals 2.2 U.S. pounds. **Une livre** (*metric pound*) is the equivalent of half a kilogram or 500 grams.

1 | *Répondez par "vrai" ou "faux" d'après le dialogue.*

1. Les melons coûtent 15,00 francs le kilo.
2. Monsieur Gagnon trouve que les melons sont trop chers.
3. Monsieur Gagnon peut acheter deux kilos de melons pour 15,00 francs.
4. Les bananes sont moins chères que les melons.
5. Monsieur Gagnon va acheter trois kilos de bananes.
6. Les bananes vont coûter 30,00 francs.

2 | Write the names in French of two products you could buy at each of the following places. **La boulangerie** has been done for you.

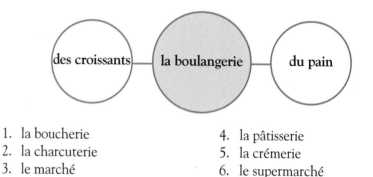

des croissants — la boulangerie — du pain

1. la boucherie
2. la charcuterie
3. le marché
4. la pâtisserie
5. la crémerie
6. le supermarché

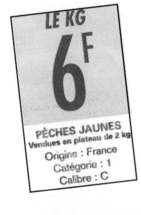

3 | What would you say in French in the following situations?

1. You want to know the price of the peaches.
2. You want to know how much the melons cost per kilogram.
3. You want to know if the bananas are more expensive than the melons.
4. The merchant has just told you that the bananas are not too ripe. You insist that they are too ripe.
5. You tell the merchant that these strawberries are too expensive.
6. You want to know if you can buy two kilograms of pears for 20 francs.

4 | *C'est à toi!*

1. Quels fruits aimes-tu?
2. Est-ce que tu préfères les bananes ou les pêches?
3. Est-ce que tu manges beaucoup de fruits?
4. Quel(s) fruit(s) vas-tu manger aujourd'hui?
5. Est-ce que ta famille achète des fruits au supermarché ou au marché?
6. Après le repas, est-ce que tu manges un fruit ou un dessert?

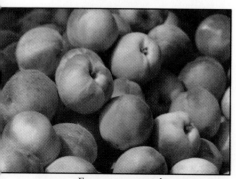

Est-ce que ces pêches sont mûres?

Structure

Comparative of adjectives

To compare people and things in French, use the following constructions:

plus (*more*)	+	adjective	+	**que** (*than*)	
moins (*less*)	+	adjective	+	**que** (*than*)	
aussi (*as*)	+	adjective	+	**que** (*as*)	

In the following examples, note how the adjective agrees with the first noun in the comparison.

La banane est plus mûre que la pêche.
The banana is riper than the peach.

Les raisins sont moins chers que les cerises.
Grapes are less expensive than cherries.

Le marchand est aussi grand qu'Abdou.
The merchant is as tall as Abdou.

Les tomates sont moins chères que les haricots verts. (Lyon)

Pratique

Compare the prices of school supplies at Monoprix with those at the Papeterie Roche. Tell whether they are more expensive, less expensive or as expensive.

	Monoprix	**Papeterie Roche**
crayons	2,95F	3,50F
stylos	14,90F	14,90F
trousses	18,00F	22,00F
cahiers	6,90F	4,90F
calendriers	39,00F	54,95F
dictionnaires	88,00F	88,00F
cartes	25,95F	21,00F

Modèle:

Les crayons à Monoprix sont moins chers que les crayons à la Papeterie Roche.

1. Les stylos à Monoprix sont... les stylos à la Papeterie Roche.
2. Les trousses à Monoprix sont... les trousses à la Papeterie Roche.
3. Les cahiers à Monoprix sont... les cahiers à la Papeterie Roche.
4. Les calendriers à Monoprix sont... les calendriers à la Papeterie Roche.
5. Les dictionnaires à Monoprix sont... les dictionnaires à la Papeterie Roche.
6. Les cartes à Monoprix sont... les cartes à la Papeterie Roche.

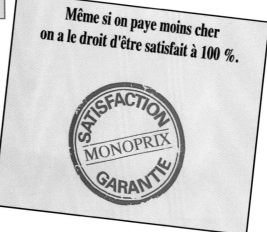

Même si on paye moins cher on a le droit d'être satisfait à 100 %.

SATISFACTION
MONOPRIX
GARANTIE

6 | Tell whether each of Robert's friends is taller, as tall as or shorter than he is. Use a form of the adjective **grand** in each of your comparisons.

Modèle:

Martine est moins grande
que Robert.

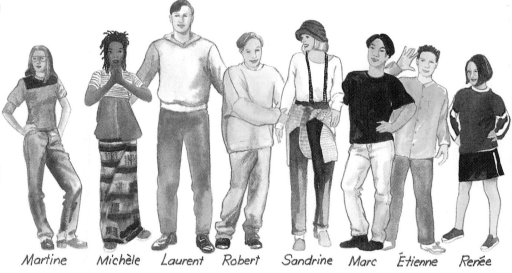

Martine   Michèle   Laurent   Robert   Sandrine   Marc   Étienne   Renée

7 | As you walk through the grocery store, comment on how the first items you see compare with the second ones. Use the appropriate form of the indicated adjective in each of your comparisons.

Modèle:

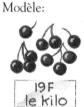

cher
Les cerises sont aussi chères que
les fraises.

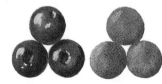

1. petit

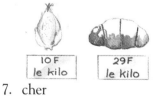

5. mûr

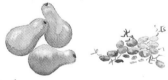

2. beau

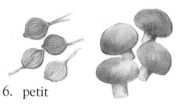

6. petit

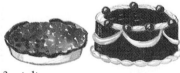

3. joli

7. cher

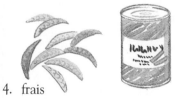

4. frais

Communication

You're planning a party for ten of your friends. Before you go grocery shopping, look at the supermarket ads that follow. Realizing that your friends don't all like to eat the same things and that you have only 150 francs to spend, write your shopping list. Be sure to specify the quantity of each item you plan to buy and its price. Then add up the total.

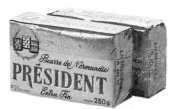

BEURRE PRESIDENT,
doux ou 1/2 sel,
le lot de 2 x 250 gr,
soit le kg : 29 F 40

14^F**70**
Le lot

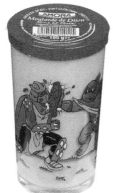

MOUTARDE DE DIJON
Amora
le verre T.V. de 195 g
soit le kg : 20.26 F

3^{F95}

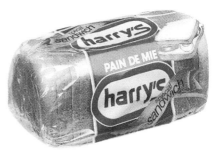

PAIN DE MIE SPECIAL SANDWICH
les 300 g soit le kg : 16.50 F

4^{F95}

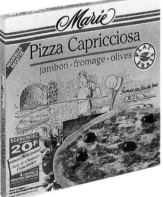

PIZZA CAPRICCIOSA
Marie
la pièce de 380 g soit le kg : 49.74 F

18^{F90}

PECHES JAUNES
Cal. A - France
le kg

7^{F95}

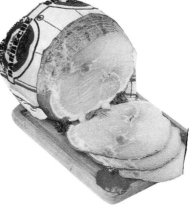

JAMBON * SUPERIEUR BARBECUE A.C.
le kg

39^{F90}

YAOURTS FRUITS
Montorval
les 8×125 g - 1 kg

9^{F95}

9 With a partner, play the roles of a person in charge of bringing a fruit salad to a family reunion and a merchant at an open-air market. The customer needs to buy enough of five kinds of fruits to make a salad for 25 people. In the course of your conversation:

1. The customer says that he or she would like some of five kinds of fruits and asks the prices.
2. The merchant tells the prices.
3. The customer comments that at least one of the fruits is too expensive.
4. The merchant gives at least one reason why that fruit is a good buy.
5. The customer complains about at least one of the fruits, saying that it is too ripe.
6. The merchant offers the customer a better price for that fruit.
7. The customer tells what he or she is going to buy and the quantity of each item.
8. The merchant totals the bill and the customer pays.

Combien coûtent les raisins?

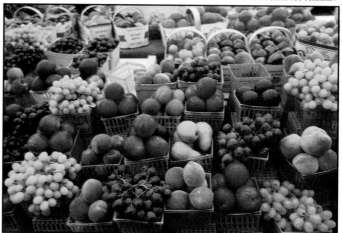

Sur la bonne piste

When you read in French, your instinct probably tells you to translate all the words into English. Because you have been reading in English since you were very young, and because English has helped you understand many things, translation may appear to be a very appealing option. However, there is one big problem with translating a French reading into English: you have to know what every French word means! Translating while you read is like riding a bicycle with training wheels while competing in the **Tour de France**—you won't tip over or crash, but you'll never win the race. Right now it may seem risky to let your mind's bicycle speed down new terrain by thinking in French. You may get the urge to put on those training wheels and translate what you read. But eventually you'll discover that thinking in French, not translating into English, is the fastest, most comfortable and most effective way to read in French.

Try to think in French as you read the following salad recipe three times. Resist the temptation to translate it word for word into English. The information in the recipe will become clearer each time you read it.

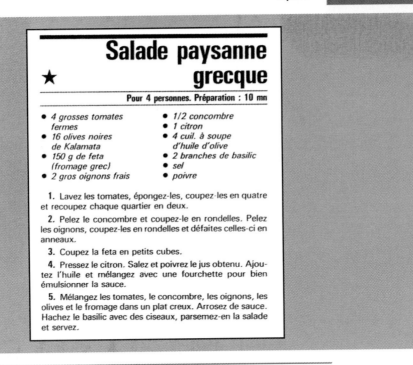

Salade paysanne grecque

★

Pour 4 personnes. Préparation : 10 mn

- 4 grosses tomates fermes
- 16 olives noires de Kalamata
- 150 g de feta (fromage grec)
- 2 gros oignons frais
- 1/2 concombre
- 1 citron
- 4 cuil. à soupe d'huile d'olive
- 2 branches de basilic
- sel
- poivre

1. Lavez les tomates, épongez-les, coupez-les en quatre et recoupez chaque quartier en deux.

2. Pelez le concombre et coupez-le en rondelles. Pelez les oignons, coupez-les en rondelles et défaites celles-ci en anneaux.

3. Coupez la feta en petits cubes.

4. Pressez le citron. Salez et poivrez le jus obtenu. Ajoutez l'huile et mélangez avec une fourchette pour bien émulsionner la sauce.

5. Mélangez les tomates, le concombre, les oignons, les olives et le fromage dans un plat creux. Arrosez de sauce. Hachez le basilic avec des ciseaux, parsemez-en la salade et servez.

Answer the following questions.

1. How long does it take to make this salad?
2. Should you buy green or black olives?
3. Do you need French cheese?
4. Which ingredients could you buy at a fruit and vegetable market? Which could you buy at a dairy store?
5. After you wash and dry the tomatoes, how should you cut them?
6. Should you grate the cheese?
7. What part of the lemon do you use?
8. Does this salad appeal to you? Why or why not?

Nathalie et Raoul

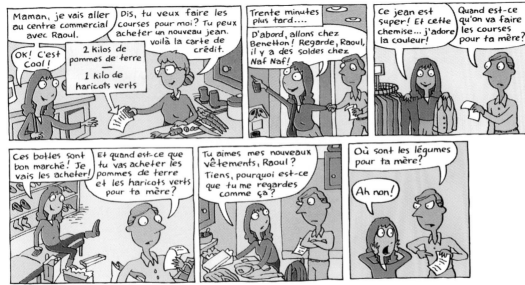

C'est à moi!

Now that you have completed this unit, take a look at what you should be able to do in French. Can you do all of these tasks?

➤ I can ask for and give information about what someone can and wants to do.

➤ I can tell what I like.

➤ I can agree with someone.

➤ I can point out specific things.

➤ I can ask for permission.

➤ I can ask for, state and compare prices.

➤ I can make a complaint.

➤ I can insist on something.

➤ I can negotiate prices.

➤ I can choose and purchase various things.

Here is a brief checkup to see how much you understand about French culture. Decide if each statement is **vrai** or **faux**.

1. Marseille is France's oldest city and largest seaport.
2. Some well-known French foods are named after the provinces they come from: **quiche lorraine** comes from Lorraine and **bœuf bourguignon** is from Burgundy.
3. Regional specialties, such as **bouillabaisse** and **pâté de foie gras**, can be purchased in French grocery stores and ordered in restaurants.
4. French grocery stores rarely stock reduced-calorie or low-fat products since the French are well known for their heavy sauces and rich pastries.
5. The long, thin loaf of bread with the crisp crust that we often call "French bread" is called a **croissant** in French.
6. Camembert, Brie and Roquefort are three of the more than 300 different kinds of yogurt produced in France.

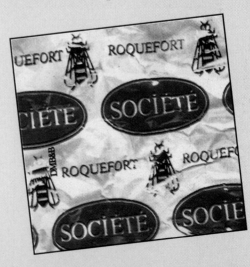

7. French teenagers drink as much milk as American teens do.
8. French people now do all of their grocery shopping in large supermarkets instead of going to small shops and markets.

Since French people generally drink more mineral water than Americans, they often buy enough for one or two weeks.

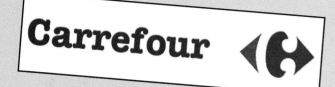

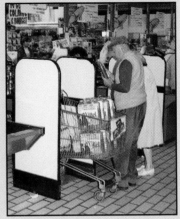

9. French supermarkets sell more bottled water and usually have a smaller variety of cold cereal than American supermarkets.
10. Because of its climate, Guadeloupe must buy most of its fresh fruits and vegetables from France.

Communication orale

With a partner, play the roles of a student who is planning to have a party to celebrate his or her friend's birthday and a grocer at the corner store. The student is going to order by phone several trays of party food and some beverages. During the course of your phone conversation, turn away from each other and talk as though you are on the phone.

1. The student dials the number of the grocery store, saying the numbers out loud in pairs.
2. The grocer answers the phone by saying hello and giving the name of the store.
3. The student identifies himself or herself and explains that he or she needs to buy some meat and cheese, fruits and vegetables, desserts and beverages for a party.
4. The grocer asks what day the party is.
5. The student gives the date of the party and then asks for the prices of specific items.
6. The grocer gives the prices.
7. The student orders the amount of the kinds of meat and cheese, fruits and vegetables, desserts and beverages that he or she wants.
8. The grocer gives the price of each item and then gives the total.
9. The student thanks the grocer and both say good-bye.

Communication écrite

Imagine that you are going to give a party to celebrate a special event. The first step in getting ready for your party is to design and write an invitation to send to your guests. On the invitation say that you're having a party and what special event you're celebrating. Be sure to mention what day and where the party is and at what time. Also include the foods and beverages you'll be serving. Remember to add RSVP and your name and phone number at the end of the invitation.

Communication active

To ask for information, use:

Qu'est-ce que tu veux manger ce soir?   *What do you want to eat tonight?*

Tu peux faire une bouillabaisse?   *Can you make fish soup?*

To give information, use:

Il veut toujours un fruit après le repas.   *He always wants (a piece of) fruit after a meal.*

Nous pouvons aussi aller à la charcuterie.   *We can also go to the delicatessen.*

To say what you like, use:

Moi, j'aime aussi le pâté.   *Me, I like pâté, too.*

To agree with someone, use:

OK.   *OK.*

Ouais.   *Yeah.*

To identify objects, use:

Je vais acheter **ces** tomates et **cet** oignon pour la soupe.   *I'm going to buy these tomatoes and this onion for the soup.*

To ask for permission, use:

Nous pouvons acheter des oranges aussi?   *Can we buy oranges, too?*

To ask for a price, use:

Combien coûte la pastèque?   *How much does the watermelon cost?*

Combien coûtent les melons?   *How much do the melons cost?*

Combien coûtent ces haricots verts? (Lyon)

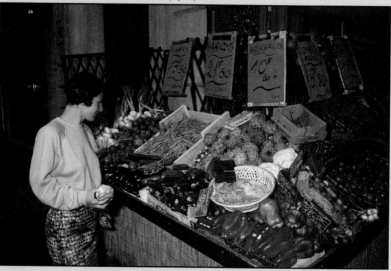

To state prices, use:

Ils/Elles coûtent 15,00 **francs** le kilo.   *They cost 15 francs per kilo.*

To compare prices, use:

Le fromage est **plus cher que** le beurre.   *Cheese is more expensive than butter.*

Les raisins sont **aussi chers que** les pastèques.   *Grapes are as expensive as watermelons.*

Les pommes sont **moins chères que** les cerises.   *Apples are less expensive than cherries.*

To make a complaint, use:

Les melons sont **déjà mûrs**.   *The melons are already ripe.*

Je trouve que c'est trop cher.   *I think it's too expensive.*

Les cerises sont déjà mûres.

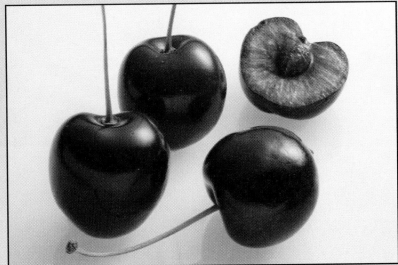

To insist on something, use:

Si!   *Yes!*

To negotiate a price, use:

Est-ce que je peux acheter deux kilos de melons **pour 15,00 francs?**   *May I buy two kilos of melons for 15 francs?*

To choose and purchase items, use:

Je vais acheter trois kilos de bananes.   *I am going to buy three kilos of bananas.*

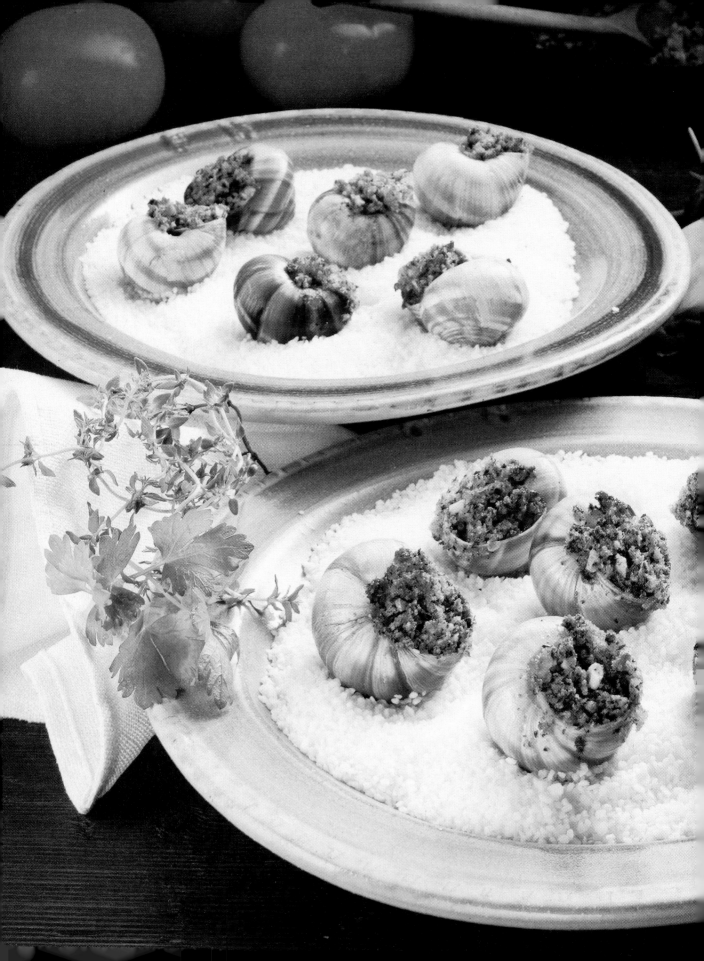

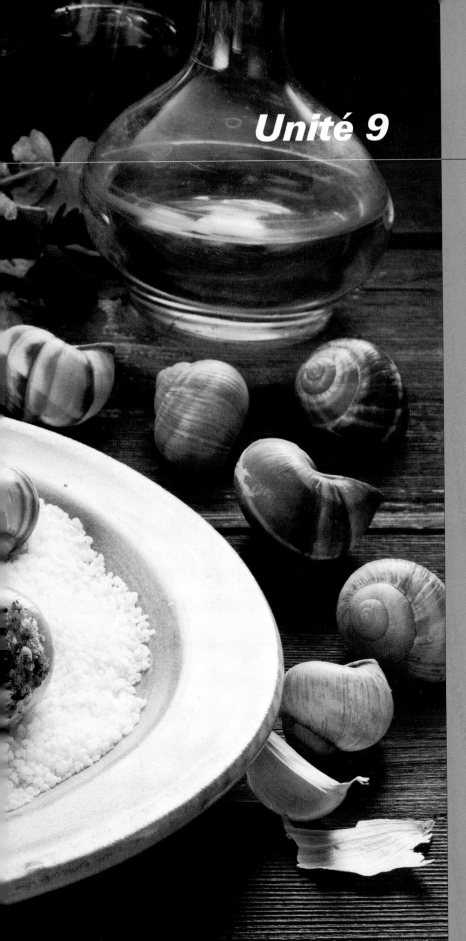

Unité 9

À la maison

In this unit you will be able to:

➤ invite

➤ accept and refuse an invitation

➤ greet someone

➤ greet guests

➤ introduce someone else

➤ offer and accept a gift

➤ identify objects

➤ describe daily routines

➤ tell location

➤ express intentions

➤ agree and disagree

➤ offer food and beverages

➤ excuse yourself

Leçon A

In this lesson you will be able to:

➤ invite

➤ identify objects

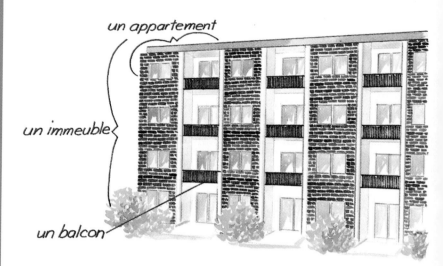

un appartement

un immeuble

un balcon

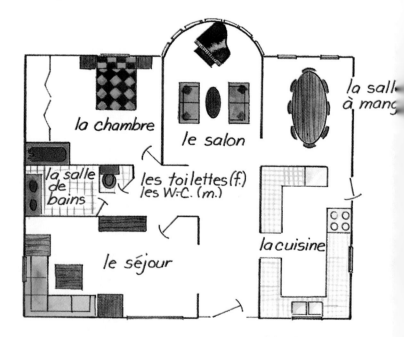

la chambre

le salon

la salle à manger

les toilettes (f.)
les W.-C. (m.)

la salle de bains

la cuisine

le séjour

les pièces (f.)

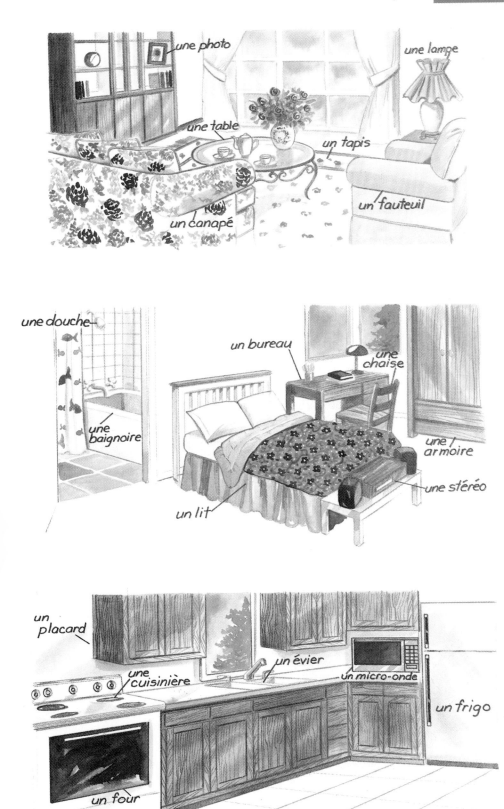

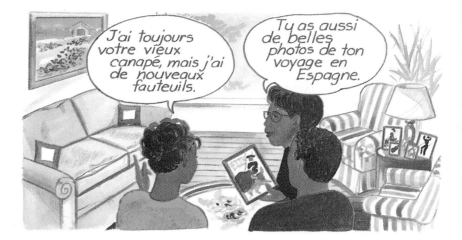

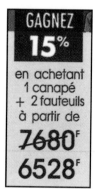

GAGNEZ
15%
en achetant
1 canapé
+ 2 fauteuils
à partir de
7680^F
6528^F

Nadine Mairet is giving her parents a tour of her new apartment.

Nadine: Vous voulez faire le tour de mon appartement maintenant? Voici le salon. J'ai toujours votre vieux canapé, mais j'ai de nouveaux fauteuils.

Mme Mairet: Tu as aussi de belles photos de ton voyage en Espagne.

Nadine: Et voici la cuisine. J'ai même un micro-onde.

M. Mairet: Avec la chambre, la salle de bains et les W.-C., cet appartement est assez grand. Tu aimes bien habiter ici?

Nadine: Oui, pour moi, ça va bien.

🔍 *Enquête culturelle*

It usually costs more to live in **le centre-ville** (*downtown*) of a French city than in **la banlieue** (*suburbs*). Many people reside in apartment buildings which surround **une cour** (*central courtyard*). They frequently purchase, rather than rent, their apartments. Single people often prefer living in a studio apartment, consisting of

PROCHE CENTRE VILLE
maison de 8 pièces, salon, sc
à manger, séjour de famille,
cuisine, 5 chambres, 2 bains,
jardin agréable
PRIX : 1 580 000 F

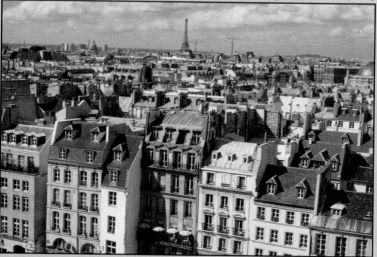

Living in *le centre-ville* usually costs more than living in *la banlieue*. (Paris)

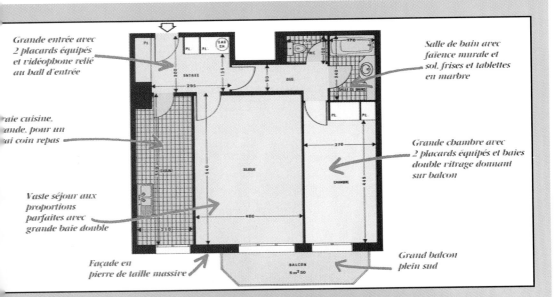

Grande entrée avec
2 placards équipés
et vidéophone relié
au hall d'entrée

...raie cuisine.
...ande. pour un
...ai coin repas

Vaste séjour aux
proportions
parfaites avec
grande baie double

Façade en
pierre de taille massive

Salle de bain avec
faïence murale et
sol. frises et tablettes
en marbre

Grande chambre avec
2 placards équipés et baies
double vitrage donnant
sur balcon

Grand balcon
plein sud

only a kitchenette, a main room and a bathroom. Even for a small studio apartment in the heart of a large city, the cost is high since rent is based on the apartment's location, not on its facilities.

Apartment buildings are protected from both noise and intruders by an outer wall. To enter the buildings, residents often use a numbered security system rather than a key. They punch in a code number in a box which is installed near the front door.

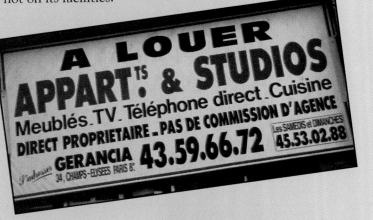

Although some bedrooms have closets, many French people keep their clothes in a tall, free-standing piece of furniture called **une armoire**.

What do French teens have in their bedrooms? According to a recent survey, 100% have a desk and a lamp. Over 80% own a stereo, stuffed animals, books and posters. About 40% have a TV and video games. One in five French teens has a computer.

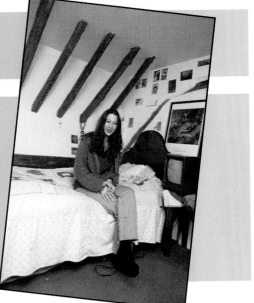

Annick, like almost half of all French teens, has a TV in her bedroom.

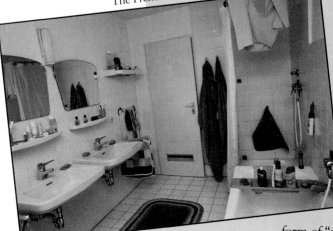

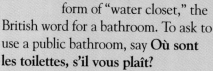

The French *salle de bains* doesn't have a toilet.

Most French houses and apartments have two separate bathrooms. **La salle de bains** contains a bathtub, a sink, a bidet and a vanity. **Un bidet** is a small, toilet-shaped tub where you sit to take a sponge bath. Hand-operated showers are often attached to the bathtub faucet. Instead of a washcloth, people use **un gant de toilette** (*bath mitt*). The second bathroom, **les W.-C.**, is smaller and has only a toilet and a sink. **W.-C.** (often pronounced "vay-say") is the abbreviated form of "water closet," the British word for a bathroom. To ask to use a public bathroom, say **Où sont les toilettes, s'il vous plaît?**

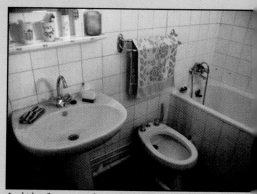

Le bidet (between the sink and the tub) is used for personal hygiene.

When counting the rooms of a house or an apartment, the French do not include the bathroom.

In public places a variety of words may appear on restroom doors. The word **Hommes** or **Messieurs** or a picture of a man designates the men's restroom; the word **Femmes** or **Dames** or a picture of a woman shows which restroom is for women. You may also see the word **Toilettes** or **W.-C.**, which refers to facilities that may be used by either sex.

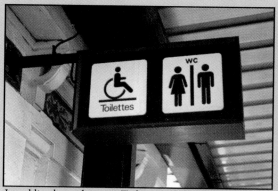

In public places the signs *Toilettes* and *W.-C.* indicate the restrooms.

MORIZET
agréable 3 pièces, 80 m2 environ, 2ème étage dans immeuble ravalé, entrée spacieuse, grand séjour ouvert sur balcon, 2 belles chambres, cuisine équipée, parking sous-sol
PRIX : 1 600 000 F

1 | *Répondez en français.*

1. Qui fait le tour de l'appartement de Nadine?
2. Où est-ce que le tour commence?
3. Qu'est-ce qu'il y a dans le salon?
4. Est-ce que Nadine a aussi des photos de son voyage en Allemagne?
5. Qu'est-ce qu'il y a dans la cuisine de Nadine?
6. Combien de pièces est-ce qu'il y a dans l'appartement?
7. Est-ce que l'appartement est petit?
8. Est-ce que Nadine aime son appartement?

Trouvez dans la liste suivante le mot qui complète correctement chaque phrase.

cuisine	séjour
chambre	photos
immeuble	fauteuils
magnétoscope	four
frigo	lampe

1. Nadine habite dans un appartement. Son appartement est dans un....
2. Il y a quatre... dans la pièce.
3. On trouve un micro-onde dans la....
4. Est-ce qu'il y a une vidéocassette dans le...?

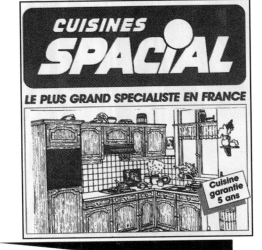

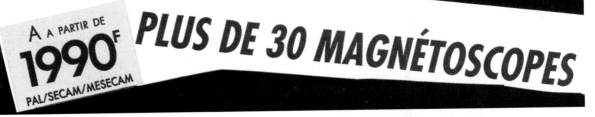

5. On regarde la télé au....
6. J'ai un grand lit dans ma....
7. Nous avons beaucoup de... de notre voyage en Italie.
8. J'aime lire, mais j'ai besoin d'une....
9. Maman fait un gâteau. Le gâteau est maintenant dans le....
10. Pierre veut du lait. Le lait est dans le....

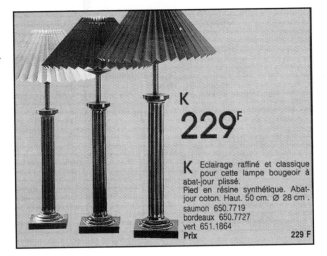

3 | *C'est à toi!*

1. Est-ce que tu habites dans un appartement?
2. Qu'est-ce qu'il y a dans ton salon?
3. Dans quelle pièce est-ce que tu regardes la télé?
4. Où est-ce que ta famille mange?
5. Est-ce que ta famille a un micro-onde?
6. De quelle couleur est ta chambre?
7. Est-ce que tu as des affiches dans ta chambre?
8. Est-ce que tu as un bureau dans ta chambre?

La famille Dufresne mange dans leur cuisine.

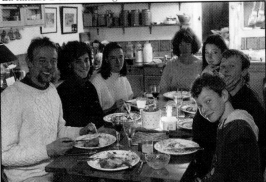

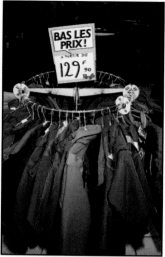

Voilà de nouveaux anoraks.
(Bayonne)

Structure

De + plural adjectives

Des becomes **de** before most plural adjectives that precede a noun.

> Tu as toujours **de** vieilles chaises?   *Do you still have (some) old chairs?*
>
> Oui, mais j'ai **de** nouvelles lampes.   *Yes, but I have (some) new lamps.*

When an adjective that precedes a noun is an inseparable part of that noun, **des** does not become **de** or **d'**.

> Je voudrais **des** petits pois.   *I would like (some) peas.*

Remember to use **des** before a noun whose plural adjective comes afterward.

> On va acheter **des** légumes frais.   *We're going to buy (some) fresh vegetables.*

Pratique

4   Last week the Ramos family went shopping for new furniture. As each delivery truck arrives at their house, tell what new things they have.

Modèle:

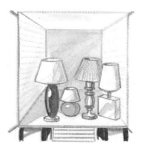

Les Ramos ont de nouvelles lampes.

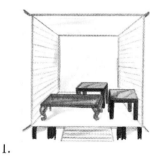

1.

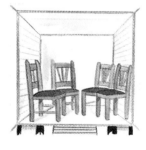

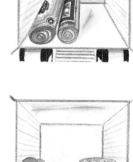

2.

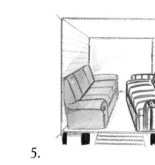

3.

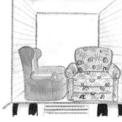

4.

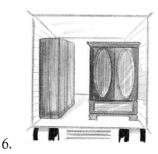

5.

6.

5 Nadine likes old things, and her favorite color is green. Tell what old or green items there are in her apartment.

Modèle:

Dans le salon il y a de vieux fauteuils, de vieux tapis et des tables vertes.

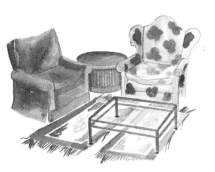
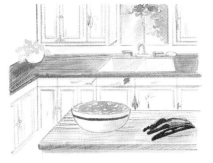

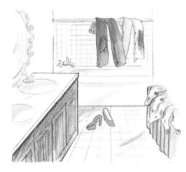
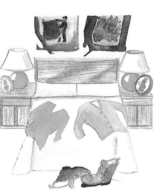

1. Dans la salle de bains il y a....
2. Dans la cuisine il y a....
3. Dans la chambre il y a....

Communication

6 Charles is going to move into his first apartment and is trying to find some inexpensive furniture. He made a list of everything he needs (on the left). His mother made a list of the things the family has but no longer needs (on the right). With a partner, play the roles of Charles and his mother. Charles tells his mother each item he needs and asks for it. Then his mother tells him whether or not he can have it.

Modèles:

Charles: J'ai besoin d'un fauteuil. Est-ce qu'on a un fauteuil?
Maman: Oui, tu peux avoir le fauteuil noir.

Charles: J'ai besoin d'une chaise. Est-ce qu'on a une chaise?
Maman: Non, on n'a pas de chaise.

J'ai besoin d'....

un fauteuil
une chaise
un lit
une stéréo
une table
un tapis
un micro-onde
un canapé
une lampe
un magnétoscope

On a....

un fauteuil noir
un bureau
une petite table
une télé
un frigo
une lampe
une vieille armoire

7 After you and your partner have completed Activity 6, make a list of the items that Charles needs to buy, based on what his family can't furnish.

8 Imagine that you and a friend are going to move into your own apartment. You've saved up 6500 francs to spend on furniture. The store where you are going to shop is advertising certain specials. Using the store's ads, make a list of each item you are going to purchase along with its price. Then total your purchases, remembering not to exceed your limit.

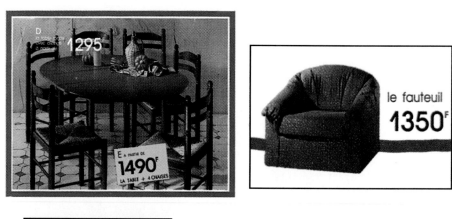

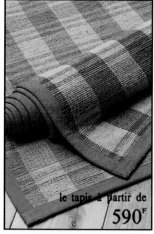

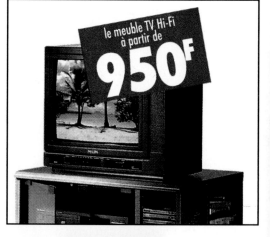

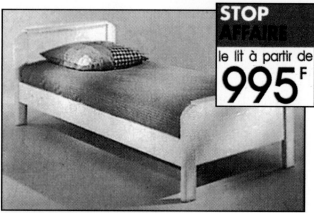

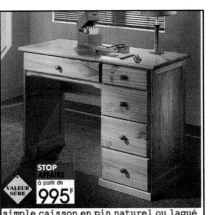

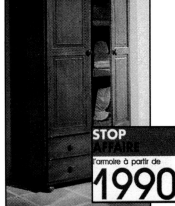

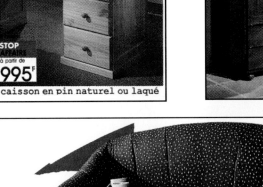

simple caisson en pin naturel ou laqué

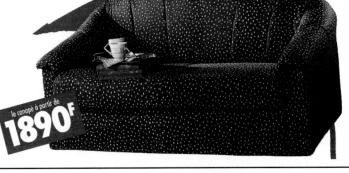

The sound [ə]

The vowel **e** without an accent mark is pronounced [ə] when it comes at the end of a one-syllable word, such as **de, je** or **le**.

It is also pronounced [ə] when it appears at the end of the first syllable in a word of more than one syllable. Say each of these words:

fenêtre	cerise
premier	devant
crevette	besoin

Silent "e"

The vowel **e** without an accent mark is usually silent, that is, unpronounced, when it comes at the end of a word containing more than two letters, such as **pièce, salle** or **immeuble**.

It is also silent when it appears after the first syllable of certain words and before the last one. Say each of these words:

maintenant	médecin
acheter	vêtements
omelette	boucherie

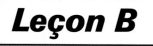

Leçon B

In this lesson you will be able to:

➤ invite

➤ accept and refuse an invitation

➤ greet someone

➤ greet guests

➤ introduce someone else

➤ offer and accept a gift

➤ excuse yourself

➤ offer food and beverages

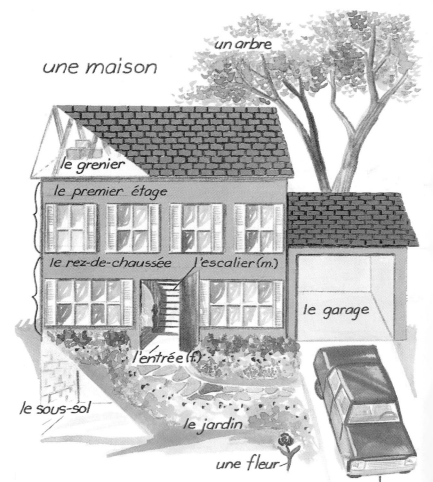

une maison

un arbre

le grenier

le premier étage

le rez-de-chaussée   l'escalier (m.)

le garage

l'entrée (f.)

le sous-sol

le jardin

une fleur

la voiture

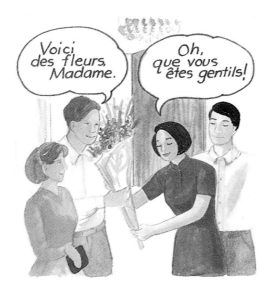

Monsieur and Madame Poitras have invited their new neighbors, Monsieur and Madame Giraud, to their home for dinner.

Mme Poitras: **Bonsoir, Monsieur. Bonsoir, Madame. Bienvenue! Je vous présente mon mari, Raymond. Raymond, Anne-Marie et Étienne Giraud.**

M. Giraud: **Enchanté. Bonsoir, Monsieur. Voici des fleurs, Madame.**

Mme Poitras: **Oh, que vous êtes gentils! Raymond, prends le vase rouge, s'il te plaît. Il est sur la table.**

M. Poitras: **Bien sûr. Entrez donc, allons au salon.**

Mme Poitras: **Euh..., pardon, j'ai encore quelques petites choses à faire dans la cuisine. Prenez des chips. Vous voulez un jus de fruit?**

Mme Giraud: **Oui, je veux bien.**

Enquête culturelle

Every region of France has its unique style of house that is constructed with building materials from that region. In the northern part of the country, many houses have stone or brick exteriors. In Normandy, dark wooden trim commonly decorates white stucco dwellings with sloped roofs. In Brittany, even contemporary houses sometimes have thatched roofs that resemble those of

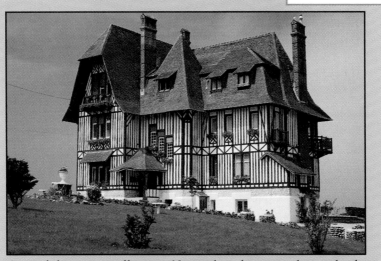

A typical characteristic of houses in Normandy is white stucco decorated with dark wooden trim in an "X" shape.

homes from the past. In the south of France, awnings as well as flat roofs made of reddish orange tiles protect houses from the hot sun. Two especially distinctive French styles of houses are the **chalet alpin**, a cottage in the Alps, and the **mas provençal,** a picturesque farmhouse in the Provence region of southern France.

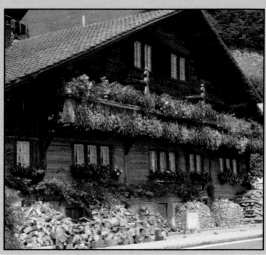

Alpine chalets have a distinctive shape and a long, flower-covered balcony.

The first or ground floor of a building in French-speaking countries is called **le rez-de-chaussée.** The floor directly above is **le premier étage,** and the next floor is **le deuxième étage.** Beneath **le rez-de-chaussée,** families store wine and other beverages and food items in **la cave** (*cellar*).

More French people own vacation homes than any other national group. Often this home is located in the region of the country where the family comes from originally. Many of these homes have been passed down from generation to generation. Other people buy vacation apartments on one of the French coasts. Many city dwellers tolerate holiday and weekend traffic jams to spend time at their vacation home.

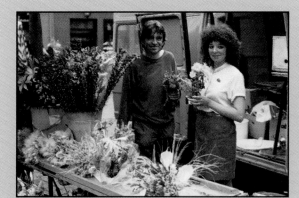

It's appropriate to take a bouquet of cut flowers when you're invited to a French home for dinner.

You've already learned that when you are invited to someone's home for a meal in a French-speaking country, you should bring a small gift for your hosts. Most guests bring flowers or have them sent the following day. However, don't choose chrysanthemums! They are appropriate only at funerals.

In French-speaking countries, **les apéros** is a general term used to refer to many kinds of small crackers (**les biscuits salés**), chips (**les chips**) and other snacks which are served to guests before a meal. Small quantities of these snacks are put in little bowls or on tiny plates for guests to munch on.

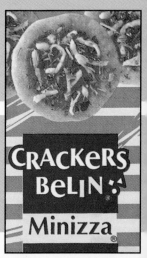

CRACKERS BELIN
Minizza

1 Reread the conversation between the Poitras and Giraud families. Then answer the following questions, telling who does what.

    1. Qui est à la porte des Poitras?

    2. Qui présente son mari?

    3. Qui a des fleurs pour M. et Mme Poitras?

    4. Qui est gentil?

    5. Qui va chercher le vase rouge?

    6. Qui invite M. et Mme Giraud à aller au salon?

    7. Qui a quelques petites choses à faire dans la cuisine?

    8. Qui veut un jus de fruit?

2 Tell exactly where certain people or things are in or around the house, depending on what's happening.

    1. M. Bouchard présente M. Duval à sa femme.

    2. Le petit oiseau est dans l'arbre.

    3. Hervé écoute un CD.

    4. La famille mange ensemble.

    5. Nathalie trouve les vieux vêtements de sa grand-mère.

    6. Les enfants regardent la télé.

    7. Le chat est sous la voiture.

Modèle:

Denise a faim.

Denise est dans la cuisine.

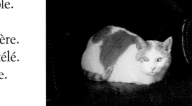

Les chats sont sur le fauteuil. Donc, ils sont dans le salon.

3 *C'est à toi!*

    1. Est-ce que tu habites dans une maison ou dans un appartement?

    2. Quelles pièces est-ce qu'il y a dans ta maison ou ton appartement?

    3. Combien de chambres est-ce qu'il y a dans ta maison ou ton appartement?

    4. Est-ce que ta maison ou ton appartement a un balcon?

    5. Est-ce que ta maison ou ton appartement a un garage?

    6. Est-ce que tu as une voiture?

    7. À qui est-ce que tu donnes des fleurs?

    8. Est-ce que tu manges souvent des chips?

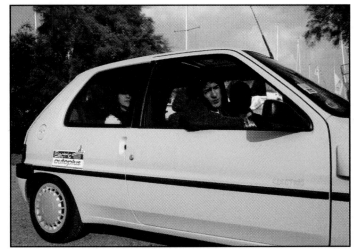

La famille Aknouch a une nouvelle voiture. (La Rochelle)

Structure

Present tense of the irregular verb *prendre*

The verb **prendre** (*to take*) is irregular. Note that it can also mean "to have" when referring to something to eat or drink.

prendre			
je	**prends**	Je **prends** la voiture.	*I'm taking the car.*
tu	**prends**	Tu **prends** des photos?	*Are you taking (some) pictures?*
il/elle/on	**prend**	Il **prend** le vase rouge.	*He takes the red vase.*
nous	**prenons**	Nous **prenons** des chips.	*We're having (some) snacks.*
vous	**prenez**	Qu'est-ce que vous **prenez**?	*What are you having?*
ils/elles	**prennent**	Ils **prennent** du café.	*They're having (some) coffee.*

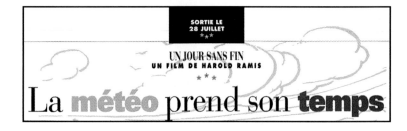

SORTIE LE 28 JUILLET ★★★
UN JOUR SANS FIN
UN FILM DE HAROLD RAMIS
★ ★ ★
La **météo** prend son **temps**

The **d** is pronounced [t] in the inverted forms of **il/elle/on:**
Prend-on une glace?
    [t]

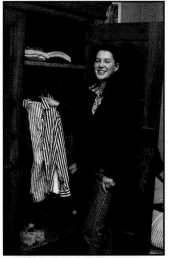

Claire prend une chemise de son armoire. (Strasbourg)

Pratique

4 | At Ariane and Raoul's wedding dinner, the guests have a choice of fish or beef. Tell what the people at your table are having to eat.

Modèles:

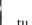

Florence
Florence prend du poisson.

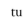

Benjamin
Benjamin prend du bœuf.

1. 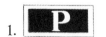 Clémence

2. je

3. Abdou

4. Florence et moi

5.  Cécile et Sébastien

6. tu

7. Alexandre et Karine

8. Benjamin et toi

5 You and your relatives are meeting in La Rochelle for a family reunion. Tell whether or not certain people are driving there, based on what you see.

Modèles:

ma tante Élise
Ma tante Élise prend la voiture.

1. ma belle-sœur

4. mon oncle Raoul

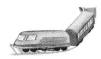

2. ma grand-mère et mon grand-père

5. ma sœur et sa fille

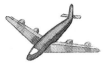

mon cousin Laurent et sa femme
Mon cousin Laurent et sa femme ne prennent pas la voiture.

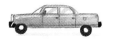

3. je

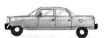

6. mon père, ma belle-mère et moi

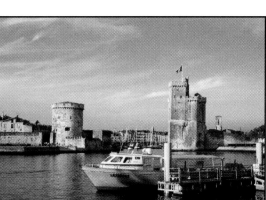

La Rochelle, en Charente-Maritime, est un port sur l'Atlantique.

6 With a partner, play the roles of a server in a restaurant and a customer who has ordered a meal at a fixed price. Student A, the server, asks Student B, the customer, what he or she wants to have for each course.

Modèle:

Student A: Vous prenez le pâté ou la salade de tomates?

Student B: Je prends la salade de tomates.

Menu à 100 francs

pâté ou salade de tomates
porc ou bœuf
petits pois ou carottes
fromage ou yaourt
gâteau ou glace

Les enfants prennent le bœuf. (Urcuit)

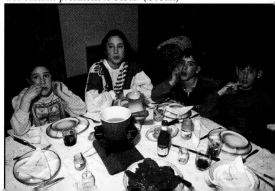

The imperative

Imperative verb forms are used to give commands and make suggestions. Each French verb has three imperative forms whose subjects are understood to be **tu, vous** and **nous.** These subjects, however, are not used with commands. Compare the following present tense forms of the verb **étudier** with their corresponding commands.

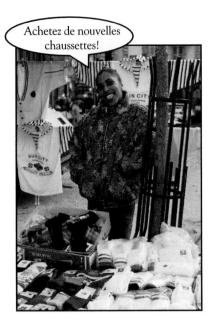

Achetez de nouvelles chaussettes!

Present Tense	Imperative	
tu étudies	**Étudie!**	*Study!*
vous étudiez	**Étudiez!**	*Study!*
nous étudions	**Étudions!**	*Let's study!*

As you can see, the **nous** and **vous** imperative forms of verbs ending in **-er** are exactly the same as their corresponding present tense forms. However, the **tu** imperative form does not end in **-s.**

The imperative forms of verbs ending in **-ir** and **-re** are exactly the same as their corresponding present tense forms: **Finis! Finissez! Finissons!** and **Vends! Vendez! Vendons!**

The **nous** form of the imperative is used to make a suggestion and means "Let's + *verb.*"

Form the negative imperative by putting **ne** before the verb and **pas** afterward.

    Ne va **pas** chez les Giraud!   *Don't go to the Girauds!*

Pratique

7   As guests arrive at your party, make sure they have a good time by telling them to do the following things.

1. donner vos blousons à ma belle-mère
2. aller au salon
3. parler avec tout le monde
4. manger des chips
5. prendre des boissons
6. écouter mes nouveaux CDs
7. danser

Modèle:

entrer

Entrez!

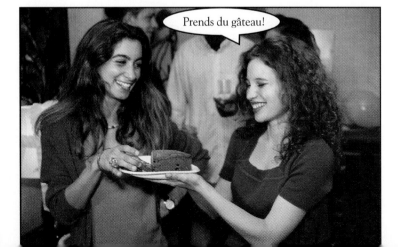

Prends du gâteau!

8   Based on what Marcel tells you, advise him to do or not to do certain things.

1. J'ai soif. (prendre de l'eau)
2. Je n'aime pas les fast-foods. (manger au Quick)
3. Je veux acheter un nouveau jean. (faire les magasins)
4. Il y a des soldes. (acheter ce pull)
5. J'ai beaucoup de vidéocassettes. (vendre le magnétoscope)
6. Je ne veux pas danser. (aller en boîte)
7. Je n'aime pas le rock. (écouter le reggae)
8. Il pleut. (entrer donc)

Modèles:

Il y a une interro demain. (étudier)
Alors, étudie!

Je n'ai pas faim. (finir le dessert)
Alors, ne finis pas le dessert!

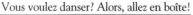

Vous voulez danser? Alors, allez en boîte!

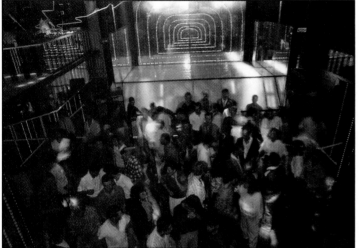

9   For each place you and your friends go to this weekend, suggest one thing to do there.

1. la maison de Jean-Christophe
2. le centre commercial
3. le fast-food
4. le grand magasin
5. la pâtisserie
6. le cinéma
7. la boum de Sylvie
8. le café

Modèle:

la boîte
Dansons!

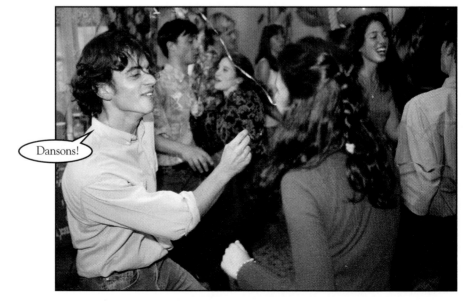

Dansons!

Communication

10 Imagine the house or apartment of your dreams! On a separate sheet of paper, draw the floor plan of your ideal residence, labeling all the rooms in French. It may have one or two floors. Then choose any room in this house or apartment and make a larger drawing of it on another piece of paper, adding whatever you would buy to decorate and furnish the room. You may either draw the decorations and furniture or find pictures of them in back issues of magazines to cut out and attach to your drawing.

11 After you have completed the drawing of your ideal house or apartment, write a paragraph in French describing it. Also write about the specific room you chose to draw in detail, mentioning what decorations and furniture are in it. You may also want to tell the colors of various items.

12 In reading the classified ads for houses and apartments in French newspapers, you notice that many of the names of rooms and related expressions are abbreviated. Write one abbreviation used for each of the expressions that follow.

> **11ᵉ REPUBLIQUE:** très bel imm., grd, 2 pces 42m², cuis. 710.000F

> Réf 410 - **BLANC-MESNIL** - Appt F4, à rénov., entrée, cuis., séj., 3 chbres, sdb, wc, cft, cave, gar. + park. priv. 560.000F

> 30m Paris Nord, pavillon 4 pièces, cuisine, RdC douche wc, 1ᵉʳ ét. bains wc, 508m² terrain, s/sol cave 620.000F 16.44.24.81.92

> **GAGNY** pr. ctre. Pav. Ind. 300m² de terr., s/sol tot. av. cuis. d'été + chem., dche, wc, cave. RdC: dble séj. + chem. sur terrasse, cuis. amén., 1 ch., bureau, SdB + wc. Etage: 3 ch., cab. de toil., wc, plac. gge 2 voit. A saisir 860,000F

1. chambre
2. salle de bains
3. cuisine
4. rez-de-chaussée
5. douche
6. immeuble
7. premier étage
8. garage
9. pièces
10. sous-sol
11. séjour

13 Now that you know how French classified ads in the real estate section look, write your own ad in French for the house or appartment of your dreams that you designed and described in Activities 10 and 11. Remember to use appropriate abbreviations as seen in Activity 12.

Meals play an important part in a French person's day. He or she can relax and talk with family and friends, enjoy well-prepared food served on a beautifully set table and observe dining customs that have been handed down from generation to generation.

Mise au point sur... les repas

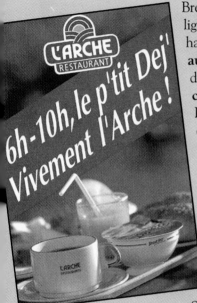

Breakfast **(le petit déjeuner)** is often a light meal. At home, adults usually have coffee, coffee with milk **(le café au lait)** or tea **(le thé)**. Children drink fruit juices or hot chocolate **(le chocolat chaud)**. Although some French people choose to eat a bowl of cereal in the morning, most of them prefer to cut crusty **baguettes** into thick slices and cover them with butter and jam. Other choices include dry toast **(les biscottes)** and toasted bread **(le pain grillé)**. Occasionally, perhaps on Sunday mornings, one member of the family goes to the bakery for fresh **croissants**. Since warm beverages are usually served in large, deep bowls, many people like to dip their bread in their coffee or hot chocolate when they are at home. People who have breakfast at a hotel eat either in their room or in a small dining area. The usual hotel breakfast consists of part of a **baguette**, a **croissant**, butter, jam and a beverage.

Laurier d'Or
de la Qualité et de la Tradition Boulangère

COPALINE

COPALINE
LA BAGUETTE DU CHEF

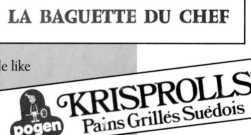

Bread usually comes with butter only at breakfast.

Lunch **(le déjeuner)** is still the largest meal of the day when families are able to get together. In the past, families gathered at home for the noon meal. Today, however, many women work outside of the home, students eat at school or at cafés, and businesses in urban areas remain open over the noon hour. Therefore, families usually reserve long lunches for weekends and special occasions.

Since the French usually don't eat dinner until 7:30 or 8:00 P.M., students often enjoy a small snack (**le goûter**) after school. Rather than just grabbing food from the cupboard or refrigerator, teenagers often stop for something sweet at a **pâtisserie** or sit down at home or at a café for a bite to eat and a beverage.

Families often spend time during the evening meal, **le dîner**, discussing what they did during the day. A typical main meal, either lunch or dinner, may last several hours and consists of various courses. First of all comes an

hors-d'œuvre, such as soup, **crudités** or **pâté**, or an **entrée**, such as a small slice of quiche. Then the main dish (**le plat principal**), usually meat and vegetables, is served. A salad of lettuce mixed with vinegar and oil dressing (**vinaigrette**) usually follows the main course, although sometimes the salad may be served before or with the main course. Different kinds of cheeses are offered next; each person takes just a small portion of his or her favorites. A dessert, such as fruit, ice cream or pastries, tops off the meal.

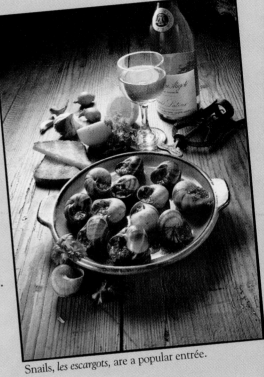

Snails, *les escargots*, are a popular entrée.

A bottle of water or mineral water accompanies most meals. Children sometimes drink fruit juices or soft drinks; adults often drink wine. Coffee is served at the end of the meal.

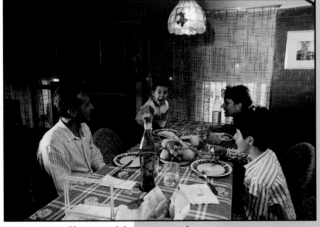

Cheese and fruit are served at the end of a meal.

Fresh bread accompanies every meal. Instead of being sliced, bread is usually broken into individual pieces and served in a basket. Bread plates are generally used only in elegant restaurants; at home, each person puts his or her bread right on the table.

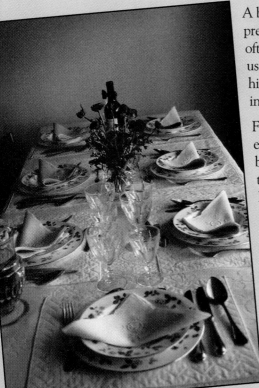

The French use a tablecloth and napkins even for ordinary meals at home. (Paris)

A beautiful table setting enhances the presentation of the food. Fresh flowers often serve as a centerpiece. Most families use cloth napkins. Each family member has his or her own napkin which may be kept in a napkin ring or a cloth holder.

French families have adopted certain eating habits and traditions that have been passed on from one generation to the next. They set the table differently in France than in the United States. Teaspoons or dessert forks go horizontally above the plate, and forks and spoons are turned face down. French silverware is slightly larger and heavier than American silverware. For formal meals the French use different dishes for each course. They usually cut and eat each piece of meat separately, keeping the fork, tines down, in the left hand. They even scoop up vegetables, such as peas, on the fork. Instead of leaving one hand in their lap, they keep both hands above or resting on the table during the meal. At the end of the meal, they place the fork and knife horizontally across the plate.

French cooking is famous throughout the world, and the opportunity to relax and talk at the table, the presentation of the food and the chance to maintain family traditions are as important to the French as a well-prepared meal.

4 Answer the following questions.

1. What is a typical French breakfast for an adult?
2. When French people eat breakfast at home, how do they serve warm beverages?
3. What is a typical French breakfast served at a hotel?
4. When is lunch still the largest meal of the day?
5. At what time do most French people eat their evening meal?
6. At a French dinner, what might be served as an **hors-d'œuvre**?
7. What is the French expression for the main course of a meal?
8. What are two desserts that might be served in France?
9. What kind of napkins do the French use?
10. How is a French table setting different from a table setting in the United States?
11. Do the French switch the fork from one hand to the other while eating?
12. How can you tell that someone has finished eating in France?

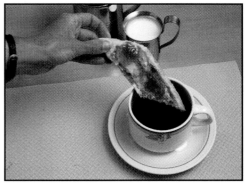

A typical French breakfast is a *baguette*, butter, jam and coffee.

15 | Look at the menus from an international flight between the United States and France. Answer the questions that follow.

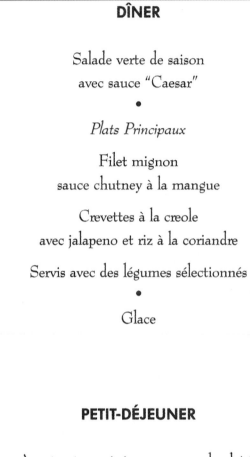

DÎNER

Salade verte de saison
avec sauce "Caesar"
•
Plats Principaux

Filet mignon
sauce chutney à la mangue

Crevettes à la creole
avec jalapeno et riz à la coriandre

Servis avec des légumes sélectionnés
•
Glace

PETIT-DÉJEUNER

Avant votre arrivée nous avons le plaisir
de vous offrir des jus de fruits rafraîchis,
la pâtisserie du jour, confiture et beurre.

1. Which is the larger of the two meals that are served on this flight?
2. Based on the order in which the two meals are served, at approximately what time of day does this flight arrive in Paris?

In the first meal:
   1. What is the first course?
   2. What are the two choices for the main course?
   3. What is served with either main course?
   4. What is the dessert?

In the second meal:
   1. What beverages are offered?
   2. What accompanies the pastries?

le couvert

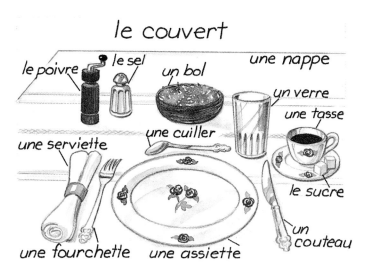

le poivre   le sel   un bol   une nappe

un verre

une tasse

une cuiller

une serviette

le sucre

un couteau

une fourchette   une assiette

La fourchette est à gauche de l'assiette.

Le couteau est à droite de l'assiette.

La cuiller est au-dessus de l'assiette.

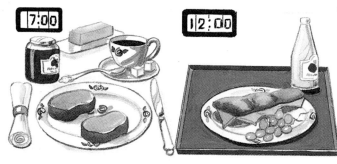

7:00   **12:00**

le petit déjeuner   le déjeuner

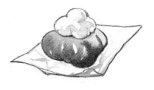

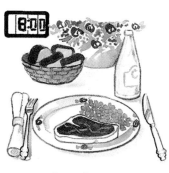

4:30   **8:00**

le goûter   le dîner

Leçon C

In this lesson you will be able to:

➤ **express intentions**

➤ **describe daily routines**

➤ **tell location**

➤ **agree and disagree**

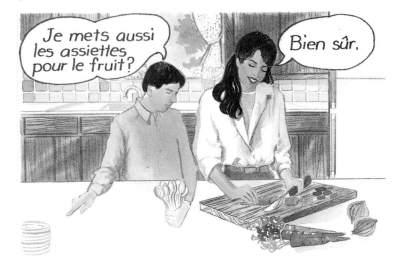

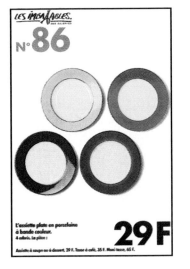

Arabéa Mamoudi and her younger brother, Djamel, live in Rabat, Morocco. They are helping their parents get ready to entertain luncheon guests to celebrate the end of Ramadan. Djamel is going to set the dining room table while Arabéa finishes preparing the meal.

Djamel: **Qu'est-ce que j'ai besoin de mettre sur la table pour le déjeuner?**

Arabéa: **On va manger du couscous. Mets les verres, les serviettes et les cuillers, s'il te plaît.**

Djamel: **Je mets aussi les assiettes pour le fruit?**

Arabéa: **Bien sûr.**

👁 *Enquête culturelle*

Le Maroc (*Morocco*), **l'Algérie** (*Algeria*) and **la Tunisie** (*Tunisia*) make up a region in North Africa called **le Maghreb**. Each year thousands of tourists flock to this sunlit area. They explore the markets and the Muslim sections (**les médinas**) of the cities in **le Maghreb**, admire the artwork, stonecuttings and ancient fortresses of the region and relax at its beaches on the Mediterranean Sea.

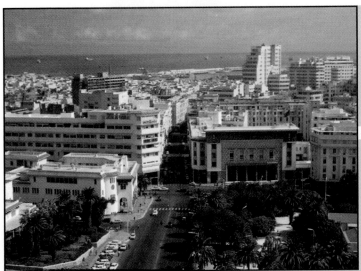

Casablanca is the largest North African city west of Egypt.

Morocco's two largest cities are Casablanca and the capital, Rabat. They both lie on the Atlantic Ocean. The country gained its independence from France in 1956. Arabic is the official language of Morocco, yet many people also speak French and Spanish.

Ramadan is the ninth month of the Islamic year. During this sacred month, Muslims don't eat or drink from sunrise to sunset. On the day after the end of Ramadan, **l'Aïd el-Fitr**, people celebrate by eating from morning until night. The noon meal often consists of **couscous**, which is served in a large bowl placed in the

Eating *couscous* marks the end of Ramadan. (La Rochelle)

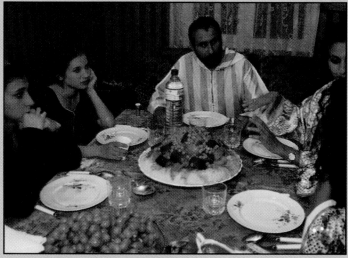

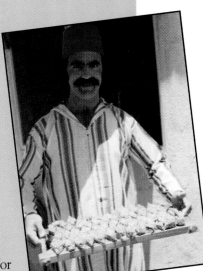

Baklava is a sweet made of thin pastry, honey and nuts. (Morocco)

middle of the table. Everyone eats out of the same bowl with spoons. For dessert, people have fruit, often watermelon. In the afternoon, young people visit their friends and relatives. Even if they stay for only a few minutes, they have time to enjoy mint tea, the national beverage of Morocco, and cookies, cakes or baklava, a honey and nut pastry.

*Choisissez la bonne réponse d'après le dialogue et l'***Enquête culturelle.**

1. Qui parle?
   a. une femme et son mari
   b. une sœur et son frère
   c. deux amis

2. Où habite la famille Mamoudi?
   a. en France
   b. à Casablanca
   c. à Rabat

3. Quelle heure est-il?
   a. 11h30
   b. 15h00
   c. 20h00

4. Où est-ce que Djamel travaille?
   a. dans le séjour
   b. dans la salle à manger
   c. dans la salle de bains

5. Où est-ce qu'Arabéa travaille?
   a. dans le salon
   b. dans la cuisine
   c. dans le grenier

6. Comment est-ce qu'on mange du couscous?
   a. avec les cuillers
   b. avec les verres
   c. avec les serviettes

7. Le dessert, c'est quoi?
   a. du fromage
   b. de la glace
   c. de la pastèque

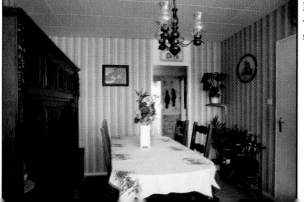

La famille Mamoudi va manger dans la salle à manger.

2 | Tell what serving dish or container the following items are served in or on and what utensils are used, if any, to eat or drink them.

Modèle:

le steak
une assiette; une fourchette, un couteau

1. le jambon
2. le couscous
3. le café
4. les haricots verts
5. la pizza
6. le lait
7. la glace

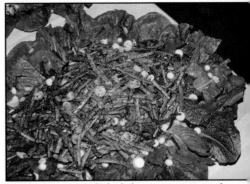

Pour manger une salade de haricots verts, on a besoin d'une assiette et d'une fourchette.

3 | *C'est à toi!*

1. Qu'est-ce que tu prends au petit déjeuner?
2. Est-ce que tu préfères un grand déjeuner ou un grand dîner?
3. Où est-ce que tu prends le goûter?
4. À quelle heure est-ce que tu prends le dîner?
5. Est-ce que tu mets souvent la table?
6. Est-ce que tu veux manger du couscous?

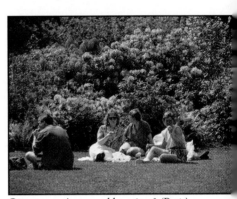

Où est-ce qu'on prend le goûter? (Paris)

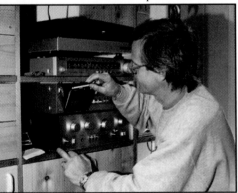

Où est-ce qu'il met la cassette?

Structure

Present tense of the irregular verb *mettre*

The verb **mettre** (*to put, to put on, to set*) is irregular.

		mettre	
je	**mets**	Je **mets** la table.	*I'm setting the table.*
tu	**mets**	Où **mets**-tu les cuillers?	*Where are you putting the spoons?*
il/elle/on	**met**	Il **met** le sel avec le poivre.	*He puts the salt with the pepper.*
nous	**mettons**	Nous **mettons** des baskets.	*We're putting on hightops.*
vous	**mettez**	**Mettez**-vous un jean?	*Are you putting on jeans?*
ils/elles	**mettent**	Ils **mettent** les fleurs dans le vase.	*They put the flowers in the vase.*

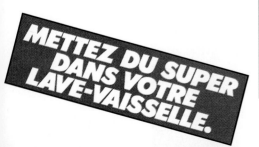

METTEZ DU SUPER DANS VOTRE LAVE-VAISSELLE.

Pratique

4 It's Claude Garnier's birthday. Tell who's putting what on the table to get ready for his party.

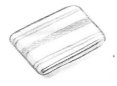

Modèle:

la grand-mère de Claude
La grand-mère de Claude met la nappe.

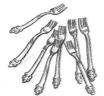

1. M. Garnier

5. vous

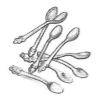

2. je

6. Mme Garnier et Daniel

3. nous

7. tu

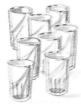

4. les sœurs de Claude

Everyone bought something at the grocery store. Tell whether they're putting what they bought in the refrigerator or in the cupboard.

1. Zakia et Karima/les yaourts
2. nous/les boîtes de petits pois
3. je/les œufs
4. M. Baribeau/le steak
5. tu/le poulet
6. Diane/le poivre
7. M. et Mme Charpentier/ le fromage
8. vous/les chips

Modèles:

Mme Surprenant/le lait
Madame Surprenant met le lait dans le frigo.

Daniel et Alain/le sel
Daniel et Alain mettent le sel dans le placard.

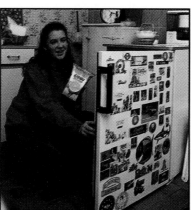

Claire met le jus d'orange dans le frigo. (Strasbourg)

Modèle:

le lit/la stéréo

Student A: Où est-ce que je mets le lit?

Student B: Mets le lit dans la chambre. Où est-ce que je mets la stéréo?

Student A: Mets la stéréo dans le salon.

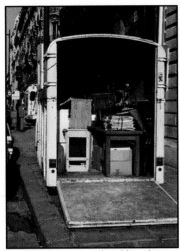

Où est-ce qu'on met la table et les chaises?

Modèle:

Student A: On a besoin de combien de fourchettes?

Student B: On a besoin de 16 fourchettes.

Modèle:

Student A: Où est-ce que je mets les deux fourchettes?

Student B: Mets les deux fourchettes à gauche de l'assiette.

6 Imagine that you and your partner are helping a friend move into an apartment. Take turns asking and telling whether you should put certain appliances and pieces of furniture in the living room, the kitchen or the bedroom.

1. le bureau/l'armoire
2. la table/le fauteuil
3. le canapé/le micro-onde
4. la lampe/le tapis
5. les chaises/la télé

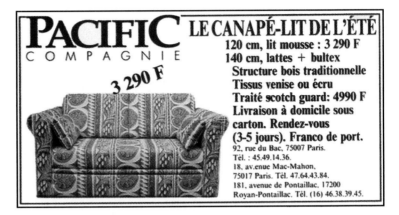

Communication

7 Imagine that you and your partner are in charge of setting the table for a formal dinner party for eight people. Talk about exactly what you need to set the table with, decide how many of each item you need and write down this information.

8 Before you and your partner set the table for your formal dinner, see if you can remember what a typical French place setting looks like by drawing it. On a separate sheet of paper, draw a plate. Then take turns asking and telling each other where each item goes in relation to another. As you determine the correct placement of each item, add it to your drawing.

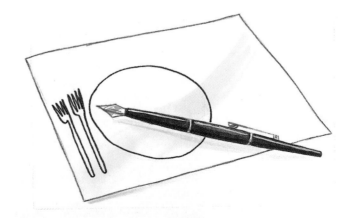

9   Review the information you learned about French eating habits in the **Mise au point sur... les repas** section on pages 299-301. Then form small groups of four or five students. With your group members, make one list of French eating habits and another list of American ones. Use only vocabulary words and expressions that you have already learned in French. For example, you might write **À la maison les Français prennent le café ou le chocolat dans un bol** and **Les Américains prennent le café ou le chocolat dans une tasse.** When your group has written as many sentences as possible, put them in graphic form. Draw two intersecting circles. Then write the sentences that describe only the French in one circle, the sentences that describe only Americans in the other circle, and the sentences that describe both the French and Americans where the circles intersect.

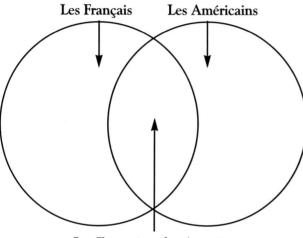

Les Français   **Les Américains**

Les Français et les Américains

Sur la bonne piste

When you read, how do you figure out the meaning of words you don't know? One way is to take advantage of the clues their context provides. In the following plot summary, certain words are underlined. Some of them may be new to you. See if you can use the context of the summary to find a synonym—a word that has the same meaning—to logically replace each one.

> What a <u>Utopian</u> place for an adventure—the French Riviera—with its eternal sunshine, sandy beaches, and that wonderful <u>azure</u> of the Mediterranean! But our friends' summer <u>escapades</u> happen to lead them to the exact <u>locale</u> of a plutonium-smuggling <u>rendezvous</u>! And who happens to be at the meeting? Their host, Monsieur Cau. Is this man a spy, a foreign agent involved in smuggling atomic products? What happens to him <u>hinges</u> entirely on the <u>proficiency</u> of our young friends.

You probably found synonyms for at least some of the underlined words without too much difficulty. Although the summary is in English, you can use this technique when you read in French, too. In the reading that follows, taken from a brochure on vacation housing, the underlined words are ones you probably haven't seen before. The rest are either words you already know or obvious cognates. As you read the passage, practice the technique of inference—that is, using the context of the words you *do* know to help you understand the ones you *don't* know.

Le logement

Cent appartements <u>répartis</u> dans 13 chalets sur 2 ou 3 étages sont regroupés <u>autour</u> du <u>pavillon</u> central. Vous <u>serez</u> <u>logé</u> dans un trois-pièces pour 5 ou 6 personnes.

<u>Chaque</u> <u>logement</u> <u>comprend</u>: une salle de séjour-chambre des parents <u>meublée</u> de 2 lits ou d'un canapé-lit, d'une table et de chaises; une chambre d'enfants avec 2 lits <u>superposés</u>; un <u>coin</u>-cuisine équipé d'un bloc-évier-réfrigérateur-<u>plaque</u> 2 <u>feux</u> incorporés et placard de <u>rangement</u> du matériel de cuisine; une salle d'eau avec w.-c. séparé.

10 | Draw a floor plan of the apartment described in the reading, using the context of the words you know to infer the meaning of the others. Be sure to include in your floor plan the furniture and appliances that are mentioned.

Nathalie et Raoul

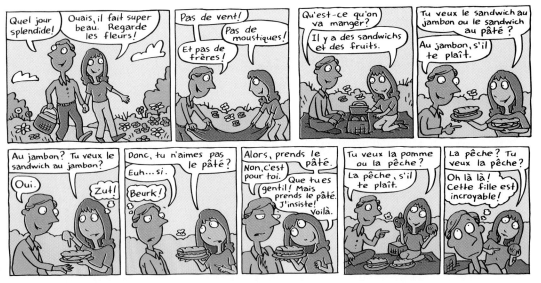

C'est à moi!

Now that you have completed this unit, take a look at what you should be able to do in French. Can you do all of these tasks?

➤ I can invite someone to do something.

➤ I can accept an invitation.

➤ I can greet someone by saying good evening.

➤ I can welcome guests.

➤ I can introduce people to each other.

➤ I can offer and accept a gift.

➤ I can identify objects, including types of housing, rooms, pieces of furniture and appliances.

➤ I can describe daily routines.

➤ I can tell where things are located, such as items in a place setting.

➤ I can say what someone is going to do.

➤ I can agree with someone.

➤ I can offer someone something to eat and drink.

➤ I can excuse myself.

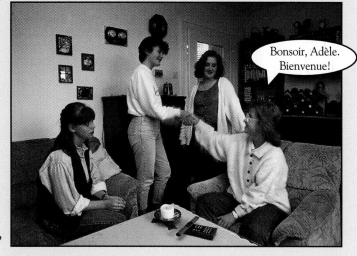

Bonsoir, Adèle. Bienvenue!

Here is a brief checkup to see how much you understand about French culture. Decide if each statement is **vrai** or **faux**.

1. Many people in France live in apartment buildings and often buy their apartments.
2. Most French homes and apartments have two different types of bathrooms.
3. To ask to use the bathroom in French, you say **Où est la salle de bains, s'il vous plaît?**
4. The style of houses in France differs from region to region depending on construction materials.
5. The second floor of a French building is called **le premier étage**.
6. If you are invited to a French home for a meal, it's appropriate to bring or send chrysanthemums to your hosts.
7. A typical French breakfast consists of eggs, bacon, pancakes and fruit juice.
8. The French often serve the salad and cheese courses after their main course.
9. **Le Maghreb** is a region in North Africa that includes **le Maroc, l'Algérie** and **la Tunisie**.
10. Muslims celebrate the month of Ramadan by eating **couscous**, fruit and desserts for their noon meal.

Communication orale

With a partner, play the roles of a French-speaking exchange student and an American host student. It's the day the exchange student arrives in the American student's home town. Begin your conversation at the airport where the American student greets the exchange student and welcomes him or her to the United States. Then continue your conversation on the way home. The exchange student, curious to find out what his or her new home is like, asks questions about his or her room and what's in it. The American student answers, giving as much specific information as possible.

Communication écrite

Imagine that Abdel-Cader Mamoude, a French-speaking Moroccan exchange student, is coming to live with your family for the year. Before arriving in the United States, he writes you a letter asking what his room in your home or apartment is like. Write a response to Abdel-Cader in French. Describe his room, saying where each piece of furniture and electronic appliance is in relation to something else. You may also want to enclose a floor plan of his room to help him visualize his new surroundings.

Communication active

To invite someone to do something, use:

Vous voulez faire le tour de mon appartement? — *Do you want to take a tour of my apartment?*
Entrez donc! — *Then come in!*
Allons au salon. — *Let's go to the living room.*

To accept an invitation, use:
Oui, je veux bien. — *Yes, I'm willing.*

To greet someone, use:
Bonsoir! — *Good evening!*

To greet guests, use:
Bienvenue! — *Welcome!*

To introduce someone else, use:
Je vous présente.... — *Let me introduce you to . . . .*
Raymond, Anne-Marie. — *Raymond, this is Anne-Marie.*

To offer a gift, use:
Voici des fleurs, Madame. — *Here are some flowers, Ma'am.*

To accept a gift, use:
Oh, que vous êtes gentil! — *Oh, how nice you are!*

Bienvenue!

Voici le canapé.

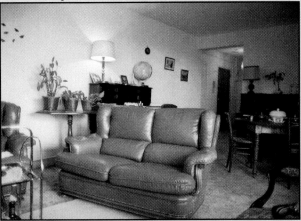

To identify objects, use:

Voici la cuisine. *Here's the kitchen.*

To describe daily routines, use:

Je mets les verres, les serviettes et les assiettes. *I'm putting the glasses, napkins and plates on (the table).*

To tell location, use:

La fourchette est **à gauche** de l'assiette. *The fork is (to the) left of the plate.*

Le couteau est **à droite** de l'assiette. *The knife is (to the) right of the plate.*

To express intentions, use:

On va manger du couscous. *We're going to eat couscous.*

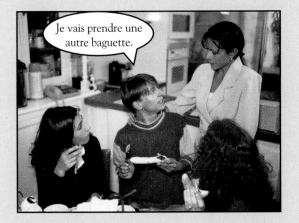

Je vais prendre une autre baguette.

To agree, use:

Bien sûr. *Of course.*

To offer food, use:

Prenez des chips. *Have some snacks.*

To offer a beverage, use:

Vous voulez un jus de fruit? *Do you want fruit juice?*

To excuse yourself, use:

Pardon, j'ai encore quelques choses à faire. *Excuse me, I still have some things to do.*

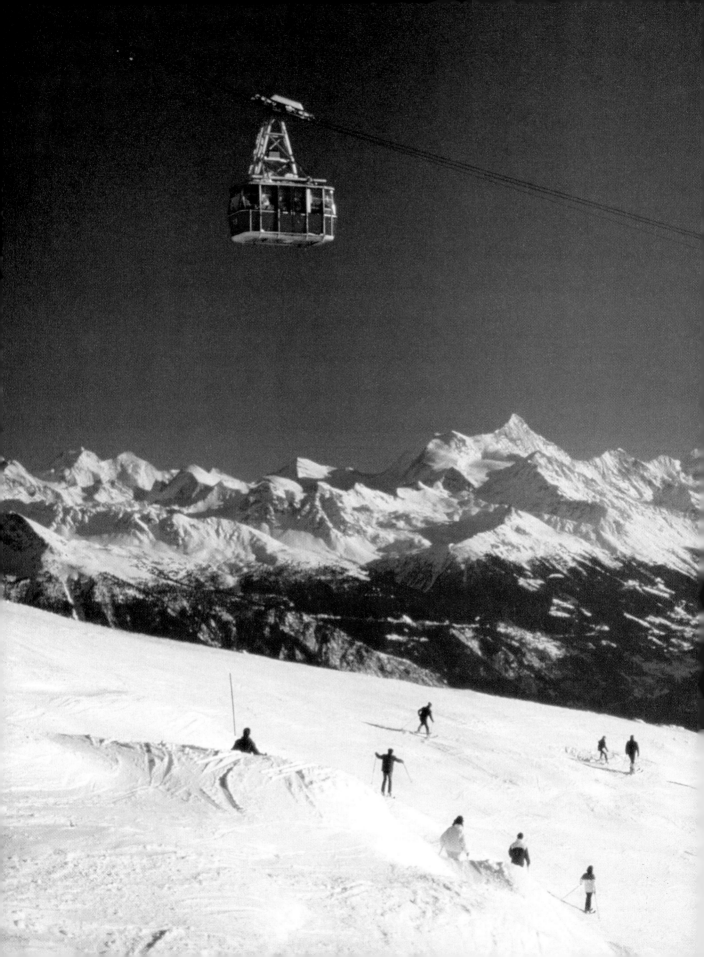

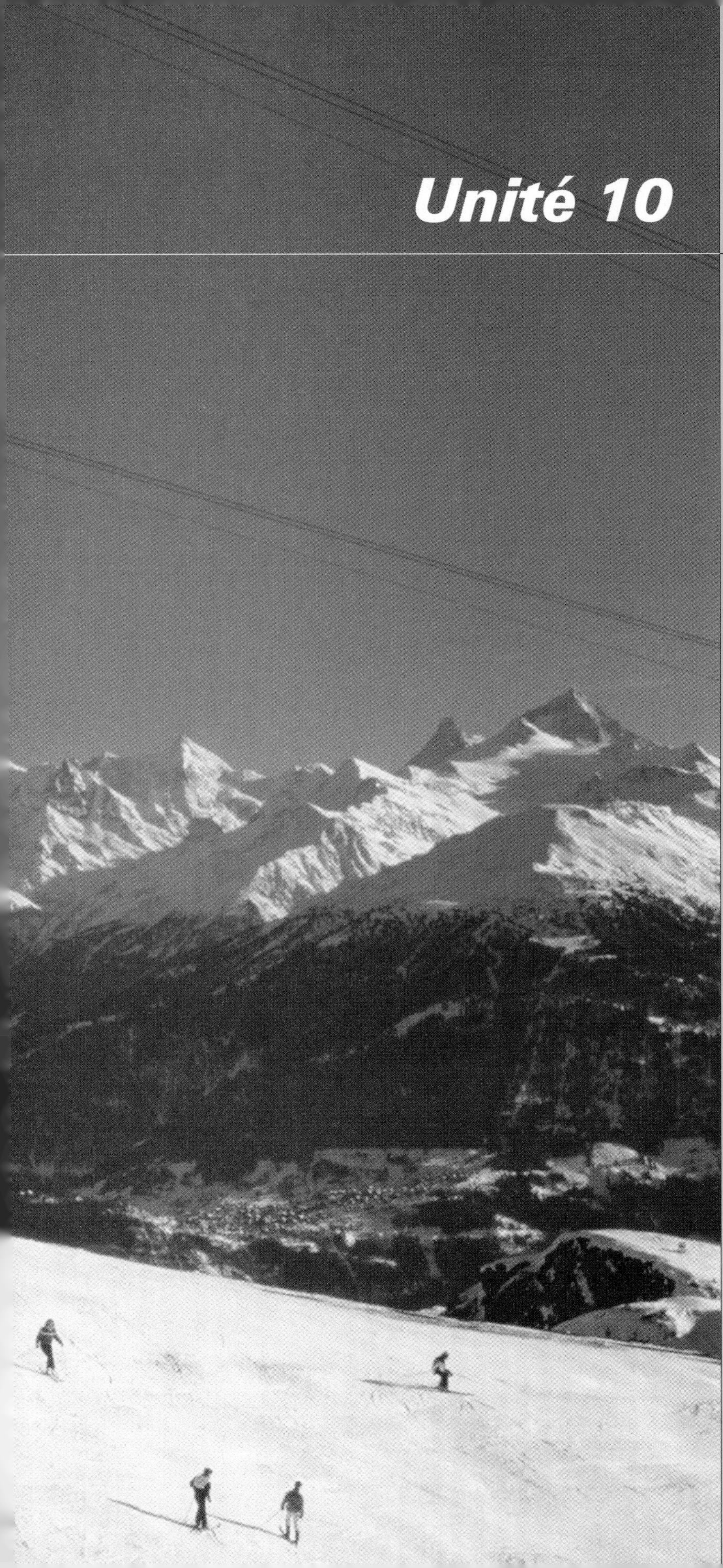

Unité 10

La santé

In this unit you will be able to:

➤ **express astonishment and disbelief**

➤ **express emotions**

➤ **point out something**

➤ **make a complaint**

➤ **explain a problem**

➤ **congratulate and commiserate**

➤ **express concern**

➤ **express need and necessity**

➤ **give advice**

➤ **express reassurance**

➤ **make a prediction**

➤ **make an appointment**

➤ **state exact and approximate time**

➤ **give information**

Leçon A

In this lesson you will be able to:

➤ express astonishment and disbelief

➤ express emotions

➤ express reassurance

➤ point out something

➤ express need and necessity

➤ give advice

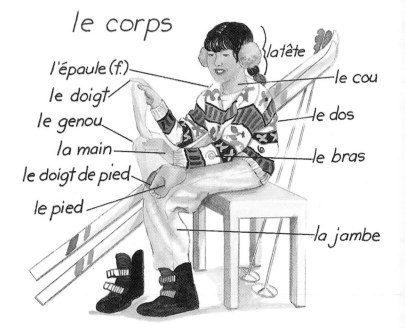

le corps

la tête

l'épaule (f.)

le doigt

le genou

la main

le doigt de pied

le pied

le cou

le dos

le bras

la jambe

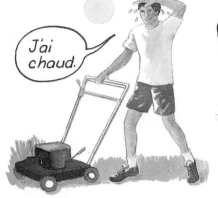

J'ai chaud.

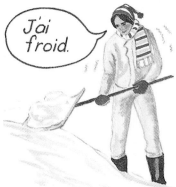

J'ai froid.

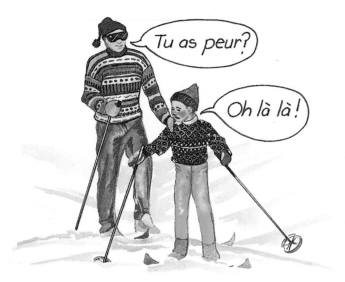

Sébastien's older brother, Francis, is teaching him how to ski near the city of Chamonix in the Alps.

Sébastien:	**Oh là là!**
Francis:	**Tu as froid?**
Sébastien:	**Non, ce n'est pas ça.**
Francis:	**Alors, tu as peur?**
Sébastien:	**Oui, un peu.**
Francis:	**Mais non, c'est facile. Regarde! Il faut prendre les bâtons dans les mains et garder les jambes solides.**
Sébastien:	**Il faut baisser la tête?**
Francis:	**Oui, mais pas trop. Allons-y!**
Sébastien:	**Au secours!**

Enquête culturelle

The French capital of mountain climbing and a popular international winter sports resort, Chamonix is situated in **les Alpes** in the eastern part of the country. From Chamonix, the highest cable car (**le téléphérique**) in the world carries people several thousand meters up the slopes of the **Aiguille du Midi**, one of the highest peaks in **les Alpes**, to ski, hike and enjoy the spectacular view.

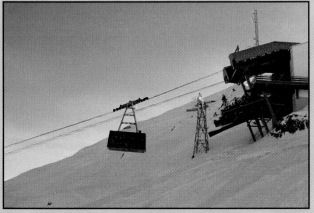

Skiers take *un téléphérique* to the top of a mountain. (Cauterets)

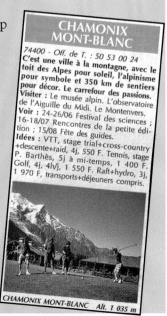

CHAMONIX MONT-BLANC

74400 - Off. de T. : 50 53 00 24
C'est une ville à la montagne, avec le toit des Alpes pour soleil, l'alpinisme pour symbole et 350 km de sentiers pour décor. Le carrefour des passions.
Visiter : Le musée alpin. L'observatoire de l'Aiguille du Midi. Le Montenvers.
Voir : 24-26/06 Festival des sciences ; 16-18/07 Rencontres de la petite édition ; 15/08 Fête des guides.
Idées : VTT, stage trial+cross-country +descente+raid, 4j, 550 F. Tennis, stage P. Barthès, 5j à mi-temps, 1 400 F. Golf, 4j, 4h/j, 1 550 F. Raft+hydro, 3j, 1 970 F, transports+déjeuners compris.

CHAMONIX MONT-BLANC   Alt. 1 035 m

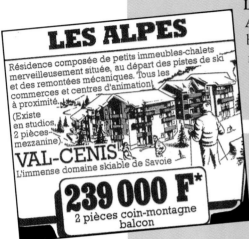

Le Mont Blanc, the highest mountain in **les Alpes**, rises over 15,000 feet and stands on the border of France, Switzerland and Italy. This mountain received its name (in English, "White Mountain") because its peak remains snow covered the entire year.

When French schools are closed for a week during winter vacation in February, many students go skiing in **les Alpes** and **les Pyrénées**. During the regular school year some schools offer organized

Le ski alpin is a popular sport in a country with five major mountain ranges.

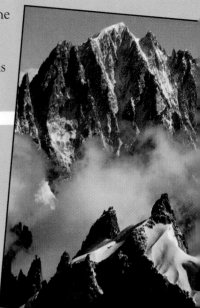

Many mountain peaks in France are named *aiguilles* because they resemble needles. (Chamonix)

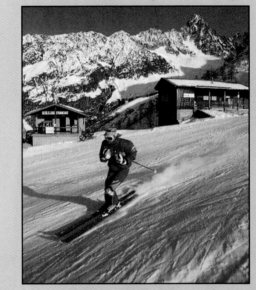

excursions, such as **les classes de neige**, where students have academic classes in the morning and ski in the afternoon. Most teenagers in France would rather downhill ski (**le ski de piste** or **le ski alpin**) than cross-country ski (**le ski de fond**). Skiing is also a popular winter sport in Switzerland, the site of many world-class ski slopes.

The French proverb **Mains froides, cœur chaud** means "Cold hands, warm heart." This proverb suggests that the way the body feels does not always reflect a person's emotions. Therefore, you may be cold on the outside, but still have a warm and friendly personality.

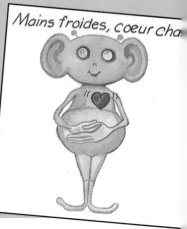

Mains froides, cœur cha...

Répondez par "vrai" ou "faux" d'après le dialogue.

1. Francis et Sébastien sont à Paris.
2. Chamonix est en Italie.
3. Sébastien a froid.
4. Sébastien a peur.
5. Francis trouve que skier, c'est facile.
6. Il faut prendre les bâtons dans les mains.
7. Il faut beaucoup baisser la tête.

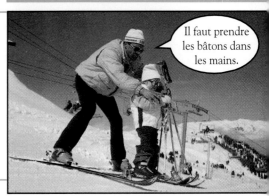

Il faut prendre les bâtons dans les mains.

Match the letter of the object with the part of the body it is associated with.

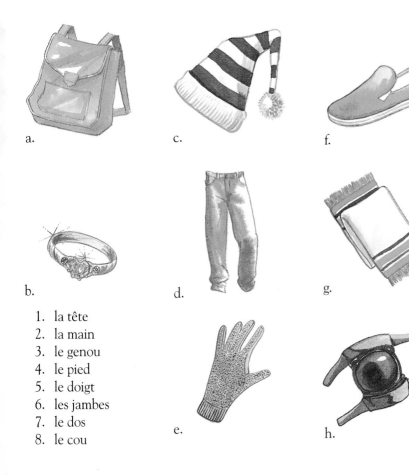

a.

c.

f.

b.

d.

g.

1. la tête
2. la main
3. le genou
4. le pied
5. le doigt
6. les jambes
7. le dos
8. le cou

e.

h.

Monsieur Belanger porte un anorak quand il skie.

C'est à toi!

1. Tu trouves qu'il est facile de skier?
2. Est-ce que tu skies bien ou mal?
3. Qu'est-ce que tu portes quand tu skies?
4. Quand est-ce que tu as peur?
5. Est-ce que tu as chaud ou froid maintenant?
6. Est-ce que tu étudies trop?
7. Est-ce que tu manges de la pizza avec les doigts ou avec une fourchette?

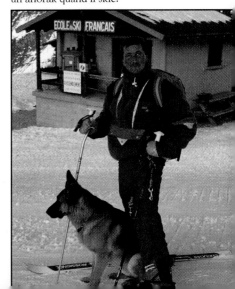

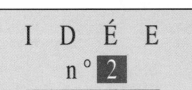

I D É E

n° 2

Il faut toujours profiter des bonnes opportunités.

Structure

Present tense of the irregular verb *falloir*

The verb **falloir** (*to be necessary, to have to*) has only one present tense form. **Il faut** means "it is necessary," "one has to/must" or "we/you have to/must." **Il faut** usually is followed by an infinitive.

Il faut garder les jambes solides.   *You have to keep your leg steady.*

Il ne faut pas baisser la tête.   *You must not lower your head.*

Pratique

4   For each of Ariane's statements, tell her one thing she should do.

1. J'ai faim.
2. Je voudrais faire une quiche.
3. Il n'y a pas de légumes dans le frigo.
4. Je veux regarder le nouveau film de Gérard Depardieu.
5. J'ai besoin de nouvelles chaussures.
6. Il fait très froid.
7. J'ai une interro demain.

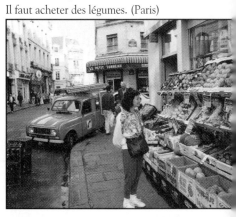

Il faut acheter des légumes. (Paris)

Modèle:

J'ai soif.
Il faut prendre une boisson.

5   With a partner, take turns asking and telling whether or not you need certain items in order to make certain things.

1. de la mayonnaise/une pizza
2. des pommes de terre/des frites
3. des raisins/du jus d'orange
4. de la moutarde/un gâteau
5. du pain/un sandwich
6. du poisson/une bouillabaisse
7. des pêches/une tarte aux fraises
8. de l'eau/du café

Modèles:

des œufs/une omelette

Student A: Est-ce qu'il faut des œufs pour faire une omelette?

Student B: Oui. Pour faire une omelette, il faut des œufs.

de la confiture/une salade

Student B: Est-ce qu'il faut de la confiture pour faire une salade?

Student A: Non. Pour faire une salade, il ne faut pas de confiture.

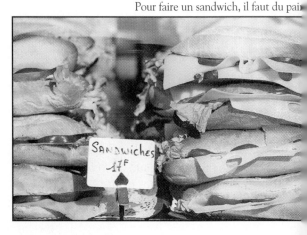

Pour faire un sandwich, il faut du pain.

Communication

You and one of your classmates have volunteered to visit elementary schools during National Foreign Language Week to present a short program in French. With your partner, create a song, rap or poem in French about parts of the body. In your song, rap or poem, name as many parts of the body as you can, using only words and expressions that you have already learned. Finally, perform your song or rap or read your poem, pointing to each part of the body as it is mentioned.

With a partner, play the roles of an American student who is spending spring break skiing in the Laurentian Hills in Quebec and a French-Canadian student who is also skiing there. Their conversation begins when the two students meet on the slopes, introduce themselves and say where they're from. Then the American confesses that he or she can't ski very well. The French Canadian asks if the American is afraid. The American admits that he or she is, but just a little. The French Canadian offers reassurance and gives the American several helpful suggestions and encouragement.

The sounds [s] and [z]

Prononciation

The French **s** is pronounced either [s] or [z] depending on what comes before or after it.

Pronounce **s** as [s] when it begins a word. Say each of these words:

solide	serviette
santé	sous-sol
Sylvie	seize

Pronounce **s** as [s] when it is followed by a consonant. Say each of these words:

escalier	disquette
pastèque	espagnol
baskets	costume

Pronounce **s** as [s] when it is doubled. Say each of these words:

baisser	assez
rez-de-chaussée	bouillabaisse
croissant	tasse

Pronounce **s** as [z] when it comes between vowels. Say each of these words:

cuisine	blouson
maison	chose
vase	magasin

Leçon B

In this lesson you will be able to:

➤ make an appointment

➤ state exact and approximate time

➤ explain a problem

➤ congratulate and commiserate

➤ give information

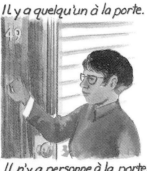

Il y a quelqu'un à la porte.

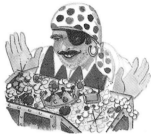

Il trouve quelque chose.

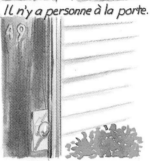

Il n'y a personne à la porte.

Il ne trouve rien.

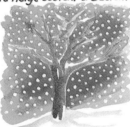

Il neige souvent à Boston.

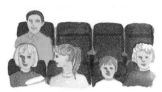

Il y a toujours de la place.

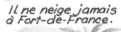

Il ne neige jamais à Fort-de-France.

Il n'y a plus de place.

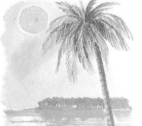

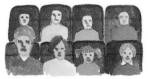

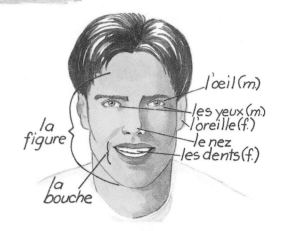

la figure
la bouche
l'œil (m.)
les yeux (m.)
l'oreille (f.)
le nez
les dents (f.)

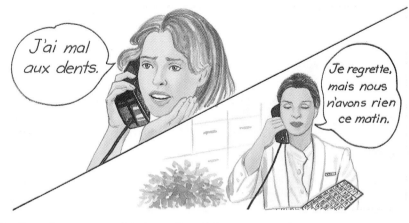

It's Thursday morning. Madame Graedel wants to make an appointment with her dentist in Lausanne, Switzerland.

La réceptionniste:	**Allô? Cabinet du docteur Odermatt.**
Mme Graedel:	**Bonjour, Madame. Je voudrais prendre rendez-vous avec Monsieur Odermatt, s'il vous plaît.**
La réceptionniste:	**Oui, Madame. Quand est-ce que vous voulez venir?**
Mme Graedel:	**Aussitôt que possible. J'ai mal aux dents.**
La réceptionniste:	**Je regrette, mais nous n'avons rien ce matin.**
Mme Graedel:	**Alors, cet après-midi?**
La réceptionniste:	**Monsieur Odermatt n'est jamais ici le jeudi après-midi. Est-ce que vous pouvez venir demain matin à 9h30?**
Mme Graedel:	**Bien sûr.**

The city of Lausanne sits on the hills overlooking the north shore of Lake Geneva in Switzerland. Of glacial origin, beautiful Lake Geneva attracts many tourists. Also called **le lac Léman**, Lake Geneva is approximately 70 kilometers long. On the western side of the lake, close to France, lies the city of Geneva (Genève). Many organizations, such as the Red Cross, the World Health Organization and the European headquarters of the United Nations, have their main offices here.

The waterspout in Lake Geneva shoots 130 meters into the air. (Genève)

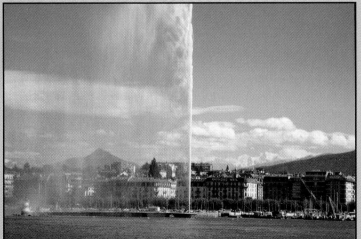

Enquête culturelle

Even though Switzerland is not a member of the United Nations, its *Palais des Nations* is the seat of the UN in Europe.

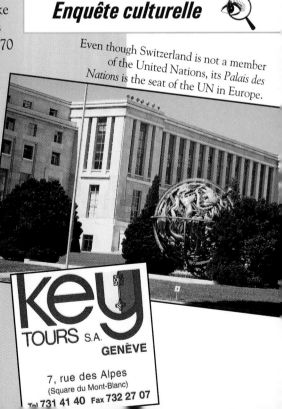

key
TOURS S.A.
GENÈVE
7, rue des Alpes
(Square du Mont-Blanc)
Tel 731 41 40 Fax 732 27 07

Switzerland has four official languages. About 20 percent of the Swiss speak French; most of these people live in western Switzerland near the French border. German is the language of the majority of people in northern Switzerland. Almost all of those in the south of the country speak Italian, while a small portion of the population in the eastern part of the country uses Romansch.

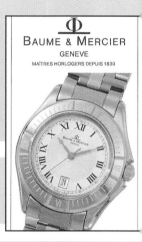

In addition to its spectacular scenery, Switzerland is famous for its watch industry, its delicious chocolates and its stable banking system.

1 Write a five-sentence paragraph in French that summarizes the conversation between the dentist's receptionist and Madame Graedel. Begin by telling the dentist's name. Then say why Madame Graedel needs to make an appointment with him. Next explain why she is unable to see him this morning. Then tell why she is unable to see him this afternoon. Finally, give the time when she is able to schedule an appointment.

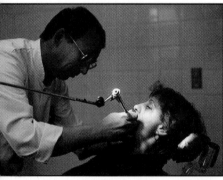

Mme Robin a mal aux dents.

2 *Complétez les phrases avec le mot convenable.*

tête	oreilles	jambes	dents	yeux	bouche	doigts	pieds

1. On écoute avec les....
2. On porte un chapeau sur la....
3. On parle avec la....
4. On regarde la télé avec les....
5. On fait du footing avec les... et les....
6. On joue aux jeux vidéo avec les....
7. On téléphone au dentiste quand on a mal aux....

3 *C'est à toi!*

1. Quand est-ce que tu prends rendez-vous avec le/la dentiste?
2. Est-ce que tu as souvent mal aux dents?
3. Est-ce que tu as peur de prendre rendez-vous avec le/la dentiste?
4. Ton/ta dentiste, il/elle s'appelle comment?
5. De quelle couleur sont tes yeux?
6. Quand il n'y a plus de place dans un café, est-ce que tu attends ou est-ce que tu vas à un autre café?

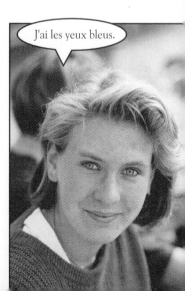

J'ai les yeux bleus.

Structure

Verbs + infinitives

Many French verbs may be followed directly by an infinitive. Here is a list of the verbs you have already learned that may be followed by an infinitive.

adorer	J'**adore faire** du shopping.
aimer	**Aimez**-vous **prendre** rendez-vous avec le dentiste?
aller	Maman **va téléphoner** à la réceptionniste.
désirer	Nous **désirons finir** aussitôt que possible.
falloir	Il ne **faut** pas **baisser** la tête.
pouvoir	Est-ce que vous **pouvez venir** demain matin?
préférer	Mes amis **préfèrent faire** du roller.
venir	Mes cousins **viennent regarder** mes photos.
vouloir	Qu'est-ce que tu **veux faire** maintenant?

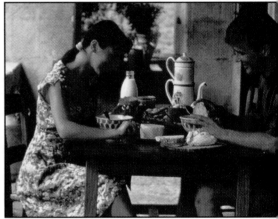

Qu'est-ce que M. et Mme Barde préfèrent prendre pour le petit déjeuner?

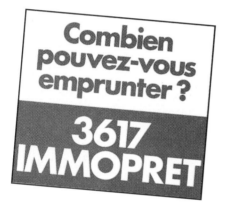

Pratique

1 Get to know your partner better. Take turns asking and answering questions.

1. aller/étudier le français aujourd'hui
2. pouvoir/sortir avec tes amis ce soir
3. aller/faire du shopping samedi
4. vouloir/être médecin
5. aimer/voyager
6. désirer/aller en vacances à Chamonix
7. adorer/skier
8. préférer/jouer au foot ou faire du footing

Modèles:

adorer/faire du roller

Student A: Est-ce que tu adores faire du roller?

Student B: Oui, j'adore faire du roller.

aimer/aller au cinéma

Student B: Est-ce que tu aimes aller au cinéma?

Student A: Non, je n'aime pas aller au cinéma.

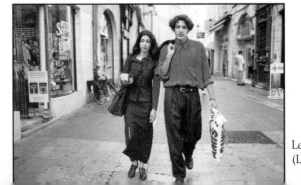

Leïla et son cousin vont faire du shopping. (La Rochelle)

Modèle:

jouer au tennis
Je n'aime pas jouer au tennis.
Je préfère jouer au basket.

5 You've been asked to take part in a survey about the typical activities of teenagers. Express your feelings about the activities on the survey, using the appropriate form of the verbs in the following list. Use each of the verbs at least once.

| adorer   aimer   falloir   préférer |

1. aller aux boums
2. écouter le rock
3. danser
4. aller au cinéma
5. manger de la pizza
6. faire les magasins
7. travailler
8. regarder la télé
9. faire les devoirs
10. étudier pour les interros

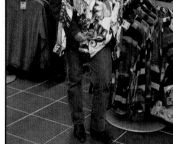

Claire adore faire les magasins.
(Strasbourg)

Negative expressions

You've already learned one French expression used to make a verb negative: **ne (n')... pas**. There are other negative expressions that follow the same pattern as **ne (n')... pas**. Compare the following expressions.

Affirmative	Negative
souvent (*often*) **toujours** (*always*)	**ne (n')... jamais** (*never*)
toujours (*still*)	**ne (n')... plus** (*no longer, not anymore*)
quelqu'un (*someone, somebody*)	**ne (n')... personne** (*no one, nobody, not anyone*)
quelque chose (*something*)	**ne (n')... rien** (*nothing, not anything*)

Il n'y a personne dans la voiture.

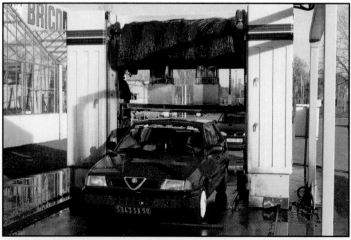

Tu vas **souvent** au cinéma avec tes parents?	*Do you often go to the movies with your parents?*
Non, je **ne** vais **jamais** au cinéma avec mes parents.	*No, I never go to the movies with my parents.*
Vous avez **toujours** de la place?	*Do you still have room?*
Non, nous **n'**avons **plus** de place.	*No, we don't have room anymore.*
Il y a **quelqu'un** devant toi?	*Is there someone in front of you?*
Non, il **n'**y a **personne** devant moi.	*No, there's no one in front of me.*
Tu prends **quelque chose**?	*Are you having something (to eat)?*
Non, je **ne** prends **rien**.	*No, I'm not having anything (to eat).*

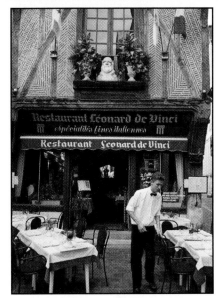

Ce restaurant a toujours de la place. (Tours)

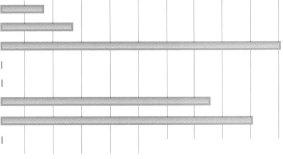

"On n'est jamais séparés plus d'une semaine"

Ne m'invitez plus à la **campagne!**

Note that in each of these negative expressions, **ne (n')** comes before the verb and **jamais, plus, personne** or **rien** follows the verb.

Remember that indefinite articles (**un, une, des**) and partitive articles (**du, de la, de l'**) become **de** or **d'** in a negative sentence.

Ton père fait toujours **du** sport?	*Does your father still play sports?*
Non, il **ne** fait **plus de** sport.	*No, he no longer plays sports.*

Personne may also be used after a preposition.

Je **ne** parle **à personne**.	*I'm not talking to anyone.*

Pratique

For two weeks Élodie kept track of how often she did certain things. Then she plotted her findings on a bar graph. Make a general statement about the frequency of each of Élodie's activities, using **toujours, souvent, ne (n')... pas souvent** or **ne (n')... jamais**.

Modèle:
Élodie ne prend pas souvent le petit déjeuner.

0% 10% 20% 30% 40% 50% 60% 70% 80% 90% 100%

- prendre le petit déjeuner
- porter des baskets
- aller à l'école
- regarder la télé après les cours
- faire du shopping au centre commercial
- téléphoner aux amis après le dîner
- finir les devoirs
- faire du sport

7 Pied-à-terre is going out of business. Student A plays the role of a customer and Student B plays the role of a salesperson who works at this store. Student A asks whether or not the store still has some of each item listed in the newspaper ad that follows. Student B answers, knowing that the only things left are sports equipment and dinnerware.

Modèles:

Student A: Vous avez toujours des stéréos?

Student B: Non, je regrette, nous n'avons plus de stéréos.

Student A: Vous avez toujours des assiettes?

Student B: Oui, nous avons toujours des assiettes.

> # *Pied-à-terre*
>
> ## SOLDES! LIQUIDATION TOTALE!
>
> | | |
> |---|---|
> | stéréos | assiettes |
> | CDs | bâtons |
> | fauteuils | lampes |
> | vélos | tapis |
> | magnétoscopes | |
> | verres | armoires |
>
> 31, RUE R. DELAGNES
> TÉL: 93.24.86.02

8 You're in a bad mood. Answer each question negatively using **ne (n')... rien** or **ne (n')... personne**.

1. Tu cherches quelque chose dans le grenier?
2. Tu veux quelque chose?
3. Tu achètes quelque chose au supermarché?
4. Tu invites quelqu'un à la boum?
5. Tu fais quelque chose ce soir?
6. Tu présentes quelqu'un à tes parents?
7. Tu ressembles à quelqu'un dans ta famille?
8. Tu étudies avec quelqu'un?

Modèles:

Tu manges quelque chose?

Non, je ne mange rien.

Tu attends quelqu'un?

Non, je n'attends personne.

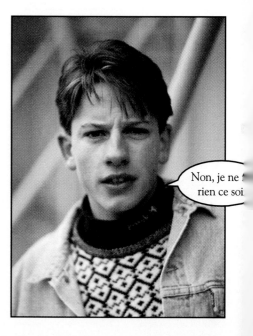

Non, je ne ? rien ce soi?

Communication

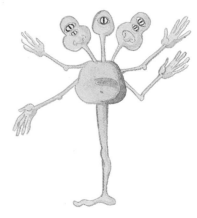

Using your imagination, draw a monster with various parts of the body that are unusual, for example, three small heads, one long leg, five eyes, etc. Next write a description in French of your monster, for example, **Il a trois petites têtes, une jambe très longue, cinq yeux...** etc. Then form groups of three. Each group member reads his or her description while the other two draw this monster based on what they hear. Afterward, students compare the original monsters with the drawings the other two group members have made and note similarities and differences.

Write a paragraph about your activities. Name five things that you never do, five things that you used to do but don't do any more and five things that you always do. You might begin to organize your thoughts by writing lists that have the following headings: **ne (n')... jamais, ne (n')... plus** and **toujours**. Use the information from your three lists to write your paragraph.

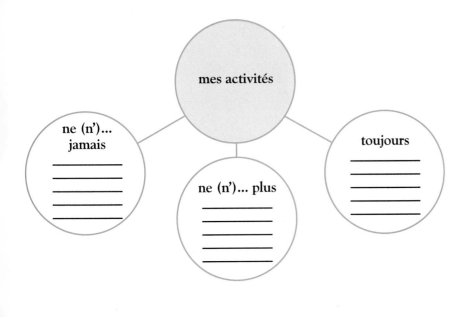

With a partner, have a phone conversation about a patient making an appointment to see a dentist. Student A plays the role of someone with a toothache and Student B plays the role of the dentist's receptionist. The patient calls the dentist's office, begins the conversation by saying hello, states his or her problem and then asks for an appointment. The receptionist and the patient discuss various times and days. They finally decide on a time that is convenient for both the dentist and the patient.

Mise au point sur... la santé

Like Americans, French people are increasingly conscious of physical fitness. By receiving adequate health care, watching their eating habits and exercising on a regular basis, **garder la ligne** (*keeping in shape*) has become a way of life for the French.

The French system of national health care provides medical treatment for everyone who needs it. All taxpayers contribute to the social security system (**la Sécurité sociale,** or **"la sécu"**), which covers most of the costs of visits to doctors and dentists, as well as prescription medicines. To avoid serious illnesses, many people try to keep healthy by eating nutritious foods and exercising.

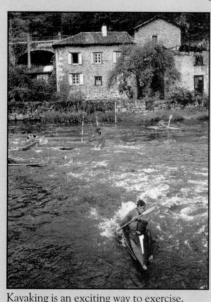

Kayaking is an exciting way to exercise. (Limousin)

The cost of most doctors' visits is covered by the social security system.

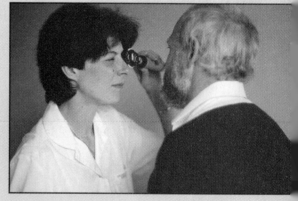

In recent years French cooking has changed to reflect a growing interest in healthy foods. In many French kitchens, products that are low in fat and high in fiber have replaced traditional heavy sauces and rich dairy products. Although a typical French meal normally consists of several courses, the portions tend to be quite small. Also, most French people snack very little between meals. When they do have **une petite faim** (*a little hunger*), they usually reach for a piece of fruit rather than for an artificially sweetened or salty snack.

Exercise is another way for the French to maintain physical well-being. Rather than relying on cars for transportation, many people choose to walk to their destinations. Health clubs provide aerobics and dance classes, as well as weight training equipment. Some people work out in their own homes with the help of exercise videos and TV programs. Many people exercise by taking advantage of inexpensive community facilities, such as public tennis courts and swimming pools. Soccer, cycling and martial arts clubs are popular with teenagers. Common family vacation activities offer other forms of exercise, such as mountain climbing (**l'alpinisme**), skiing, and windsurfing (**la planche à voile**). French people of all ages play **boules** (called **pétanque** in southern France), a form of lawn bowling.

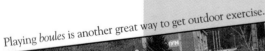

Playing *boules* is another great way to get outdoor exercise.

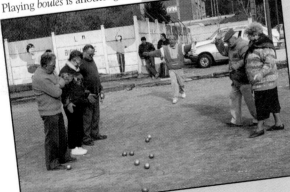

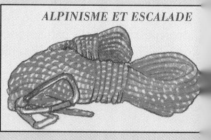

ALPINISME ET ESCALADE

Many French adults visit health spas to receive treatments for various ailments, such as liver, heart and digestive problems. During their stay, they rest, diet, drink mineral water and take thermal baths. The Romans were the first to recognize the benefits of the warm waters of the French city of Digne-les-Bains in the department of Alpes-de-Haute-Provence. The spas of this city, open from March to November, are famous for treating rheumatism and respiratory illnesses. Often people supplement a cleansing, relaxing visit to a health spa with more vigorous exercise during the rest of the year.

Yet, with all their efforts to stay fit, the French face significant health-related issues. The increasing number of fast-food restaurants and their popularity with teenagers worry people who are concerned with nutrition. Smoking is also a serious problem for this age group. The French government has a monopoly on the sale of cigarettes. Nevertheless, strict laws have been passed limiting tobacco advertising and forbidding smoking in certain places. Strong anti-smoking campaigns have been launched to reduce the number of people who smoke.

At school or work and during their leisure hours, many French people spend both time and energy on maintaining good health. Regular medical and dental visits, participation in sports and a healthy diet all contribute to the goal of physical well-being.

EUROTHERMES
LE RENDEZ-VOUS SANTE

Onze stations thermales

AIX-EN-PROVENCE - BAGNERES-DE-BIGORRE - LA BOURBOULE
CAPVERN-LES-BAINS - CAUTERETS - CHATEL-GUYON - CILAOS - DIGNE-LES-BAINS
LES EAUX-BONNES - ROCHEFORT-SUR-MER - CALDAS-DA-FELGUEIRA

Une agence à Paris

Onze indications thérapeutiques

Rhumatologie - Phlébologie - O.R.L. voies respiratoires - Appareil digestif
Maladies métaboliques - Affections psychosomatiques
Appareil réno-urinaire - Gynécologie - Dermatologie - Stomatologie
Troubles du développement chez l'enfant

87, av. du Maine - 75014 PARIS
(1) 43 27 12 50 Pour en savoir plus :   consultez l'Annuaire Electronique   Nom. EUROTHERMES Loc. PARIS Dépt. 75

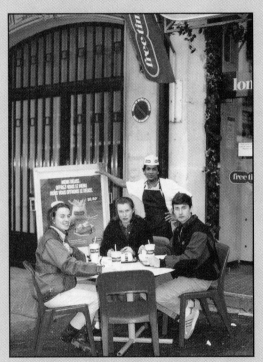

Nutritionists agree that many fast-food items have a high fat content and "empty" calories.

2   Answer the following questions.

1. How do French people keep in shape?
2. Who is covered under the French national health care system?
3. What health-related expenses are covered by the French social security system?
4. How big are the portions of food in a typical French meal?
5. Do the French often snack between meals?
6. Rather than relying on cars, how do many French people get to their destinations?
7. What are three sports in which the French participate to maintain physical well-being?
8. What is **boules**?
9. What are four things people do at a health spa?
10. What are two concerns about the health of French teenagers in general?

13 Here are ten ways to keep your heart healthy. After reading the suggestions and looking at the pictures, answer the questions that follow.

Pour votre cœur...
dix conseils-santé.

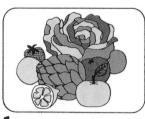

1 Mangez des fruits et des légumes pour les vitamines.

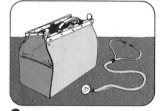

2 Voyez votre médecin une fois par an.

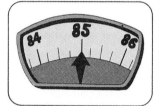

3 Contrôlez votre poids: l'excès fatigue le cœur.

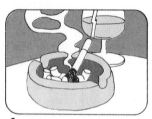

4 Réduisez tabac et alcool.

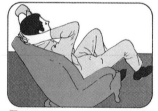

5 Ménagez-vous chaque jour quelques pauses-détente.

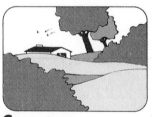

6 Faites le plein d'air pur pendant le week-end.

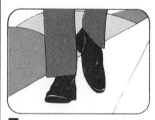

7 Pratiquez tous les jours une demi-heure de marche.

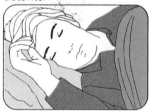

8 Dormez au moins huit heures par nuit.

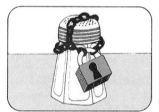

9 Ne consommez pas trop de sel.

10 Evitez l'excès de cholestérol.

1. Why should you eat a lot of fruits and vegetables?
2. How many times a year should you schedule a visit to your doctor?
3. What part of your body tires easily as a result of excess weight?
4. What two products should you avoid?
5. How long should you walk each day?
6. How many hours of sleep should you get each night?
7. Should you season your food with lots of salt?
8. How many of these suggestions do you follow?

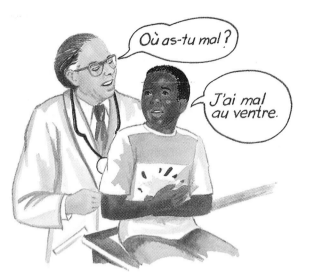

Où as-tu mal?

J'ai mal au ventre.

Leçon C

Il a mal à la tête.

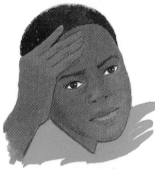

Il a mal au cœur.

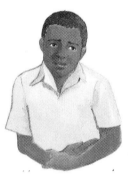

In this lesson you will be able to:

➤ express concern

➤ make a complaint

➤ explain a problem

➤ express need and necessity

➤ make a prediction

➤ give advice

Il a mal aux dents.

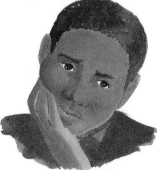

Il a mal au dos.

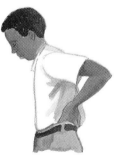

Il a mal à la gorge.

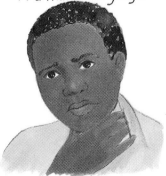

Il a mal aux oreilles.

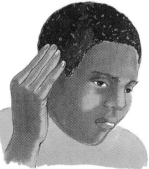

Elle est malade.

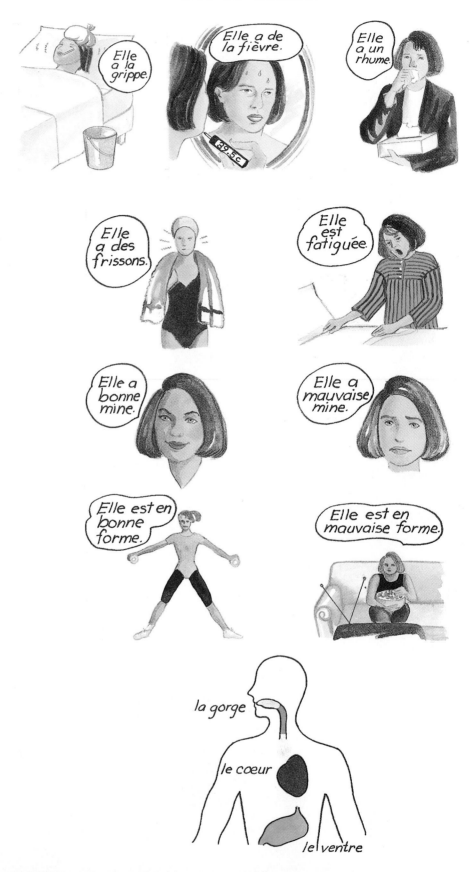

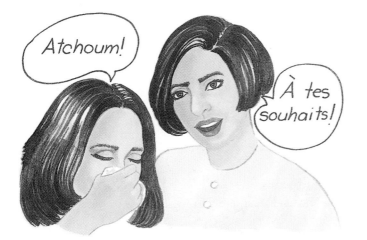

Martine Bekhechi doesn't feel well, and her mother asks her what's wrong.

Martine:	**Atchoum!**
Mme Bekhechi:	**À tes souhaits! Qu'est-ce que tu as?**
Martine:	**Je ne suis pas en bonne forme. J'ai mal au cœur.**
Mme Bekhechi:	**Tu as de la fièvre? Je dois prendre ta température.**
Martine:	**J'ai des frissons aussi.**
Mme Bekhechi:	**C'est peut-être la grippe. Tu dois rester au lit. Moi, je vais téléphoner au médecin.**

Enquête culturelle

Most stomachaches in France are blamed on the liver. When someone says that he or she has **une crise de foie** (literally, a liver attack), everyone understands that the person probably is experiencing indigestion rather than serious liver trouble.

The French use many colorful expressions to describe their health. Here are a few samples.

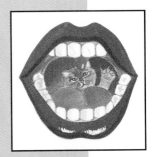

Il a les jambes en compote.	*His legs feel like jelly.*
Elle n'est pas dans son assiette.	*She's not feeling well.*
Elle a une fièvre de cheval.	*She has a very high temperature.*
Il a des fourmis dans les jambes.	*He has pins and needles in his legs.*
Elle est clouée au lit.	*She has to stay in bed.*
Il a un chat dans la gorge.	*He has a frog in his throat.*
Son estomac fait des nœuds.	*Her stomach is tied in knots.*

In French-speaking countries, a pharmacy (**une pharmacie**) has a bright green cross on the front of the building. When the cross is lit, the pharmacy is open.

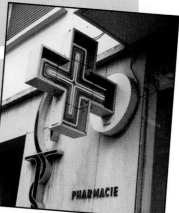

To find a pharmacy, look for the bright green cross.

Because many French people believe that certain plants can help relieve some aches and pains, most specialty stores and markets have herbal sections. Herbal teas are often given to people who don't feel well. Any tea made with natural herbs is called **une infusion.**

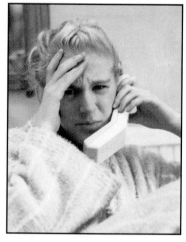

The French sometimes use alternative medical treatments to complement traditional medicine. In one such treatment, **l'homéopathie** (*homeopathy*), a person takes small doses of a remedy which provokes the same symptoms as the sickness that the patient wants to fight. By taking these pills, the person eventually builds up a resistance to the illness. Although many people believe in this type of cure, others think that this form of medicine is largely psychosomatic. Stomach ailments, colds and headaches might all be treated by **l'homéopathie.** Sections of some pharmacies and entire specialty stores are devoted to this form of treatment.

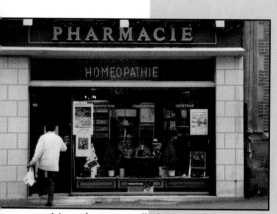

Many pharmacies offer homeopathic treatments. (Angers)

---

1   *Répondez en français.*

1. Qui est malade?
2. Martine, qu'est-ce qu'elle a?
3. Où a-t-elle mal?
4. Qui va prendre la température de Martine?
5. Est-ce que Martine a des frissons?
6. Où est-ce que Martine va rester?
7. Mme Bekhechi va téléphoner à qui?

Clémence a des frissons et elle a mal à la tête. Donc, elle téléphone au médecin.

---

2   According to the descriptions of the following people, tell what is probably wrong with them.

1. Chloé a une température de 39°.
2. Laurent Fignon finit le Tour de France.
3. Khaled mange trop de chocolat.
4. Sonia étudie beaucoup pour l'interro de maths.
5. Robert ne peut pas parler.
6. Mme Graedel prend rendez-vous avec le dentiste.

Modèle:

Le nez de Joël est très rouge.
Il a un rhume.

C'est à toi!

1. Comment vas-tu aujourd'hui?
2. Tu es fatigué(e) aujourd'hui?
3. Tu as souvent mal à la tête?
4. Est-ce que tu as beaucoup de rhumes en hiver?
5. Quand tu as de la fièvre, qui prend ta température?
6. Ton médecin, il/elle s'appelle comment?
7. Quand tu es malade, est-ce que tu aimes regarder la télé?

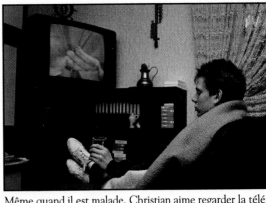

Même quand il est malade, Christian aime regarder la télé.

Structure

Present tense of the irregular verb *devoir*

The verb **devoir** (*to have to*) is irregular. It is often followed by an infinitive to express obligation.

devoir			
je	**dois**	Je **dois** téléphoner au médecin.	*I have to call the doctor.*
tu	**dois**	Tu **dois** rester au lit.	*You must stay in bed.*
il/elle/on	**doit**	Il **doit** prendre sa température.	*He must take his temperature.*
nous	**devons**	Nous **devons** étudier.	*We have to study.*
vous	**devez**	Vous **devez** prendre quelque chose.	*You should eat something.*
ils/elles	**doivent**	Qu'est-ce qu'ils **doivent** faire?	*What do they have to do?*

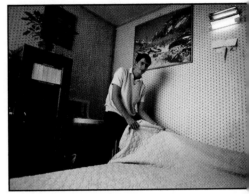

Laurent doit faire son lit.

UN PARFUM DOIT ÊTRE UNE ŒUVRE D'ART

Pratique

4 You work in Docteur Odermatt's dental office. It's time to send out reminders to people who haven't seen the dentist in the past six months. Based on how long it's been since their last checkup, tell whether or not the following patients have to make an appointment.

Modèle:

Sophie et David Tulipe doivent prendre rendez-vous avec le dentiste.

Sophie et David Tulipe	deux ans
M. et Mme Chevalier	un mois
Benjamin Robillard	trois semaines
Mlle Parsy	dix mois
Nadia et Myriam Vernon	cinq jours
M. Vega	quatre ans
Normand et Robert Bouchard	une semaine
Mme Picot	sept mois
Philippe Nino	un an

5 | Tell which two items the indicated people should buy at the **marché aux puces** in order to spend all the money they have with them.

Modèle:

la prof (37F)
La prof doit acheter le pot et la robe.

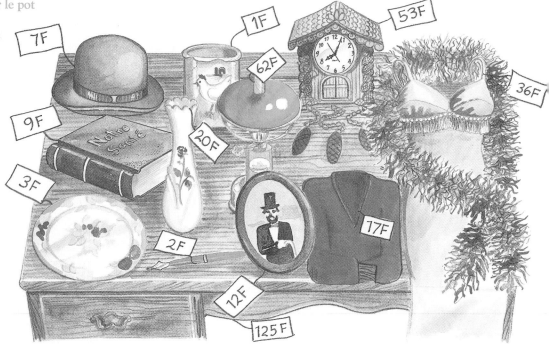

1. nous (74F)
2. tu (60F)
3. les parents de Martine (128F)
4. je (22F)
5. vous (26F)

Communication

6 | You want to know how your classmates are feeling today. On a separate sheet of paper, copy the seven indicated expressions that deal with health concerns. Then poll five of your classmates to determine whether or not they have any of these problems. As a classmate answers each of your seven questions, make a check if the answer is affirmative. After you have finished asking questions, count how many people are experiencing each of these problems and be ready to share your findings with the rest of the class.

Modèle:

Marie-Hélène:	Tu as mal à la tête?
Abdou:	Oui, j'ai mal à la tête.

. . . .

Marie-Hélène:	Deux élèves ont mal à la tête....

mal à la tête	✔✔
mal au ventre	
mal à la gorge	
mal aux dents	
un rhume	
fatigué(e)	
malade	

7 To observe Health Education Week, you and your classmates are having a contest to see who can create the best poster in French to promote good health. Choose any five of the health concerns listed in Activity 6. Then write two sentences for each one that tell what you should do or what you should not do to avoid that problem.

Modèle:

mal aux dents
Je dois prendre rendez-vous avec le dentiste.
Je ne dois pas manger beaucoup de chocolat.

When you were young, before you learned how to read, you probably spent a lot of time looking through storybooks. Even though you couldn't read the words, you were able to figure out what the stories were about. How? By looking at the pictures, of course! In fact, over time you could probably tell the stories yourself, just by referring to the illustrations or photos that accompanied them. Taking advantage of information contained in visual references can help you do two things: 1) predict what you will be reading about, and 2) figure out the meaning of unknown words. Examining pictures before you begin a French reading will put your mind on the right track; referring to them while you read will help keep it there.

Before you read the magazine article that follows, use the illustrations to predict the main idea. Then, as you read the article, use them to figure out the meaning of words you don't know in order to understand the details.

Sur la bonne piste

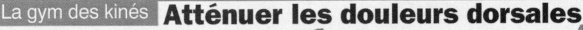

La gym des kinés   Atténuer les douleurs dorsales

Le conseil de M. Lanne, kiné-ostéopathe. Pour soulager le haut du dos, appuyez-le contre le dossier de votre siège en avançant le bassin.

Assise, jambes jointes tendues, dos droit incliné vers l'arrière sans creuser les reins, mains posées à plat derrière vous. En inspirant, bombez la poitrine et rentrez le menton, puis relâchez. 20 fois.

1.

Ces exercices sont indiqués pour soulager les tensions dans le haut du dos.

En tailleur, mains sur les genoux. En inspirant, tirez vos genoux vers vous tout en dégageant la poitrine et en étirant la nuque vers le ciel. Relâchez. 20 fois.

2.

Sur le ventre, en appui sur les avant-bras parallèles. Sur l'inspiration, renversez la tête en arrière en serrant les omoplates. Sur l'expiration, descendez peu à peu la tête entre les bras. 10 fois.

3.

8 │ Use the illustrations to help you answer the following questions.

1. Which exercise requires you to . . .
   a. squat?
   b. sit down?
   c. lie on your stomach?
2. Which exercise requires you to . . .
   a. tip your head backward?
   b. tip your head forward?
   c. raise your head by stretching your neck?
3. How many times should you repeat each exercise?
4. When you drop your head between your arms during exercise 3, should you do it quickly or slowly?
5. What part of the body are the exercises for?
6. What do the exercises relieve?
7. You know that the French word for "arm" is **bras.** What is the French word for "forearm"?
8. People in what occupations could benefit most from doing these exercises?

Nathalie et Raoul

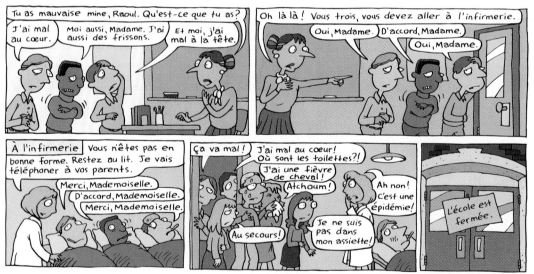

C'est à moi!

Now that you have completed this unit, take a look at what you should be able to do in French. Can you do all of these tasks?

➤ I can express astonishment.

➤ I can express emotions.

➤ I can point out something.

➤ I can make a complaint.

➤ I can explain a health-related problem.

➤ I can express sympathy.

➤ I can express concern.

➤ I can say what needs to be done.

➤ I can give advice.

➤ I can reassure someone.

➤ I can make a prediction.

➤ I can make an appointment.

➤ I can state approximate time.

➤ I can give information about various topics, using negative expressions.

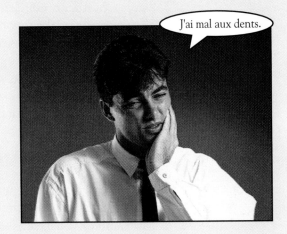

J'ai mal aux dents.

Here is a brief checkup to see how much you understand about French culture. Decide if each statement is **vrai** or **faux**.

1. Chamonix is a winter sports resort located in **les Pyrénées** in southwestern France.
2. **Le Mont Blanc** got its name because it remains snow covered all year long.
3. Cross-country skiing is more popular with French teens than downhill skiing is.
4. Geneva, Switzerland, serves as the headquarters for many international organizations.
5. Everyone in Switzerland speaks French.
6. The French have a national health care system that provides medical treatment for everyone.
7. Many French people visit health spas to treat liver, heart and digestive ailments by resting, dieting and taking thermal baths.
8. Fortunately, French teens in general do not have a serious smoking problem.
9. When people have indigestion or a stomachache in France, they usually blame it on their liver.
10. **L'homéopathie** is an alternative medical treatment in which patients build up a resistance to the illness they are suffering from.

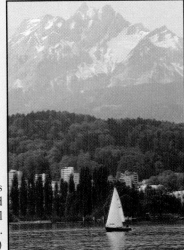

Alpine peaks are covered with snow all year long. (Switzerland)

Lausanne, a large French-speaking Swiss city, is known for its castle and cathedral.

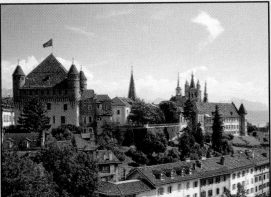

Communication orale

With a partner, play the roles of an American student and a French tour guide. The student has just arrived in France on the last stop of a ten-country, three-week European tour. The tour group encountered various weather conditions, ate many different types of food and spent long hours riding on the tour bus. The student, consequently, is not feeling at all well and begins the conversation by saying so. The tour guide asks the student what the matter is, and the student tells what symptoms he or she has. The tour guide tells the student what the problem must be, what he or she should or should not do to get better and whether or not it's necessary to make an appointment to see a doctor.

Communication écrite

Imagine that you are a French tour guide who has just spoken with a sick American student. Each night the tour company you work for requires you to write a memo telling what problems you encountered during the day. Write a report to your tour company telling which student is sick, how he or she is feeling, what the matter is, what symptoms he or she is experiencing, what problem he or she has, what he or she should or should not do to get better and whether or not the student needs to make an appointment to see a doctor.

Communication active

To express astonishment, use:

Oh là là!   *Wow! Oh no! Oh dear!*

To express emotions, use:

J'ai peur.   *I'm afraid.*

To point out something, use:

Regarde!   *Look!*

To make a complaint, use:

Je ne suis pas en bonne forme.   *I'm not in good shape.*

To explain a problem, use:

J'ai mal aux dents.   *I have a toothache.*
J'ai mal au cœur.   *I feel nauseous.*

To commiserate, use:

Je regrette.   *I'm sorry.*

To express concern, use:

Qu'est-ce que tu as?   *What's the matter with you?*

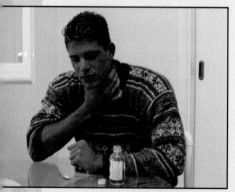

Stéphane a mal à la gorge.

To express need and necessity, use:

Il faut garder les jambes solides.   *You need (it is necessary) to keep your legs steady.*

Je dois prendre ta température.   *I need to take your temperature.*

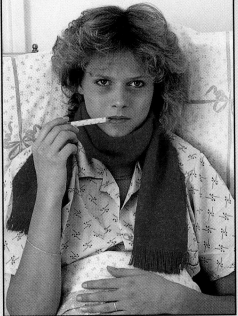

Margarette est malade; elle doit prendre sa température.

To give advice, use:

Tu dois rester au lit.   *You have to stay in bed.*
Il faut baisser la tête.   *You must lower your head.*
Mais pas trop.   *But not too much.*

To express reassurance, use:

Mais non, c'est facile.   *(But) no, it's easy.*

To make a prediction, use:

C'est peut-être la grippe.   *Maybe it's the flu.*

To make an appointment, use:

Je voudrais prendre rendez-vous avec....   *I'd like to make an appointment with . . .*

To state approximate time, use:

Aussitôt que possible.   *As soon as possible.*

To give information, use:

Nous **n'**avons **plus** de place ce matin.   *We don't have any more room this morning.*

Monsieur Odermatt **n'**est **jamais** ici le jeudi après-midi.   *Mr. Odermatt is never here on Thursday afternoon.*

Il **n'**y a **personne** ici.   *There's no one here.*

Je **ne** fais **rien.**   *I'm not doing anything.*

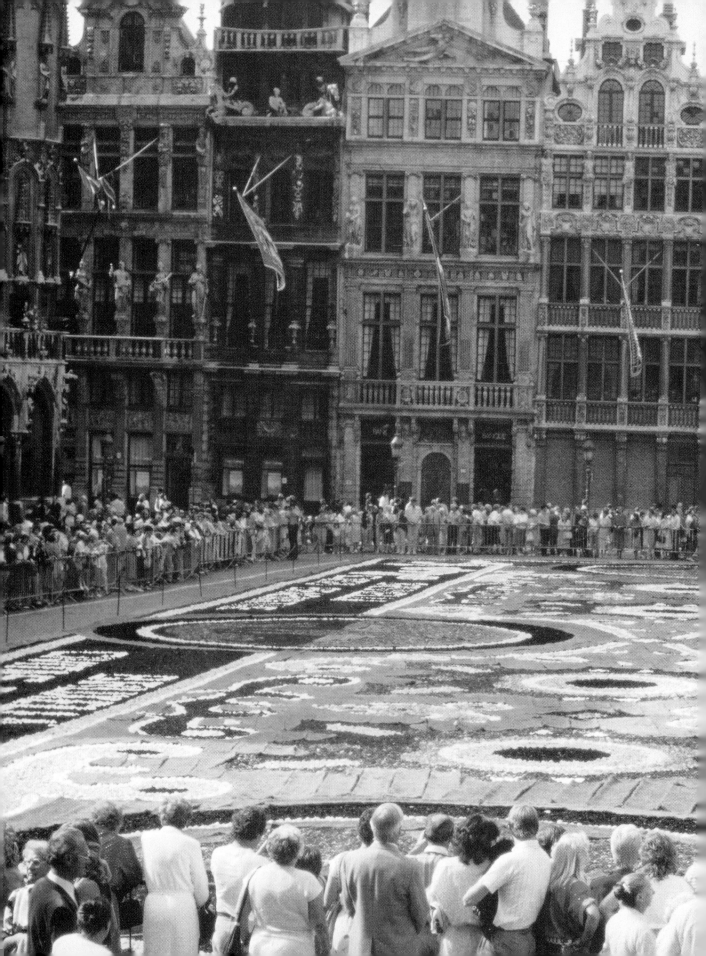

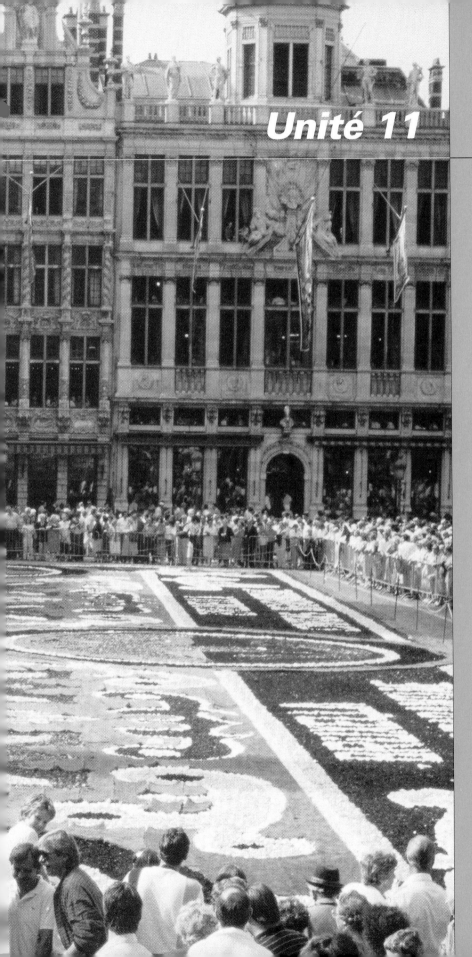

Unité 11

En vacances

In this unit you will be able to:

➤ write postcards

➤ describe past events

➤ sequence events

➤ ask for information

➤ inquire about details

➤ tell location

➤ give directions

➤ give addresses

➤ identify objects

➤ express likes and dislikes

➤ state a preference

➤ express emotions

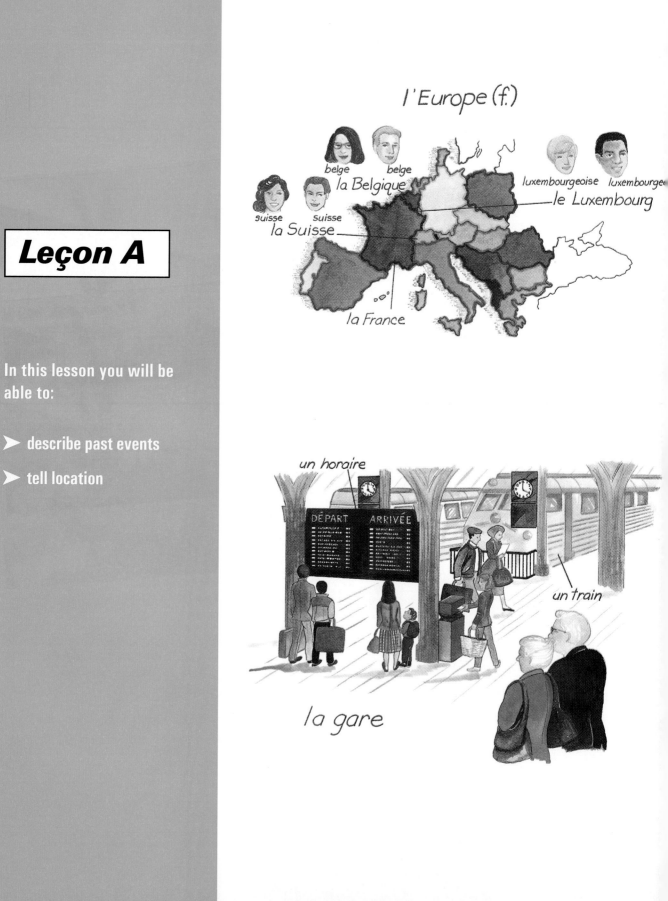

l'Europe (f.)

belge   belge
la Belgique

luxembourgeoise   luxembourge

le Luxembourg

suisse   suisse
la Suisse

la France

un horaire

un train

la gare

Leçon A

In this lesson you will be able to:

➤ describe past events

➤ tell location

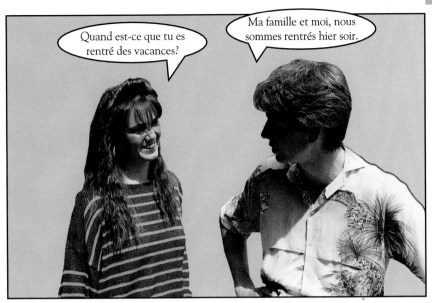

> Quand est-ce que tu es rentré des vacances?

> Ma famille et moi, nous sommes rentrés hier soir.

Diane and Nicolas are talking about what they did during vacation.

Diane: **Tiens, Nicolas! Quand est-ce que tu es rentré de vacances?**

Nicolas: **Ma famille et moi, nous sommes rentrés hier soir. Le train est arrivé à la gare à 22h05.**

Diane: **Vous êtes allés en Belgique, n'est-ce pas?**

Nicolas: **Oui, nous sommes partis pour Bruxelles le 29 octobre. C'est une belle ville. Et toi, tu es restée ici?**

Diane: **Oui, je suis sortie avec des amis la veille de la Toussaint. C'est tout.**

Enquête culturelle

Two French holidays begin the month of November: **la Toussaint** (*All Saints' Day*) on November 1 and **le jour des Morts** (*the Day of the Dead*) on November 2. On these two days the French remember their war dead as well as deceased relatives and loved ones. Flowers, especially chrysanthemums, are placed on the graves of family and friends. Students celebrate the holidays by taking a week of vacation.

Many French people travel by train. Some people who live in the suburbs of Paris take the train to work instead of drive a car. The **SNCF (Société nationale des chemins de fer français)**, a state-owned company, operates the French rail system, known for its trains that are on schedule, convenient and affordable. France has the most extensive network of tracks in Europe, and many people choose to travel by train when on vacation. France's modern **TGV (Train à grande vitesse)** runs 24 hours a day, covers all parts of France and extends into other European countries. It reaches speeds of up to 322 m.p.h., but usually goes about 186 m.p.h.

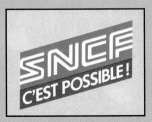

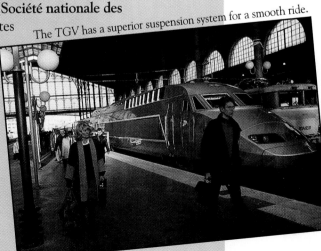

The TGV has a superior suspension system for a smooth ride.

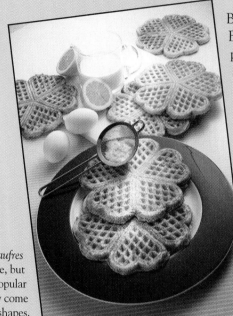

Traditional *gaufres* are square, but these popular desserts may come in various shapes.

Belgium lies northeast of France on the North Sea. Belgians are divided primarily into two groups, according to which language they speak. The French-speaking Walloons live in the southern part of the country; the Dutch-speaking Flemings live in northern Belgium. Another country known for its good food, Belgium is the capital of French fries and **gaufres,** thick waffles covered with syrup, fresh fruit or cream. Belgian chocolates have a worldwide reputation.

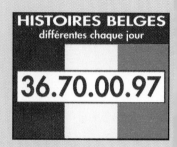

HISTOIRES BELGES
différentes chaque jour

36.70.00.97

Brussels, the capital of Belgium, is the country's economic, cultural and political center. Organizations such as the European Union (EU) and the North Atlantic Treaty Organization (NATO) have headquarters in or near the city. Ornate buildings that date from the 1500s, sidewalk cafés, and bird and flower markets decorate the city's main square (**la Grand-Place**). In 1815 Napoléon Bonaparte suffered his final defeat near Brussels in the city of Waterloo.

The historic buildings in Brussels' *Grand-Place* are in the Flemish Baroque style and decorated with gold.

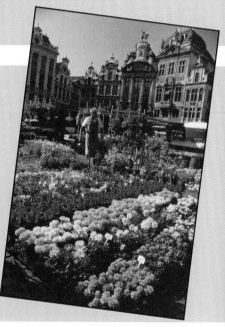

1 | *Trouvez dans la liste suivante l'expression qui complète correctement chaque phrase.*

hier soir	français	22h05	Toussaint
le 29 octobre	Nicolas	Belgique	Diane

1. ... est rentré de vacances.
2. Nicolas et sa famille sont rentrés....
3. Le train est arrivé à....
4. Nicolas est allé en....
5. Nicolas est parti....
6. En Belgique on parle....
7. ... est sortie avec des amis.
8. La... est le premier novembre.

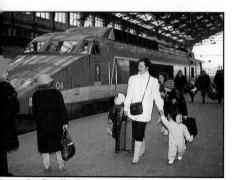

La famille Gautier est rentrée des vacances.

2   Identify each numbered country you see in the illustration.

Modèle:

C'est la France.

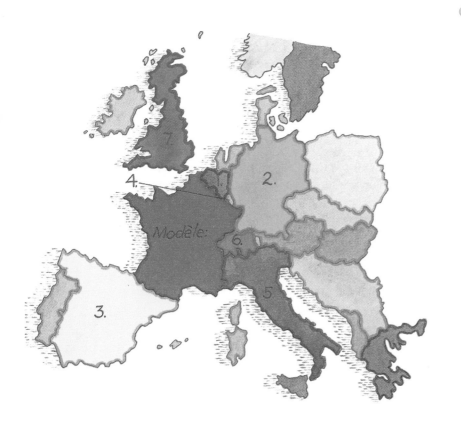

3   *C'est à toi!*

1. Est-ce que tu préfères l'école ou les vacances?
2. Est-ce que tu prends souvent le train?
3. À quelle heure est-ce que tu vas rentrer après les cours aujourd'hui?
4. Est-ce que tu vas sortir avec tes amis ce vendredi soir?
5. Est-ce que tu restes à la maison la veille de la Toussaint?
6. Qu'est-ce que tu fais la veille de la Toussaint?

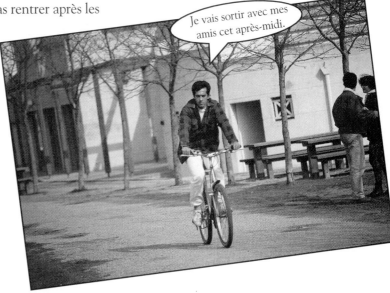

Je vais sortir avec mes amis cet après-midi.

Structure

Passé composé with être

The **passé composé** is a verb tense used to tell what happened in the past. This tense is composed of two words: a helping verb and a past participle. To form the **passé composé** of certain verbs, use the appropriate present tense form of the helping verb **être** and the past participle of the main verb.

> Vous **êtes allé** en Belgique.   *You went to Belgium.*
>
> (helping verb)   (past participle of **aller**)

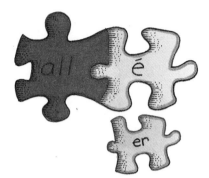

To form the past participle of **-er** verbs, drop the **-er** of the infinitive and add an **é**: **aller → allé**. The past participle of the verb agrees in gender (masculine or feminine) and in number (singular or plural) with the subject. For a masculine singular subject, add nothing to the past participle; for a masculine plural subject, add an **s**. For a feminine singular subject, add an **e**; for a feminine plural subject, add an **es**. Here is the **passé composé** of **aller**. Note in the chart that both the form of **être** and the ending of the past participle agree with the subject.

			aller	
je	suis	allé	Je **suis allé** en France.	*I went to France.*
je	suis	allée	Je **suis allée** chez moi.	*I went home.*
tu	es	allé	Marc, tu **es allé** à Paris?	*Marc, did you go to Paris?*
tu	es	allée	Nora, tu **es allée** au cinéma?	*Nora, did you go to the movies?*
il	est	allé	Ahmed n'**est** jamais **allé** en Europe.	*Ahmed has never gone to Europe.*
elle	est	allée	Elle **est allée** à la gare.	*She went to the train station.*
on	est	allé	Où **est**-on **allé**?	*Where did they go?*
nous	sommes	allés	Nous **sommes allés** en boîte.	*We went to the dance club.*
nous	sommes	allées	Nous ne **sommes** pas **allées** en Suisse.	*We didn't go to Switzerland.*
vous	êtes	allé	Monsieur Diouf, où **êtes-vous allé**?	*Mr. Diouf, where did you go?*
vous	êtes	allée	Vous **êtes allée** au centre commercial, Mme Gras?	*Did you go to the mall, Mrs. Gras?*
vous	êtes	allés	Vous n'**êtes** pas **allés** à la boulangerie?	*You didn't go to the bakery?*
vous	êtes	allées	Comment **êtes**-vous **allées** au Canada?	*How did you go to Canada?*
ils	sont	allés	Ils **sont allés** à l'école.	*They went to school.*
elles	sont	allées	Quand les filles **sont**-elles **allées** au café?	*When did the girls go to the café?*

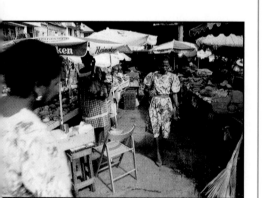

Denise est allée au marché. (Pointe-à-Pitre)

To form the past participle of most **-ir** verbs, drop the **-ir** and add an **i**: **partir** → **parti.** (For some verbs that end in **-ir,** add a **u.**)

Most of the verbs that use **être** in the **passé composé** *express motion or movement* of the subject from one place to another. Here are the verbs you have already learned that use the helping verb **être,** along with their past participles. (You will learn more of these verbs later.)

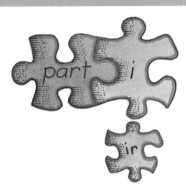

Infinitive	Past Participle
aller	allé
arriver	arrivé
entrer	entré
rentrer	rentré
rester	resté
partir	parti
sortir	sorti
but: venir	venu

To make a negative sentence in the **passé composé**, put **ne (n')** before the form of **être** and **pas** after it.

| Ma sœur n'est pas rentrée de vacances hier. | *My sister didn't come back from vacation yesterday.* |
| Le train n'est pas arrivé à la gare à 22h00. | *The train didn't arrive in the station at 10:00 P.M.* |

To ask a question in the **passé composé** using inversion, put the subject pronoun after the form of **être**.

| Thierry est-il déjà parti? | *Did Thierry leave already?* |
| Et toi, pourquoi n'es-tu pas restée à la boum? | *And why didn't you stay at the party?* |

The **passé composé** has more than one meaning in English.

| Ils sont sortis. | { *They have gone out.* *They went out.* |
| Sont-ils sortis? | *Did they go out?* |

Mme Dagorne est sortie de la boucherie.

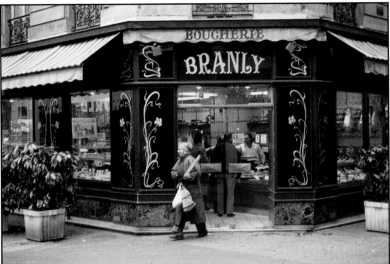

Pratique

4 | Yesterday was the first day of vacation. Tell whether the following people left for Belgium or for Switzerland.

Modèles:

Karine

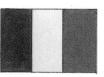

Karine est partie pour la Belgique.

M. Dumont

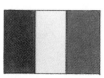

M. Dumont est parti pour la Suisse.

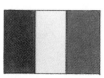

1. Bruno

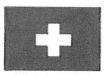

4. M. Vert

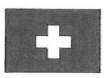

2. Mme Clerc

5. le prof de français

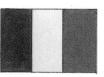

3. Amina

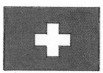

6. la prof d'allemand

5 | You took a poll to find out whether or not your classmates went out on Friday night. Give the results of your poll by completing the sentences that follow.

Modèles:

Sylvie et Salim sont sortis.
Sabrina et Nicole ne sont pas sorties.

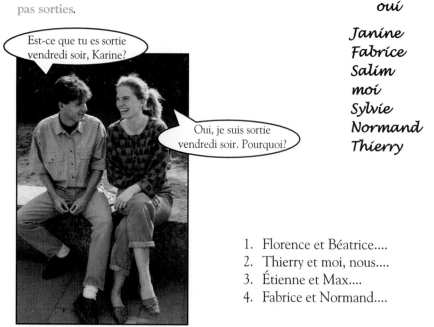

Est-ce que tu es sortie vendredi soir, Karine?

Oui, je suis sortie vendredi soir. Pourquoi?

Est-ce que tu es sorti(e) vendredi soir?

oui	*non*
Janine	*Étienne*
Fabrice	*Manu*
Salim	*Patricia*
moi	*Sara*
Sylvie	*Sabrina*
Normand	*Max*
Thierry	*Yasmine*
	Nicole
	Béatrice
	Florence

1. Florence et Béatrice....
2. Thierry et moi, nous....
3. Étienne et Max....
4. Fabrice et Normand....
5. Manu et Patricia....
6. Janine et moi, nous....
7. Sara et Yasmine....

6 When did people arrive at school this morning? To find out, complete the following short dialogues with the appropriate forms of the verb **arriver**.

1. Sonia: Tu... à sept heures et demie?
   Daniel: Non, je... à sept heures vingt.

2. Jean-François: Vous... à quelle heure, Madame?
   Mme Graedel: M. Laurier et moi, nous... à huit heures moins le quart.

3. M. Smith: Vous... à huit heures?
   Élise et Anne: Oui, nous... à huit heures.

4. Thibault: Vous... à sept heures et demie, Monsieur?
   M. Deslauriers: Non, je... à huit heures moins vingt.

5. Malick: Tu... à quelle heure?
   Margarette: Je... à sept heures vingt.

6. Ariane: Vous... à sept heures et quart, Monsieur?
   M. Pinot: Oui, je... à sept heures et quart.

Modèle:

Ahmed: Tu es arrivée à quelle heure?
Caroline: Je suis arrivée à sept heures et demie.

7 Based on their purchases, tell where the following people went shopping.

Modèle:

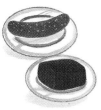

Chloé
Chloé est allée à la crémerie.

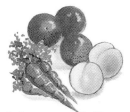

1. mon ami et moi, nous

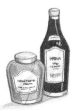

2. Frédéric et toi, vous

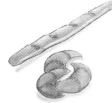

3. Isabelle et sa sœur

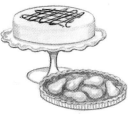

4. le beau-père de Denise

5. Mlle Paganelli

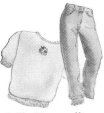

6. je

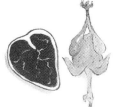

7. Mohamed et son demi-frère

8
Find out what your partner did last weekend. Take turns asking and answering questions.

Modèle:

aller au cinéma

Student A: Es-tu allé(e) au cinéma?

Student B: Oui, je suis allé(e) au cinéma. Et toi, es-tu allé(e) au cinéma?

Student A: Non, je ne suis pas allé(e) au cinéma.

1. rentrer à la maison après les cours vendredi après-midi
2. sortir avec des amis vendredi soir
3. aller à une boum
4. entrer dans une boutique
5. rester à la maison samedi soir
6. venir à l'école
7. partir en vacances

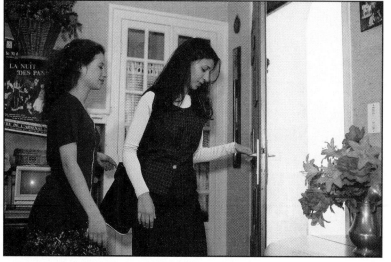

Aurélie et Leïla sont sorties samedi soir. (La Rochelle)

Communication

9
Your French teacher, Mlle Hopen, is a program coordinator for an organization that sponsors French-speaking students who visit the United States. You have offered to help her with part of her report on an international group that just arrived. Mlle Hopen has asked you to write a memo detailing each student's departure and arrival times to send to the program director in Paris. Based on the information she has given you, prepare this memo to send to France.

Modèle:

Martine Vannier est partie à 13h55 de Paris. Elle est arrivée à Chicago à 20h00.

Élève	Départ	Ville	Arrivée	Ville
Martine Vannier	13h55	Paris	20h00	Chicago
Adja Mutumbo	02h30	Dakar	16h39	Atlanta
Damien Vau	08h00	Paris	14h00	Denver
Sabine Kaas	08h25	Bruxelles	17h00	Boston
Patrick Boucher	11h45	Genève	17h45	Cincinnati
Nicole Bertrand	11h45	Nice	14h45	San Francisco
Henri Tremblay	13h45	Montréal	15h05	Salt Lake City

0 You want to know what your classmates did last weekend. On a separate sheet of paper, create a chart like the one that follows and copy the six indicated expressions. Then poll five of your classmates to determine whether or not they did any of these activities. Write the names of the five classmates at the top of your chart. As a classmate answers each of your six questions, make a check in the appropriate column if he or she answers affirmatively. After you have finished asking questions, count how many people answered each question affirmatively and be ready to share your findings with the rest of the class.

Modèle:

Myriam:	Est-ce que tu es allé chez un ami?
Théo:	Oui, je suis allé chez un ami.

. . . .

Myriam:	Trois élèves sont allés chez un ami....

	Théo	Jérémy	Sandrine	Sonia	Max
aller chez un ami	✔		✔		✔
rester à la maison vendredi soir					
aller au centre commercial					
sortir samedi soir					
aller au fast-food					
sortir dimanche avec les parents					

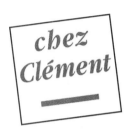

chez Clément

1 Now use the results of your survey in Activity 10 to write a report on what your classmates did last weekend. For each question you asked, specify who answered affirmatively and who answered negatively.

Modèle:

Théo, Sandrine et Max sont allés chez un ami. Jérémy et Sonia ne sont pas allés chez un ami....

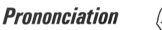

The sound [ɛ̃]

Prononciation

The nasal sound [ɛ̃] is represented by **in** when it appears before a consonant or at the end of a word. The **n** is not pronounced; the sound [ɛ̃] comes out through your nose. Say each of these words:

jar**din**   **in**firmier
pr**in**temps   mat**in**
informaticienne   magas**in**

The sound [ɛ̃] is also found in words containing the letters **ain** when they occur before a consonant or at the end of a word. Say each of these words:

tr**ain**   salle de b**ain**s
Touss**aint**   p**ain**
m**ain**tenant   mexic**ain**

The sound [jɛ̃]

Words that end in **-ien** contain the sound [jɛ̃]. The only difference between the sounds [ɛ̃] and [jɛ̃] is the **i** in the **-ien** ending. Say each of these words:

informatic**ien**   b**ien**
ch**ien**   ital**ien**
canad**ien**   comb**ien**

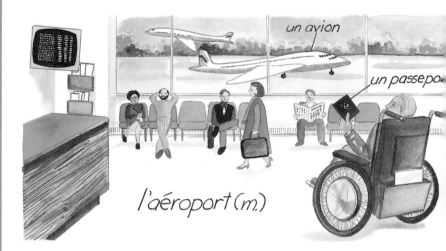

un avion

un passepo...

l'aéroport (m.)

Leçon B

In this lesson you will be able to:

➤ write postcards

➤ express emotions

➤ tell location

➤ describe past events

➤ sequence events

➤ express likes and dislikes

➤ state a preference

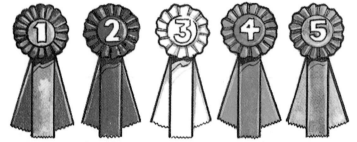

premier deuxième troisième quatrième cinquième
première

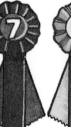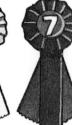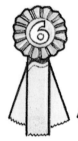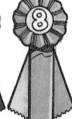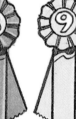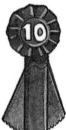

sixième septième huitième neuvième dixième

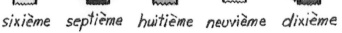

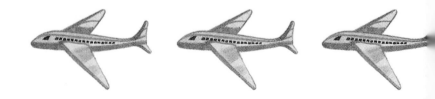

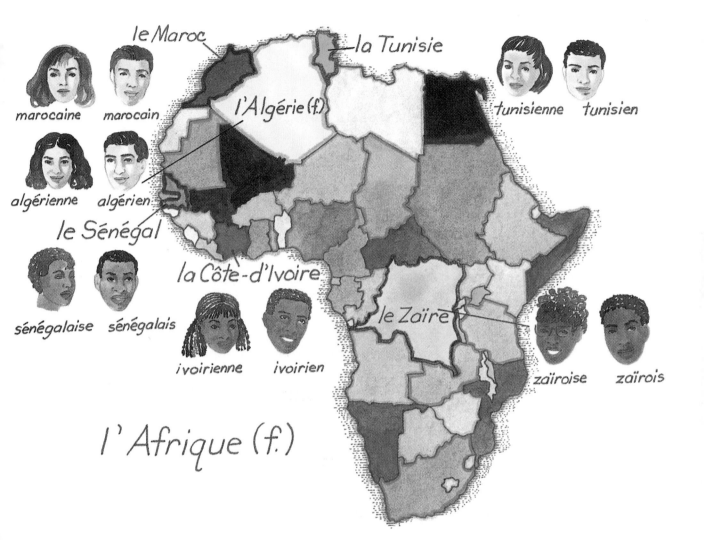

le Maroc

marocaine   marocain

l'Algérie (f.)

algérienne   algérien

le Sénégal

sénégalaise   sénégalais

la Côte-d'Ivoire

ivoirienne   ivoirien

la Tunisie

tunisienne   tunisien

le Zaïre

zaïroise   zaïrois

l'Afrique (f.)

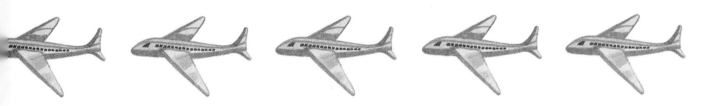

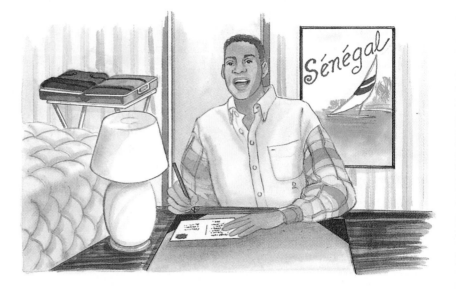

Alexandre is sending his friend Marie-Claire a postcard from his trip to West Africa with his parents.

> *Chère Marie-Claire,*
>
> *Ce petit séjour est formidable! L'avion est parti de Roissy-Charles de Gaulle, et nous sommes arrivés à l'aéroport à Abidjan en Côte-d'Ivoire. Nous sommes restés chez ma grand-mère qui est ivoirienne. Quatre jours après nous sommes partis pour Dakar. Le premier jour au Sénégal on est allé à Cayar, un petit village. Le deuxième jour nous sommes revenus à Dakar. Hier on est allé à Saint-Louis pour faire le tour de la ville. L'Afrique me plaît beaucoup! Je n'ai pas envie de rentrer!*
>
> *Grosses bises,*
> *Alexandre*

 ## Enquête culturelle

Planes from all over the world use the international airports of Roissy-Charles de Gaulle and Orly. Both on the outskirts of Paris, Roissy is to the north and Orly is to the south of the city. Air France and Air Inter are the two French nationally owned airlines.

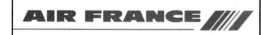

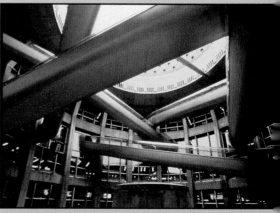

Escalators enclosed in glass tubes crisscross the center of the main terminal at Roissy-Charles de Gaulle.

The Ivory Coast received its name from French sailors who traded for ivory in this West African country in the fifteenth century. It became independent from France in 1960 and has rapidly developed into one of

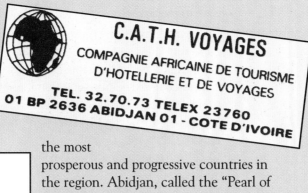

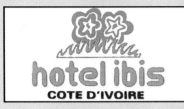

the most prosperous and progressive countries in the region. Abidjan, called the "Pearl of Africa," is the Ivory Coast's largest city and the main seaport on the Atlantic Ocean. Tourists enjoy water sports on Abidjan's beautiful beaches.

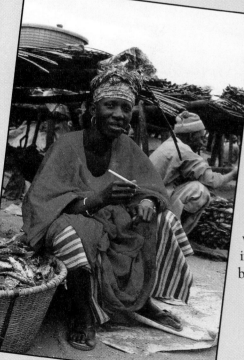

Although Senegal also became independent from France, it keeps close cultural and economic ties with the country that governed it for 300 years. About the size of South Dakota, Senegal has a landscape that varies from dry land in the north near the Sahara Desert, to grassy plains in the center, to rain forests in the southwest. Its 7 million people belong to a variety of ethnic groups. French is taught in schools and used in government, business and the media. However, most

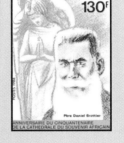

Mme Diouf speaks the Senegalese national language, Wolof.

Senegalese also speak Wolof, the national language. From the modern capital of Dakar to the seventeenth century French settlement at Saint-Louis to the tiny fishing village of Cayar, from peanut farms to wildlife preserves, Senegal is a country full of contrasts.

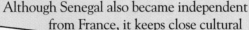

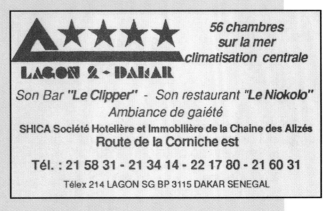

1 | *Répondez en français.*

1. Est-ce qu'Alexandre et ses parents sont allés en Afrique ou est-ce qu'ils sont allés en Europe?
2. De quel aéroport est-ce que l'avion est parti?
3. Où est-ce qu'Alexandre et sa famille sont arrivés?
4. Qui habite en Côte-d'Ivoire?
5. Où est-ce qu'Alexandre et ses parents sont allés après quatre jours en Côte-d'Ivoire?
6. Où est-ce que la famille d'Alexandre est allée le premier jour au Sénégal?
7. Est-ce qu'Alexandre aime l'Afrique?
8. Est-ce qu'Alexandre veut rentrer?

2 | Based on which country they come from, describe the following people's nationality.

Modèle:

Hanako vient du Japon.
Elle est japonaise.

1. Brigitte vient de Belgique.
2. Abdou vient de Côte-d'Ivoire.
3. Yasmine vient de Tunisie.
4. Bernard vient de Suisse.
5. Paul vient du Luxembourg.

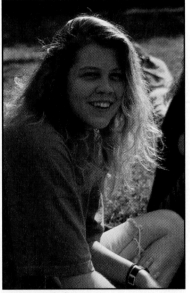

Brigitte est belge.

Amina est sénégalaise.

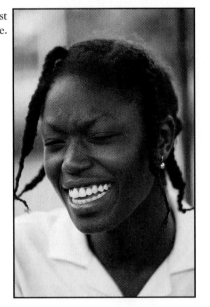

6. Malika vient du Maroc.
7. Sonia vient du Zaïre.
8. Salim vient d'Algérie.
9. Amina vient du Sénégal.

3 | *C'est à toi!*

1. Est-ce que tu as des amis sénégalais ou ivoiriens?
2. Est-ce que tu es allé(e) en Afrique?
3. Aimes-tu voyager en avion?
4. Est-ce que tu préfères voyager avec ta famille ou avec tes amis?
5. Vas-tu souvent chez ta grand-mère?
6. Ta grand-mère et ton grand-père, d'où viennent-ils?
7. Qu'est-ce que tu as envie de faire après les cours aujourd'hui?

Structure

Ordinal numbers

You have already learned cardinal (or counting) numbers in French (**un, deux, trois**, etc.). Numbers like "first," "second" and "third" are called ordinal numbers because they show the order in which things are placed. All ordinal numbers in French, except **premier** and **première**, end in **-ième**. To form most ordinal numbers, add **-ième** to the cardinal number. If a cardinal number ends in **-e,** drop this **e** before adding **-ième.** Here are cardinal numbers and their corresponding ordinal numbers from "first" through "tenth." Note that "first," "fifth" and "ninth" are formed irregularly.

un, une	→	premier (m.), première (f.)
deux	→	deuxième
trois	→	troisième
quatre	→	quatrième
cinq	→	cinquième
six	→	sixième
sept	→	septième
huit	→	huitième
neuf	→	neuvième
dix	→	dixième

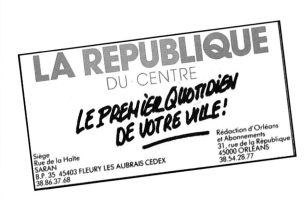

C'est mon premier voyage en Afrique.

This is my first trip to Africa.

Le deuxième jour nous sommes revenus à Dakar.

On the second day we came back to Dakar.

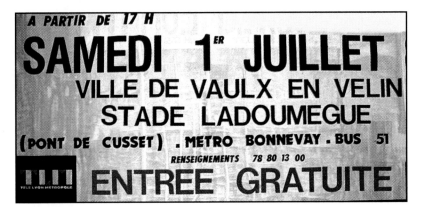

Pratique

4 Tell the order of each day of the week using the appropriate ordinal number. (Remember that Monday is the first day of the week on the French calendar.)

1. vendredi
2. dimanche
3. mercredi
4. samedi
5. jeudi
6. lundi

Modèle:

mardi
Mardi est le deuxième jour de la semaine.

5 Planes from various countries are in France for an air show. As they wait to take off, give each plane's place in line.

Modèle:

l'avion américain

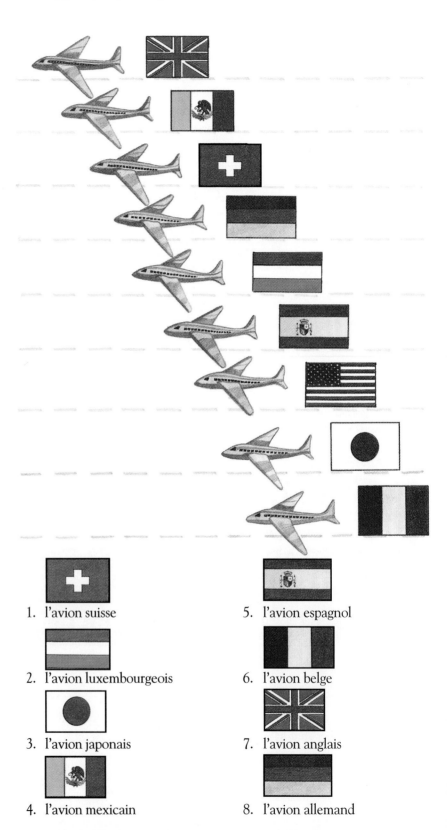

L'avion américain est le septième.

1. l'avion suisse

2. l'avion luxembourgeois

3. l'avion japonais

4. l'avion mexicain

5. l'avion espagnol

6. l'avion belge

7. l'avion anglais

8. l'avion allemand

Prepositions before cities, countries and continents

You have already learned that **au** is used to express "to" or "in" before countries with masculine names. Use **aux** if the country has a masculine plural name.

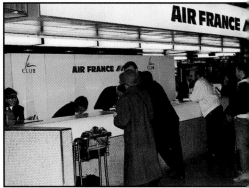

M. et Mme Foch vont aux États-Unis.

Tu vas au Sénégal?	*Are you going to Senegal?*
Non, je vais aux États-Unis.	*No, I'm going to the United States.*

Use **en** before countries or continents with feminine names.

Nous allons en Côte-d'Ivoire en Afrique.	*We're going to the Ivory Coast in Africa.*

Use **à** before the names of cities.

On est allé à Abidjan.	*We went to Abidjan.*

Pratique

5   Tell which of the following cities each person lives in, based on the country he or she is from.

Tokyo	Paris	Genève	Berlin
Boston	Toronto	Madrid	Rome

1. Mme Anderson vient des États-Unis.
2. Alejandro vient d'Espagne.
3. Monika vient d'Allemagne.
4. Mauro vient d'Italie.
5. Mlle Callaghan vient du Canada.
6. M. Hamada vient du Japon.
7. Bernard vient de Suisse.

Modèle:

M. Arnaud vient de France.
Il habite à Paris.

All the foreign exchange students are getting ready to go home at the end of the school year. Tell what country each student is returning to.

1. Tatsuo, l'élève japonais
2. Phong, l'élève vietnamienne
3. Karim, l'élève tunisien
4. Zakia, l'élève zaïroise
5. Isabelle, l'élève belge
6. Ousmane, l'élève sénégalais
7. Assia, l'élève marocaine
8. Nora, l'élève algérienne
9. Ricardo, l'élève espagnol
10. Charles, l'élève anglais

Modèle:

Fabrice, l'élève luxembourgeois
Il rentre au Luxembourg.

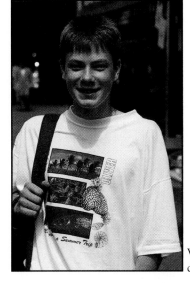

Will rentre au Canada dans une semaine.

Modèles:

Abidjan/la Côte-d'Ivoire
Student A: Abidjan est en Côte-d'Ivoire?
Student B: Oui, Abidjan est en Côte-d'Ivoire.

Paris/le Zaïre
Student B: Paris est au Zaïre?
Student A: Non, Paris est en France.

Modèle:

Le premier jour nous sommes arrivés à Dakar, au Sénégal.

8 With a partner, take turns asking and answering questions about where certain cities are located.

1. Bruxelles/le Mexique
2. Dallas/les États-Unis
3. Tours/l'Allemagne
4. Dakar/l'Italie
5. Montréal/le Canada
6. Lausanne/le Japon
7. Rabat/la Chine

Communication

9 You and your family spent 10 days traveling through Africa visiting various French-speaking countries. During your trip you kept a journal. Now that you're back home, you need to write a summary to put at the top of each day's entry to help you remember details. For each day, write where you were (city or village, and country). Use the map to help you remember your itinerary as you write your summaries. (Make sure that the order of the countries you visited and the time spent in each one are realistic.) The first day has been done for you.

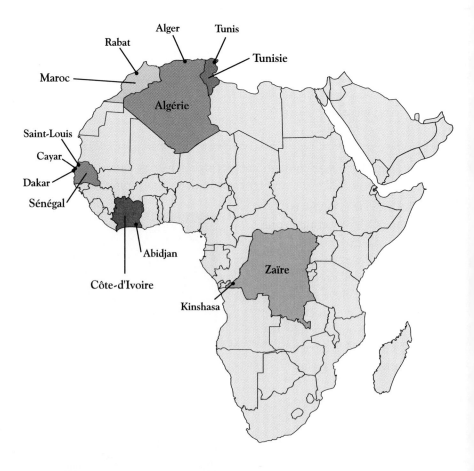

0 You didn't have time during your trip to French-speaking Africa to buy any postcards. Once you returned home, you decided to make your own. Do some research on one of the countries you visited: Senegal, the Ivory Coast, Zaire, Morocco, Tunisia or Algeria. Look for current information on this country in your school's resource center or instructional materials center. Then design an original postcard. On one side, draw something that you found interesting about this country (for example, the scenery). On the other side, write a friend's name and address and a message in French about your visit to this country. In your note, be sure to describe your drawing, tell where you went and say how much you liked what you saw and did.

Mise au point sur... le monde francophone

The rich vocabulary, colorful expressions and precise structures of the French language extend beyond the borders of France itself. During hundreds of years of colonial expansion, the French people spread their language and culture throughout the world. Today, nearly 200 million people use French in their daily lives; millions more understand this international language. Even humor, certain manners of thinking and gestures are shared by the variety of people around the globe who communicate in French.

Some French citizens, such as those in Corsica, live beyond France's borders. This Mediterranean island, near the west coast of Italy, is one of metropolitan France's 96 administrative divisions (**départements**). Outside of Europe, some French citizens live in France's overseas departments (**Départements d'Outre-Mer**): Martinique and Guadeloupe in the Caribbean, Réunion in the Indian Ocean and French Guiana in South America. Residents of these departments enjoy all the rights that mainland French citizens have.

People in France's overseas territories (**Territoires d'Outre-Mer**) also maintain close cultural and economic ties with France. Although they have no voice in French politics, the French government protects them in times of international crisis. Among these territories are French Polynesia, a group of islands in the South Pacific, and New Caledonia, an island near Australia.

In Europe, several countries bordering France have designated French as one of their official languages. People in parts of Belgium, Luxembourg and Switzerland speak French at home and when they travel or do business in neighboring countries. In the tiny principality of Monaco, near the Italian border but surrounded on three sides by France, the only official language is French.

In North America, many Canadians speak both French and English. Throughout the country, communication in government, business, schools and entertainment is usually

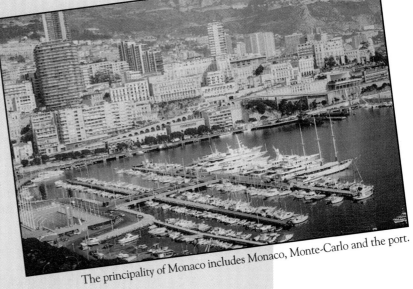

The principality of Monaco includes Monaco, Monte-Carlo and the port.

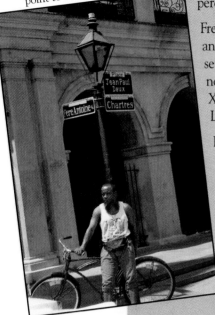

In Louisiana many street signs point to the area's French heritage.

bilingual. In the Province of Quebec, French is the native language of almost 80 percent of the population and has been named the only official language.

French and French-Canadian settlers in New England brought the French language and culture to the United States. Both Creoles, descendants of the original French settlers, and Cajuns, whose French-Canadian ancestors were called "Acadians," now live in Louisiana. In fact, Louisiana was named after the French king Louis XIV. Names of cities such as Pierre (South Dakota), Des Moines (Iowa), Saint Louis (Missouri) and Boise (Idaho) reflect the French presence in America.

France once had the largest colonial empire in Africa. People in more than 20 African countries speak French, even though all these countries have gained their independence. Because these people represent various ethnic groups, French is often used as the common language of communication. Many people in **le Maghreb** and on the large island of Madagascar off the eastern coast of Africa communicate in French on a daily basis. In West Africa, the French influence still remains strong in the Ivory Coast, Zaire and Senegal.

France's former colonial empire extended far beyond the African continent. Today many people living in Haiti in the Caribbean and in Vietnam, Cambodia and Laos in Southeast Asia also speak French.

People all over the world use French in their daily lives. As the world continues to become smaller and smaller through faster means of communication and greater travel opportunities, the French language remains a key to understanding for vast numbers of people.

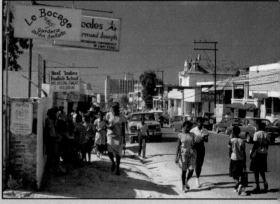

French is the official language of Haiti, but many people speak Creole. (Port-au-Prince)

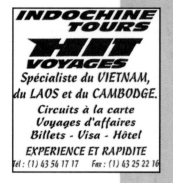

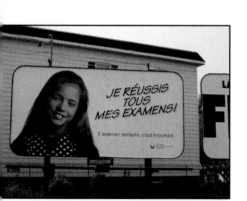

French is everywhere in Quebec, even on billboards.

11 | Answer the following questions.

1. How did the French language and culture originally spread throughout the world?
2. What French department is located in the Mediterranean?
3. Which overseas department of France is in South America?
4. What are two of the French overseas territories?
5. What are the names of three European countries (other than France) where many people speak French?
6. In what Canadian province is French the only official language?
7. What are the two major areas of the United States settled by the French and French Canadians?
8. What cities do you know in the United States that have French names?
9. Why do various ethnic groups in some African countries still use French?
10. What are three former French colonies in Southeast Asia?

2 Look at the Air France schedule of flights from Paris to five different French-speaking cities throughout the world. To answer the questions that follow, you will need to know that on the schedule the days of the week are numbered from one (Monday) to seven (Sunday), **départ** means "departure," an **A** or a **G** after the departure time indicates Roissy-Charles de Gaulle, an **S** after the departure time indicates Orly, and **arrivée** means "arrival."

1. You can fly from Paris to four of these cities every day of the week. Which city does not have daily service?
2. At what time does a flight from Paris to Casablanca leave every day of the week? From which airport does this flight leave?
3. On what two days is there only one flight from Paris to Montreal?
4. If you want to fly to Montreal on Monday, from which airport would you leave?
5. At what time does the plane for Papeete leave Paris on Friday?
6. How many flights from Paris to Dakar leave on Saturday?
7. Does the 10:15 A.M. flight from Paris to Abidjan get in earlier or later than the flight leaving Paris at 10:45 A.M.?
8. If you want to fly to Dakar on Sunday and arrive there in the early afternoon, at what time would your flight leave?
9. If you want to fly to Abidjan on a 747 but don't want to fly at night, what day would you leave?
10. The 12:30 P.M. flight from Paris to Montreal arrives at 2:05 P.M. Why is there only about an hour and a half difference between departure and arrival times for this transatlantic flight?

ABIDJAN
Côte d'Ivoire.   ABJ
Port-Bouet 16 km.   GMT
Taxi 2500 CFA
Taxe 1000 CFA
UTA/AF 11 av. Anoma.
BP 1527
☎ 33 22 31.

Jours	Départ		Arrivée		Avion		Vol	
1								
2	12	00G	X	18	50	D10	FY	RK 047	
2	08	45G	R	15	35	D10	FJY	UT 803	
3	23	59G	X	07	05a	D10	FY	RK 023	
3	10	30G	X	17	40	D10	FY	RK 081	
4	10	40G	R	19	10	747	FJY	UT 831	
4	15	30G	R	22	05	D10	FJY	UT 807	
5	23	45G	X	05	00a	747	FJY	UT 837	
5	10	15G	X	18	05	D10	FY	RK 027	
5	10	45G	X	17	30	D10	FY	RK 031	
6	22	15G	T	05	00a	D10	FJY	UT 801	
6	11	20G	R	18	15	D10	FY	RK 805	
7	22	15G	X	06	30a	AB4	FY	RK 021	
7	13	00G	X	20	50	D10	FY	RK 041	
	22	40G	T	05	30a	747	FJY	UT 809	

CASABLANCA
Maroc   CAS
Mohammed V 35 km   GMT
car 20 dirhams
15 av. de l'Armée Royale
☎ 22 41 33 - R : 27 42 42

3	09	15S	T	11	10	727	CY	AFAT2045	
12-4	09	15S	T	11	10	727	CY	AFAT2017	
5-7	09	15S	T	11	10	AB3	CY	AFAT2045	
6	09	15S	T	11	10	AB3	CY	AFAT2017	
7	15	00S	R	17	55	757	FY	ATAF781	
1-4-	15	00S	R	16	55	727	FY	ATAF703	
23-5-	15	00S	R	17	55	727	Y	ATAF781	
1234567	17	00S	R	22	00	737	FY	ATAF783	
1-4567	18	30S	R	20	25	727	FY	ATAF751	
5--	19	50S	R	22	45	727	CY	AFAT2035	
	20	00S	R	23	20	727	Y	ATAF723	

MERIDIEN ☎ 36 35 35
Telex 24692

DAKAR Sénégal   DKR
Yoff 17 km   GMT
47 av. A. Sarrault BP 142
☎ 22 29 41 - R : 22 49 49

1	09	35A	X	14	20	AB3	FY	AF 301	
1	10	00G	X	16	30	AB4	FY	RK 007	
2	07	45A	R	14	10	AB3	FY	AF 303	
2	11	00G	X	17	00	AB4	FY	RK 019	
3	07	45A	T	13	55	AB3	FY	AF 305	
3	12	00G	R	19	55	AB4	FY	RK 011	
4	11	30G	X	18	10	AB3	Y	AF 309	
4	15	00G	R	22	20	D10	FY	RK 003	
5	15	30A	X	20	50	AB3	FY	AF 315	
5	23	59G	T	04	50a	AB4	FY	RK 017	
5	15	00G	X	21	15	D10	FY	RKAF015	
6	15	50A	R	22	20	AB3	FY	AF 317	
6	23	59G	X	07	30a	DC8	FY	RK 035	
7	08	00A	P	12	45	AB3	YM	AFRK321	
7	13	40A	X	19	45	AB3	FY	RK 009	
7	18	00G	X	23	59	AB4			

MONTREAL Canada   YUL
Mirabel 53 km   - 5
car 8 dollars
979 Ouest b. de Maisonneuve
☎ (514) 284 2825

1234567	14	20G	P	15	45	747	FJY	AC 871	
23-56-	12	30A	X	14	05	74M	FJY	AF 033	
7	15	30A	X	17	05	74M	FJY	AF 033	

PAPEETE Tahiti   PPT
Faaa 6 km   - 10
c/o Air Polynésie
BP 314
☎ 42 23 33

3	19	15G	X	05	45a	D10	FJY	UT 501	
5	13	00A	X	22	55	747	FJY	AF 007	
6	19	15G	X	05	45a	D10	FJY	UT 503	

© 15790 F du 7/11 au 11/1

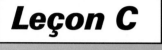

Leçon C

In this lesson you will be able to:

➤ inquire about details

➤ identify objects

➤ tell location

➤ give addresses

➤ ask for information

➤ give directions

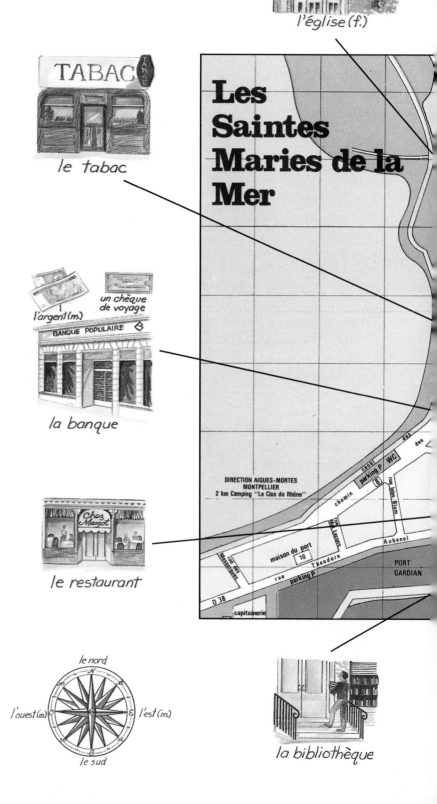

l'église (f.)

le tabac

Les Saintes Maries de la Mer

l'argent (m.) un chèque de voyage

BANQUE POPULAIRE

la banque

DIRECTION AIGUES-MORTES
MONTPELLIER
2 km Camping "Le Clos du Rhône"

Chez Margot

le restaurant

le nord

l'ouest (m.) l'est (m.)

le sud

la bibliothèque

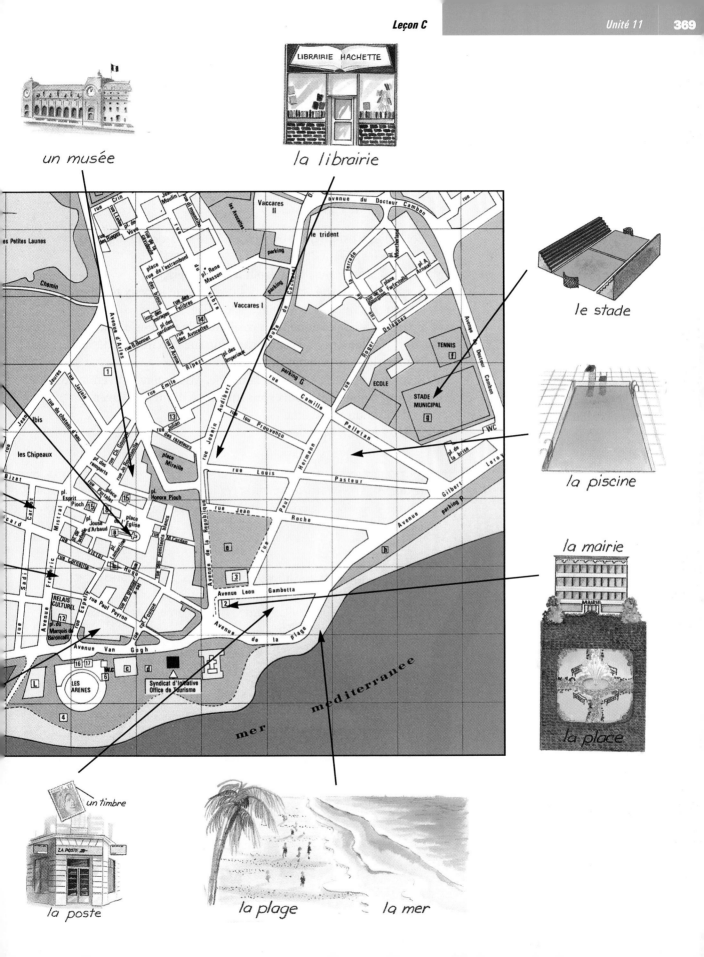

un musée

la librairie

le stade

la piscine

la mairie

la place

un timbre

la poste

la plage   la mer

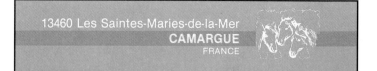

13460 Les Saintes-Maries-de-la-Mer
CAMARGUE
FRANCE

The Borde family from Luxembourg is camping near Les Saintes-Maries-de-la-Mer, the capital of the Camargue region of southern France. M. Borde questions M. Rivoire, the director of the campground, about the camping facilities and the nearby town.

M. Borde: **Qu'est-ce que vous avez à faire ici au camping pour les enfants?**

M. Rivoire: **Vous voyez, tout droit, il y a une piscine.**

M. Borde: **Oui, je vois la piscine. Et est-ce que je peux toucher des chèques de voyage dans le village?**

M. Rivoire: **Oui, la banque n'est pas loin. Elle est près d'ici... à 1,5 kilomètres à l'est du camping sur l'avenue Frédéric Mistral.**

M. Borde: **Et pour acheter des timbres?**

M. Rivoire: **La poste est près de la mairie. Vous prenez l'avenue de la République, puis vous tournez à droite sur l'avenue Léon Gambetta.**

M. Borde: **Merci, Monsieur.**

Enquête culturelle

One of Europe's oldest and smallest countries, Luxembourg lies northeast of France. Known as **le cœur vert de l'Europe** because of its landscape of thick forests and rolling hills, its capital city is also called Luxembourg.

Located in the delta formed by **le Rhône** as it enters the Mediterranean Sea, the Camargue region is famous for its environmental reserve and bird sanctuary, white horses, groups of semi-wild black bulls guarded by men on horseback, rose flamingos, marshes and vast rice paddies.

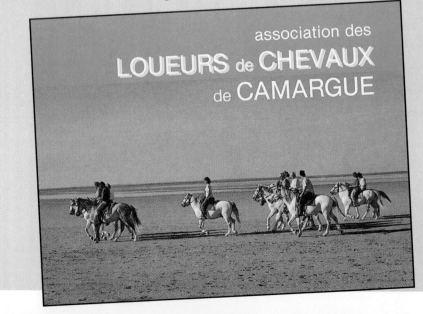

association des
LOUEURS de CHEVAUX
de CAMARGUE

Les Saintes-Maries-de-la-Mer is named after
Marie-Jacobé and Marie-Salomé, who came
across the Mediterranean Sea by boat in the
early Christian era. Residents say that the local
church contains the relics of the two Maries and
of Sara, their

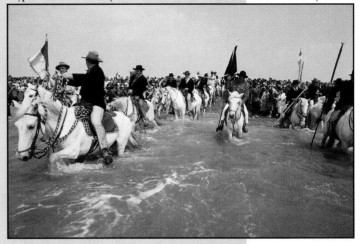

Gypsies make their way to Les Saintes-Maries-de-la-Mer twice each year.

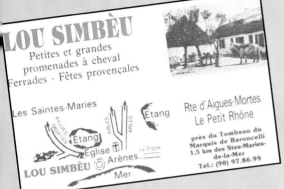

servant, who became the patron
saint of the Gypsies. Annual Gypsy
pilgrimages to the town take place in May and October.

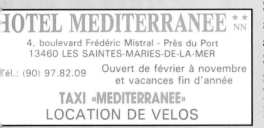

Streets in France are often named
after famous people. For example, the
avenue Frédéric Mistral in Les
Saintes-Maries-de-la-Mer honors a
famous French poet who won the
Nobel Prize in literature in 1904.
Mistral wrote in Provençal, a French
dialect spoken in southern France.

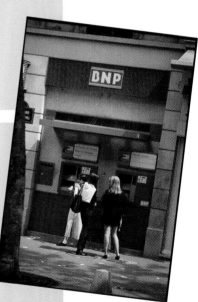

You can change money and traveler's checks in France at **la banque** or **le bureau
de change** (*money exchange*). Or, using a credit card, you can get money from an
ATM (**un distributeur**) at a more favorable
exchange rate.

An automated teller machine in
French is called *un distributeur* or *un
guichet automatique*. (Paris)

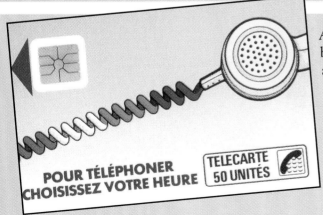

At a post office you can
buy stamps, send letters
and packages, use public
telephones, buy **télécartes**
(*phone cards to use in public
phone booths*) and use the
Minitel. Some French
people even pay their gas
and telephone bills at the
post office.

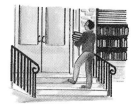

Stamps and phone cards are also sold at **le tabac (le bureau de tabac)**. A distinctive reddish-orange sign with the word **TABAC** on it makes these shops easy to recognize at a distance.

A French *tabac* usually sells newspapers, magazines, postcards, candy, lottery tickets, stamps and *télécartes*.

1 | *Qu'est-ce que c'est?* Identify the places you see in the illustrations.

Modèle:

C'est une bibliothèque.

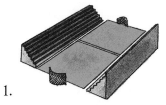
1.

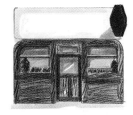
6.

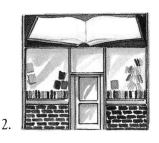
2.

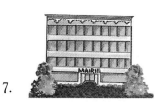
7.

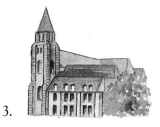
3.

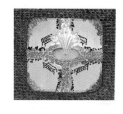
8.

9.

5.

2   Imagine that you are a teenager in the Borde family that is camping near Les Saintes-Maries-de-la-Mer. Write a postcard to your friend Yvette back home. In your postcard,

1. give the date.
2. greet Yvette.
3. tell her that your family is at the campground near Les Saintes-Maries-de-la-Mer.
4. tell her that there is a swimming pool at the campground.
5. tell her that you like camping a lot.
6. tell her that your father needs to go to the bank to cash traveler's checks.
7. tell her that he is also going to the post office to buy some stamps.
8. say that you'll see her soon.
9. give a closing and sign your name.

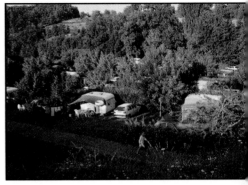

Est-ce que le camping vous plaît beaucoup? (Collonges-la-Rouge)

3   Write a sentence in French telling what you do at each of the following places.

1. l'aéroport
2. la poste
3. la banque
4. le centre commercial
5. la librairie
6. le stade
7. le restaurant
8. l'école

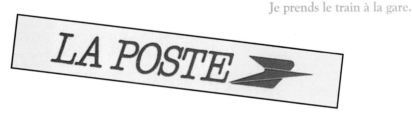

Modèle:

la gare
Je prends le train à la gare.

4   *C'est à toi!*

1. Sur quelle avenue est ta maison ou ton appartement?
2. Ton école est à combien de kilomètres de ta maison ou de ton appartement?
3. Est-ce que ton école est au nord, au sud, à l'est ou à l'ouest de ta maison ou de ton appartement?
4. Qui est à gauche de toi en cours de français?
5. Est-ce que tu préfères acheter des livres à la librairie ou lire à la bibliothèque?
6. Est-ce que tu vas souvent à la banque?
7. Est-ce que tu aimes le camping?
8. Est-ce que tu préfères nager à la piscine ou à la mer?

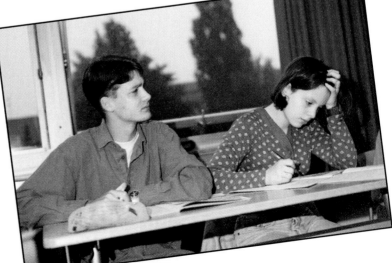

Étienne est à gauche de Joanne.

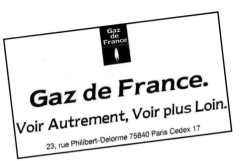

Structure

Present tense of the irregular verb *voir*

The verb **voir** (*to see*) is irregular.

voir			
je	**vois**	Je **vois** la piscine.	*I see the swimming pool.*
tu	**vois**	Tu ne **vois** pas la banque?	*Don't you see the bank?*
il/elle/on	**voit**	Elle ne **voit** jamais ses cousins.	*She never sees her cousins.*
nous	**voyons**	Nous **voyons** tout le monde.	*We see everybody.*
vous	**voyez**	Qu'est-ce que vous **voyez**?	*What do you see?*
ils/elles	**voient**	Ils **voient** le train.	*They see the train.*

Pratique

5   As you report where certain people are, tell what they see, choosing from the following list of people and things.

Modèle:

Magali est au centre commercial. Elle voit des boutiques.

des livres	beaucoup de timbres	la mer	des avions
la réceptionniste	des boutiques	une serveuse	des baguettes

1. Abdel-Cader est à la librairie. Il....
2. Vous êtes à la boulangerie. Vous....
3. M. et Mme Potvin sont au restaurant. Ils....
4. Je suis au cabinet du docteur Vaillancourt. Je....
5. Cécile est à la plage. Elle....
6. Les demi-sœurs de Catherine sont à la poste. Elles....
7. Tu es à l'aéroport. Tu....

6   You and your friends are meeting at a café in Les Saintes-Maries-de-la-Mer. Because you're all coming from different places in town, you take different routes. Tell what you see on your way to the café.

Modèle:

Béatrice et son frère/mer
Béatrice et son frère voient la mer.

1. tu/piscine
2. les garçons/stade
3. Karima et moi/plage
4. Djamel et toi/poste
5. Clarence/église
6. je/bibliothèque
7. Sara et son cousin/musée
8. Véro/banque

Communication

7 You and some of your classmates are working together on a project for French class. You're planning to all get together after school today at your house to complete it. Since these classmates have never been to your house before, write a note that you can copy and pass out to them, giving detailed directions from school to your house.

8 You and your French host family have been visiting the Camargue region and staying in Les Saintes-Maries-de-la-Mer. Since you are going to leave the area today, you have decided to take some final pictures. You're staying at a hotel near the tennis courts on the **Avenue du Docteur Cambon**. You plan to meet your family at **Les Arènes** near the center of town. Using the map, explain to them how to get from the hotel to where you will be.

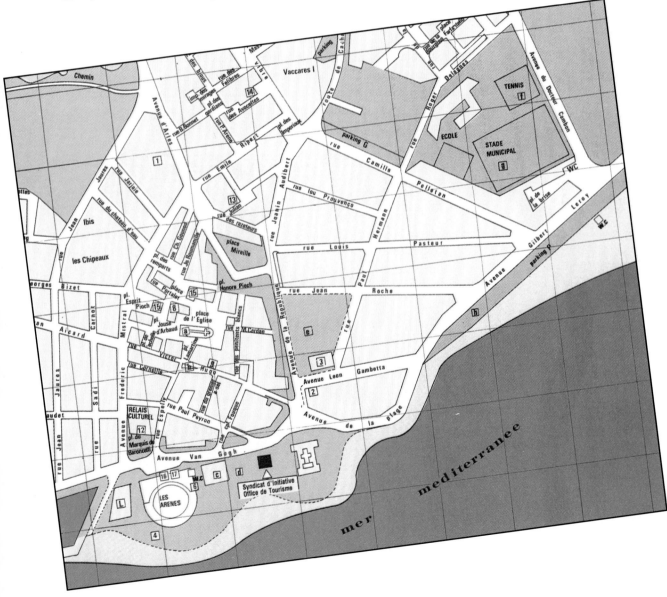

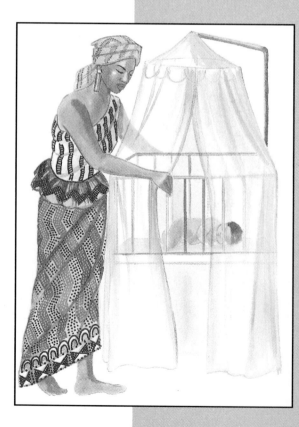

Sur la bonne piste

In previous units you learned about and practiced a variety of strategies to help you read in French. Now try to make use of all of them as you read *Dors mon enfant*, an African poem.

Cameroonian author Elalongué Epanya Yondo wrote *Dors mon enfant* during Cameroon's struggle for independence from France and England in the late 1950s and early 1960s. (Cameroon is a country in western equatorial Africa. The official languages of Cameroon are French and English.)

Use the following reading strategies to help you understand what the poem means:

1. Take advantage of the clues provided by the *illustration* to predict what the poem is about and to figure out the meaning of words you haven't seen before.
2. *Skim* the poem to figure out its context.
3. Identify *cognates* to try to make sense of the poem as a whole.
4. *Think in French* as you read the poem. Resist the temptation to translate it word for word into English.
5. Avoid "seeing" the poem through the eyes of an American. Instead, try to form mental pictures that take into account possible *cultural differences*.
6. Practice the technique of *inference*: use the context of the words you know to help you understand the ones you don't know.
7. Read the poem critically—that is, *evaluate* the information it contains.
8. *Scan* the poem to hunt for precise ideas or words that will help you answer the questions that follow it.

DORS MON ENFANT

Dors mon enfant dors
Quand tu dors
Tu es beau
Comme un oranger fleuri.

Dors mon enfant dors
Dors comme
La mer haute
Caressée par les clapotis
De la brise
Qui vient mourir en woua-woua
Au pied de la plage sablonneuse.

Dors mon enfant dors
Dors mon beau bébé noir
Comme la promesse
D'une nuit de lune
Au regard de l'Aube
Qui naît sur ton sommeil.

Dors mon enfant dors
Tu es si beau
Quand tu dors
Mon beau bébé noir dors.

Elalongué Epanya Yondo, *Kamerun! Kamerun!*

9   Scan the poem to find answers to the following questions.

1. What does the illustration suggest that the poem is about? If the poem is a song, what kind of song do you think it is?
2. Try to "see" the illustration as it would be drawn if the poem were set in the United States. What cultural differences are there between your mental picture and the illustration? Are there any similarities?
3. Can you figure out what the word **dors** means in the title of the poem? Look for clues in the illustration and use the context of the other words you already know in the title to help you. (Hint: **dors** is a form of an infinitive you've seen before.)
4. What words in the poem are cognates?
5. The poem states that the child is beautiful. Is this a fact or an opinion? If it is an opinion, whose opinion is it?
6. A simile compares two different things that share some quality. A simile often uses the word "like." In the poem the mother first compares the beauty of her son to a flowering orange tree, using the word **comme**. What two other comparisons does the mother make?
7. Cameroon is very close to the equator. What can you see in the illustration and find in the poem itself about the climate and location of the country?
8. The poem represents the hope of the mother for her son's future. Recalling the political conditions during which the author wrote the poem, do you see a relationship between the child and Cameroon? What is it?

Nathalie et Raoul

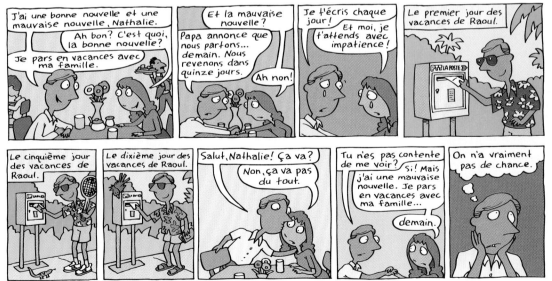

C'est à moi!

Now that you have completed this unit, take a look at what you should be able to do in French. Can you do all of these tasks?

➤ I can write a postcard.

➤ I can talk about what happened in the past.

➤ I can talk about things sequentially.

➤ I can ask for detailed information.

➤ I can tell location.

➤ I can give directions.

➤ I can give addresses.

➤ I can identify objects.

➤ I can tell what I like.

➤ I can state my preference.

➤ I can express emotions.

Here is a brief checkup to see how much you understand about French culture. Decide if each statement is **vrai** or **faux**.

1. The **SNCF**, the government-owned company that operates French trains, is well known for its prompt, affordable service.
2. Belgians are divided into four groups according to the languages they speak.
3. During the fifteenth century French sailors named the Ivory Coast for the ivory they traded there.
4. Senegal has close economic and cultural ties with France because it is one of the few African colonies still governed by France.
5. Almost 200 million people speak French around the world.
6. France is divided into nearly 100 administrative divisions called **départements**.
7. Although French is spoken in many African countries, France is the only French-speaking country in Europe.
8. In North America, the French influence is especially strong in the Province of Quebec in Canada and in Louisiana.
9. Les Saintes-Maries-de-la-Mer is a town near the mouth of the Rhône River that hosts Gypsy pilgrimages.
10. You can buy **télécartes** at the post office and at **le tabac**.

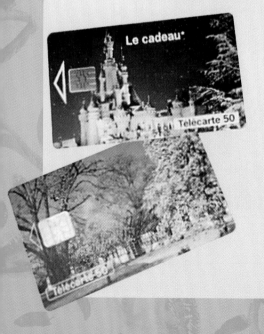

Communication orale

Imagine that you and your partner have returned from trips to a French-speaking country. One partner went to a French-speaking country in Europe, and the other partner went to a French-speaking country in Africa. Begin your conversation by greeting each other. Then ask and tell where (in what country and city) you arrived. Next ask and tell where you went in the country you visited. Finally, ask and tell when you returned home. Finish your conversation by asking and telling each other how much you like what you saw and did. (If you've already been on a trip to a French-speaking country, you will probably want to talk about this country in your conversation. Be sure to include some of your experiences there.)

Communication écrite

Your teacher overheard some of your conversation about your trips to a French-speaking country and wants to find out more information about both trips. Write out in French a description of both trips, based on the information you gave your partner and heard from your partner in your previous conversation. Also add any additional information about the places you both visited that you learned during your study of French-speaking countries. Finally, mention two other French-speaking countries you would like to see and tell why you would like to see them.

Communication active

To write postcards, use:

Cher (Chère)..., — *Dear . . . ,*
Grosses bises, — *Big kisses,*

To describe past events, use:

Je **suis sorti(e)** avec mes amis. — *I went out with my friends.*
Nous **sommes allés** au cinéma. — *We went to the movies.*
On **est revenu** à minuit. — *We came back at midnight.*
Vous **êtes rentrés** en Suisse. — *You returned to Switzerland.*
L'avion **est parti** de Roissy-Charles de Gaulle. — *The plane left Roissy-Charles de Gaulle.*
Il **est arrivé** à Genève à 20h00. — *It arrived in Geneva at 8:00 P.M.*
Chantal **est entrée** dans l'aéroport. — *Chantal entered the airport.*
Ses frères **sont venus** aussi. — *Her brothers came also.*
Pourquoi **es-tu resté** chez toi? — *Why did you stay home?*

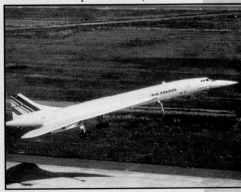

Le Concorde est parti de Roissy.

To sequence events, use:

Le premier jour.... — *The first day . . . .*
Après quatre **jours....** — *After four days . . . .*
Hier.... — *Yesterday . . . .*
Aujourd'hui.... — *Today . . . .*
Demain.... — *Tomorrow . . . .*

To ask for information, use:

Et pour acheter des timbres?

And (where do I go) to buy stamps?

To inquire about details, use:

Qu'est-ce que vous avez **à faire ici?**

What's there to do here?

To tell location, use:

Mon père est parti **pour** Bruxelles **en** Belgique.

My father left for Brussels in Belgium.

Les Caron sont arrivés **à** Boston **aux** États-Unis.

The Carons arrived in Boston in the United States.

Après une semaine, ils sont allés à la plage **au** Mexique.

After one week, they went to the beach in Mexico.

Il y a une banque **près d'ici.**

There's a bank near here.

La banque n'est pas **loin.**

The bank isn't far.

Il/Elle est à 5 kilomètres.

It's 5 kilometers.

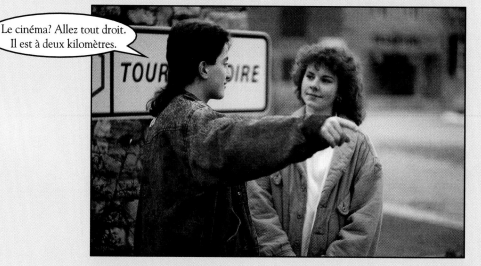

Le cinéma? Allez tout droit. Il est à deux kilomètres.

Il/Elle est au nord. — *It's (to the) north.*
Il/Elle est à l'est. — *It's (to the) east.*
Il/Elle est au sud. — *It's (to the) south.*
Il/Elle est à l'ouest. — *It's (to the) west.*
Il/Elle est à gauche. — *It's on the left.*
Il/Elle est à droite. — *It's on the right.*
Il/Elle est tout droit. — *It's straight ahead.*

To give directions, use:

Allez tout droit.

Go straight ahead.

Vous prenez l'avenue Foch.

You take Foch Avenue.

Vous tournez à droite/gauche sur l'avenue du Maine.

You turn right/left on Maine Avenue.

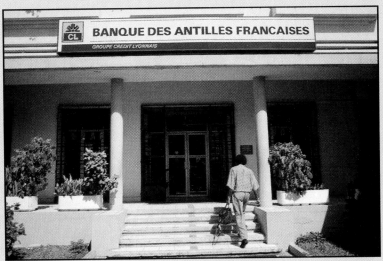

La banque est sur l'avenue du Maine. (Pointe-à-Pitre)

To give an address, use:

Il/Elle est sur l'avenue
Victor Hugo.

It's on Victor Hugo Avenue.

To identify objects, use:

Il y a une piscine.

There is a swimming pool.

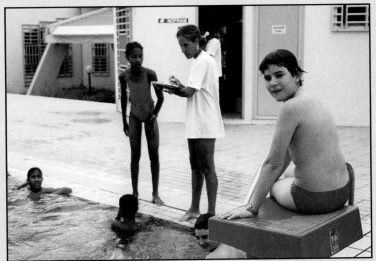

Il y a une piscine.

To say what you like, use:

L'Afrique **me plaît** beaucoup!

I like Africa a lot!

To state a preference, use:

J'ai envie de rentrer!

I want to come home!

To express emotions, use:

Ce séjour **est formidable!**

This stay is terrific!

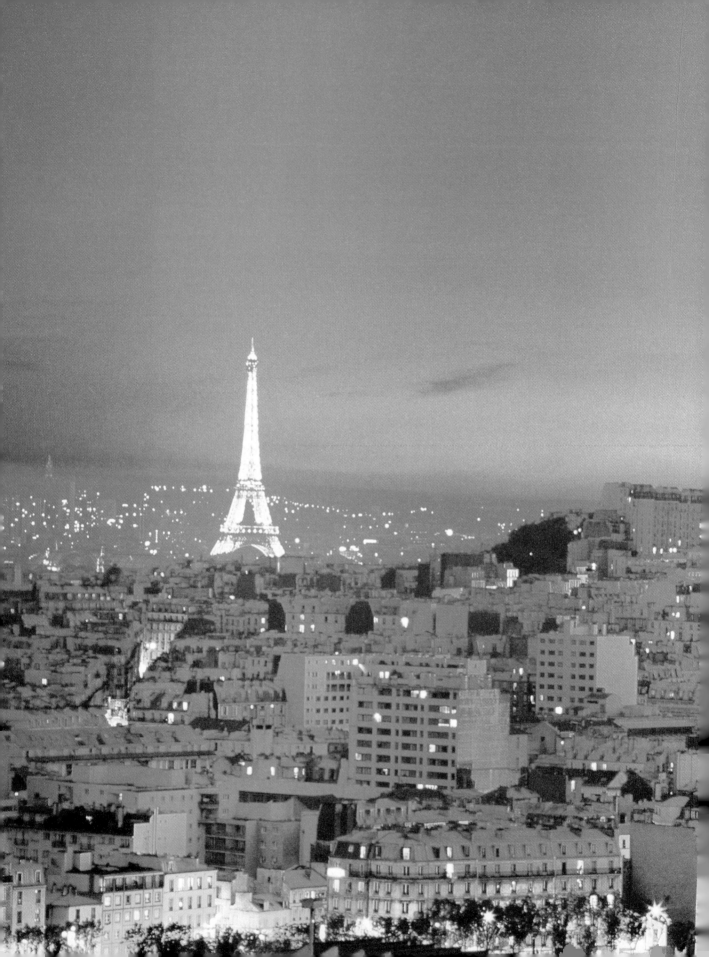

Unité 12

À Paris

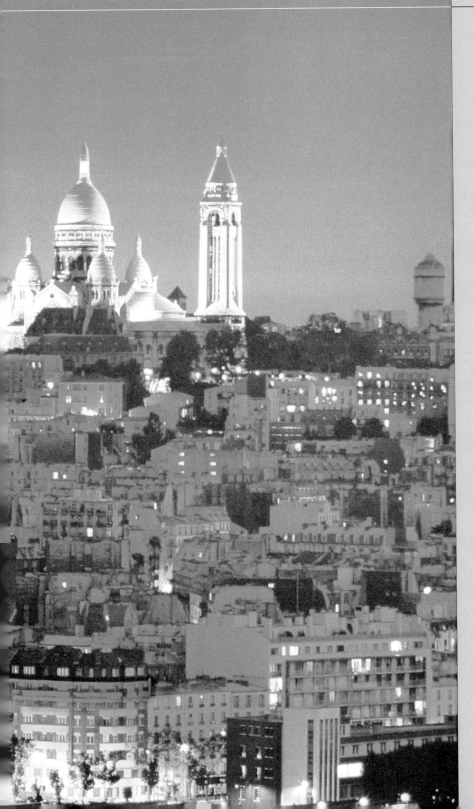

In this unit you will be able to:

➤ **write journal entries**

➤ **describe past events**

➤ **sequence events**

➤ **express need and necessity**

➤ **ask for information**

➤ **give opinions**

➤ **compare things**

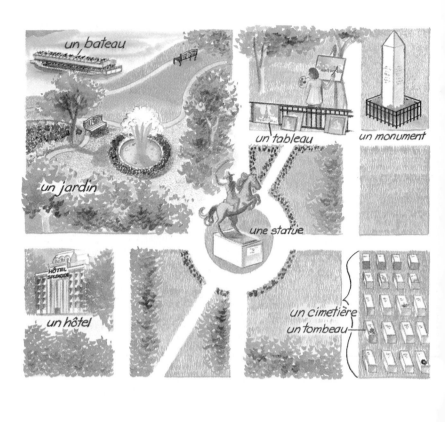

Leçon A

In this lesson you will be able to:

➤ write journal entries

➤ describe past events

➤ sequence events

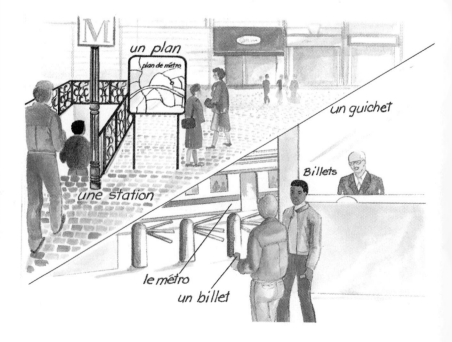

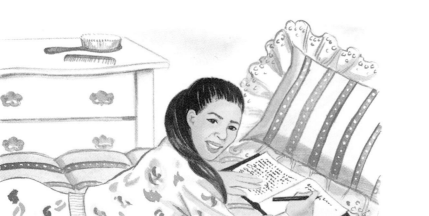

Karine Couty, a student from Papeete, Tahiti, is spending the month of July in France. In her journal she describes some of her experiences in Paris.

le 5 juillet

Ce matin j'ai quitté l'hôtel à neuf heures. D'abord, j'ai marché sur l'avenue des Champs-Élysées de l'arc de triomphe au Drugstore. Là, j'ai mangé, puis, j'ai continué mon chemin jusqu'au Louvre où j'ai regardé de beaux tableaux. J'aime <u>la Joconde</u> de Léonard de Vinci. Puis, j'ai décidé de prendre le métro pour voir le tombeau de Jim Morrison au cimetière du Père-Lachaise, mais j'ai perdu mon plan de métro. Alors je suis allée au guichet du métro, et j'ai demandé un nouveau plan.

Paris est vraiment la "Ville lumière"! J'ai fini la journée en bateau sur la Seine d'où j'ai regardé beaucoup de beaux monuments : la tour Eiffel, Notre-Dame, les jardins des Tuileries, et même la petite

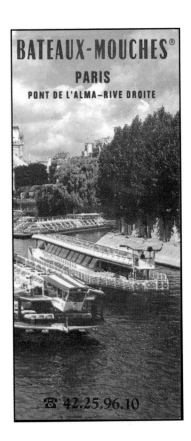

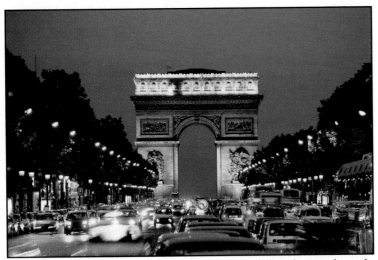

Karine a regardé l'arc de triomphe sur la place Charles de Gaulle. (Paris)

statue de la Liberté. Quel paradis! D'après mon professeur de français, il faut venir à Paris au moins trois fois : une fois quand on est jeune, une fois quand on est amoureux et une fois quand on a de l'argent et qu'on peut vraiment vivre bien! Imagine, c'est seulement ma première fois ici....

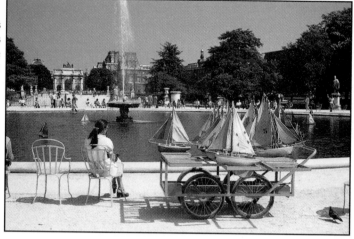

Aux jardins des Tuileries on voit souvent des enfants qui jouent avec de petits bateaux. (Paris)

Enquête culturelle

Papeete, the largest city on the South Pacific island of Tahiti, is the capital of French Polynesia. Many Tahitians work in tourism, the island's major industry. Blessed with luxuriant vegetation and spectacular waterfalls, Tahiti has been portrayed as a tropical paradise by many painters and writers, including the French artist Paul Gauguin and the American author James Michener.

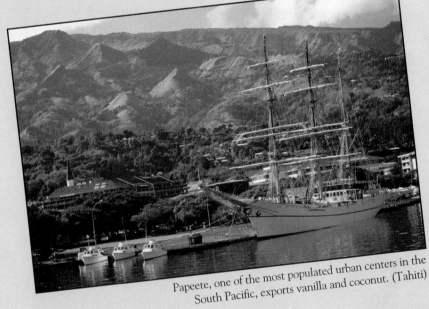

Papeete, one of the most populated urban centers in the South Pacific, exports vanilla and coconut. (Tahiti)

As its name implies, **le Drugstore** in Paris sells some over-the-counter products, such as aspirin. However, this contemporary café primarily serves light meals and American-style ice cream specialties.

The French name for the *Mona Lisa*, a painting by the Italian artist Leonardo da Vinci, is *la Joconde*. Probably the best-known painting in the **Louvre**, it became famous because of the woman's mysterious smile. The French

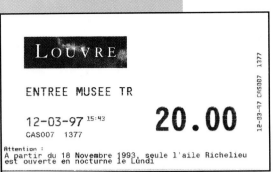

king François I not only brought the painting back from Italy, but the artist as well. Da Vinci spent the last years of his life in France.

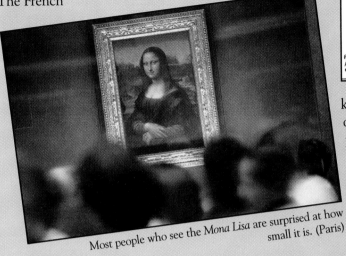

Most people who see the *Mona Lisa* are surprised at how small it is. (Paris)

The Paris subway system, called the **métro** (the shortened form of **métropolitain**), is known for its efficiency, speed, cleanliness and reasonable fares. The first **métro** line opened in 1900; today, over 300 stations dot the city. Most of them are named after streets, squares, monuments, famous people, historical places and the former gates (**portes**) to the city. Modern express lines, called **R.E.R.**, have recently been added to the **métro** system. They

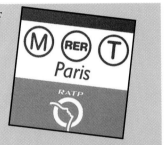

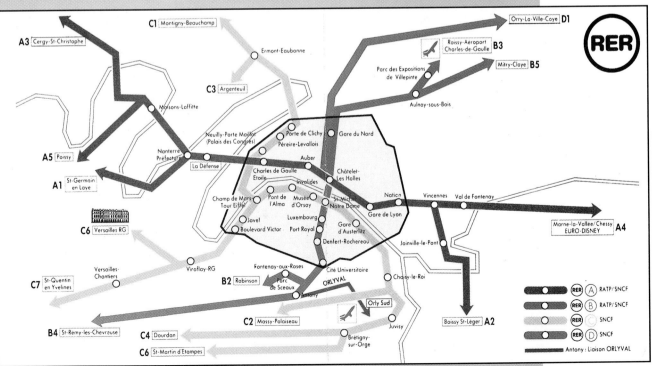

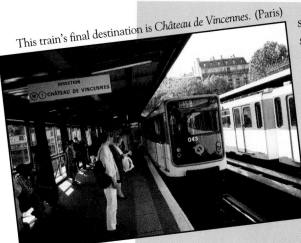

This train's final destination is *Château de Vincennes.* (Paris)

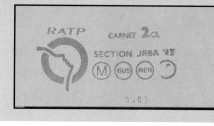

serve the suburbs and make fewer stops in the center of Paris than do the other lines. To ride the subway, you first buy a ticket or **un carnet** (a group of ten tickets). Although each **métro** line has a number, you refer to the line by the stations at each end of it. Follow the signs for the end point in the direction in which you are going. To transfer from one line to another, follow the **correspondance** signs. The **métro** runs from 5:00 A.M. to 1:00 A.M.

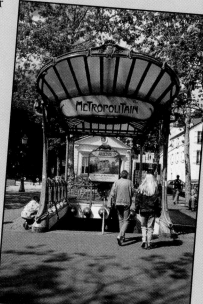

You're never more than 500 yards from a *métro* station in Paris.

Le cimetière du Père-Lachaise is the largest cemetery in Paris. Here lie the remains of such famous people as the composer

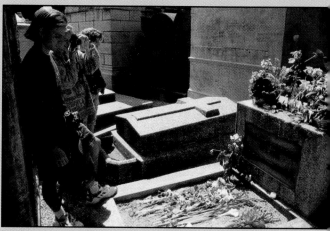

Jim Morrison's tomb, the most popular site in *Père-Lachaise,* is still frequently decorated by people who appreciate his music. (Paris)

Frédéric Chopin and the playwright Molière. Many American tourists visit the tomb of Jim Morrison, a singer with the rock group the Doors. He died in Paris in 1971.

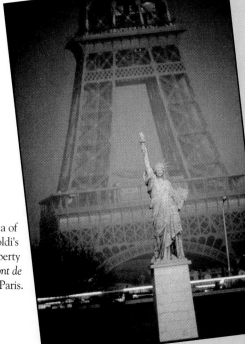

A replica of Bartholdi's Statue of Liberty is on the *pont de Grenelle* in Paris.

The French gave the United States the Statue of Liberty in 1886. A small copy of the statue stands in Paris as a continuing reminder of the friendship between the two countries.

1 *Répondez par "vrai" ou "faux" d'après le journal de Karine.*

1. Karine est en vacances à Tahiti.
2. Karine a quitté l'hôtel à dix heures.
3. L'arc de triomphe est sur l'avenue des Champs-Élysées.
4. Karine aime *la Joconde* de Léonard de Vinci.
5. Le tombeau de Jim Morrison est au Louvre.
6. Karine a perdu son plan de métro.
7. Karine a fini la journée en bateau sur le Rhône.
8. C'est la troisième fois que Karine est à Paris.

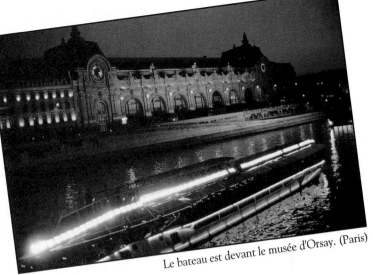

Le bateau est devant le musée d'Orsay. (Paris)

2 Choose where certain people are going, according to what they want to do.

1. François veut voir le tombeau de Molière.
2. Julien veut faire un tour en bateau.
3. Mathieu et ses parents veulent mettre leurs vêtements dans l'armoire.
4. Grégoire veut faire les magasins.
5. Marguerite veut regarder des tableaux.
6. M. Dupleix veut acheter un billet.
7. Les enfants veulent jouer.

a. la Seine
b. le musée
c. le guichet
d. l'avenue des Champs-Élysées
e. le cimetière
f. le jardin
g. l'hôtel

3 *C'est à toi!*

Voulez-vous voir le Louvre? (Paris)

1. Combien de fois est-ce que tu es allé(e) au cinéma ce mois?
2. Est-ce que tu préfères aller au musée ou au cinéma?
3. Quels tableaux aimes-tu?
4. Est-ce que tu préfères aller en vacances à Tahiti ou à Paris? Pourquoi?
5. Quel monument à Paris veux-tu voir?
6. L'avenue où tu habites s'appelle comment?
7. À quelle heure est-ce que tu quittes la maison pour aller à l'école?

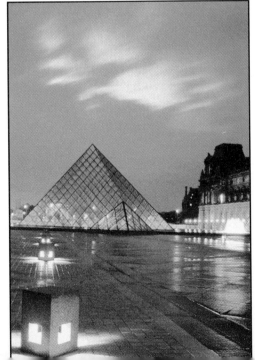

Structure

Passé composé with *avoir*

You have learned that the **passé composé** expresses what happened in the past. This tense is made up of a helping verb and the past participle of the main verb. You use the appropriate present tense form of the helping verb **être** with certain verbs. But the majority of verbs form their **passé composé** with the helping verb **avoir**.

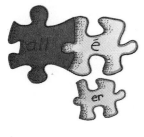

> J'ai regardé des monuments.   *I looked at some monuments.*

(helping verb)   (past participle of **regarder**)

Remember that to form the past participle of **-er** verbs, drop the **-er** of the infinitive and add an **é**: **regarder → regardé**.

The past participle of verbs that use **avoir** in the **passé composé** does not agree with the subject. Therefore, the past participle stays the same while the form of **avoir** changes according to the subject. Here is the **passé composé** of **regarder**.

regarder				
j'	**ai**	**regardé**	J'**ai regardé** mon plan.	*I looked at my map.*
tu	**as**	**regardé**	As-tu **regardé** la télé?	*Did you watch TV?*
il/elle/on	**a**	**regardé**	Malika **a regardé** l'affiche.	*Malika looked at the poster.*
nous	**avons**	**regardé**	Nous **avons regardé** la tour Eiffel.	*We looked at the Eiffel Tower.*
vous	**avez**	**regardé**	Qu'est-ce que vous **avez regardé**?	*What did you watch?*
ils/elles	**ont**	**regardé**	Ils **ont regardé** les tableaux.	*They looked at the paintings.*

Remember that to form the past participle of most **-ir** verbs, drop the **-ir** and add an **i**: **finir → fini.**

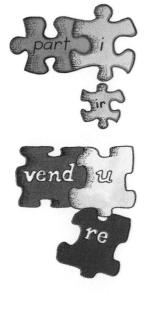

Most infinitives that end in **-re** form their past participles by dropping the **-re** and adding a **u**: **vendre → vendu, perdre → perdu, attendre → attendu.**

To make a negative sentence in the **passé composé**, put **n'** before the form of **avoir** and **pas** after it.

> Les élèves n'ont pas fini le tour.   *The students didn't finish the tour.*

To ask a question in the **passé composé** using inversion, put the subject pronoun after the form of **avoir**.

> Quand le prof a-t-il perdu son plan de Paris?   *When did the teacher lose his Paris map?*

Pratique

4 Tell what the following tourists lost while they were on vacation.

1. Amina/des CDs
2. les parents d'Amina/de l'argent
3. je/mon sac à dos
4. M. Smith/son passeport
5. Fabrice et toi, vous/des chèques de voyage
6. tu/une chaussette
7. M. et Mme Orgeval/leur plan de la ville
8. ma famille et moi, nous/nos billets d'avion

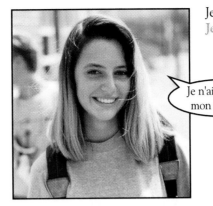

Je n'ai pas perdu mon sac à dos.

Modèle:

Jean-François/un tee-shirt
Jean-François a perdu un tee-shirt.

5 Some tourists chose to walk while they were in Paris. Others bought **métro** tickets and took the subway. Tell whether or not the following people walked.

1. Amina
2. les parents d'Amina
3. je
4. M. Smith
5. Fabrice et toi, vous
6. tu
7. M. et Mme Orgeval
8. ma famille et moi, nous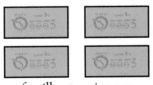

Modèle:

Jean-François
Jean-François n'a pas marché.

6 Tell what certain people did last Friday, based on where they went. Choose from the activities in the following list.

finir les devoirs	nager
attendre le train	danser
acheter des timbres	manger un hamburger
toucher des chèques de voyage	regarder des tableaux

1. Khadim est allé au fast-food.
2. Les Dupont sont allés au Louvre.
3. Florence et sa sœur sont allées à la plage.
4. Mlle Wang est allée à la banque.
5. Luc et Patrick sont allés à la bibliothèque.
6. Mme Lannion et sa fille sont allées à la gare.
7. Marc est allé au tabac.

Modèle:

Sophie est allée en boîte.
Elle a dansé.

Florence et sa sœur ont nagé à la plage. (Canet-Plage)

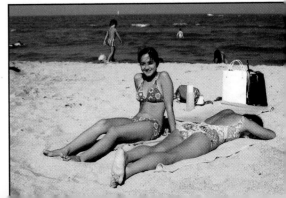

7 The teachers at your school attended a workshop on Monday. Describe what you and some of your friends did each day of your three-day weekend. The first description has been started for you.

Modèle:

Le premier jour Raoul a skié. Le deuxième jour il....

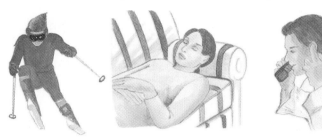

1. Raoul

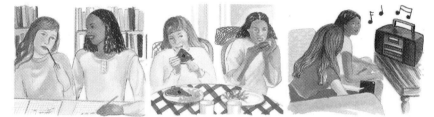

2. Christine et Saleh

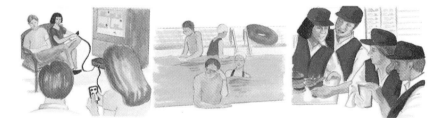

3. mes amis et moi, nous

8 With a partner, take turns asking and telling whether or not you did certain things yesterday. (Remember that some verbs use **être** as their helping verb in the **passé composé**.)

1. venir à l'école
2. finir tes devoirs
3. jouer au foot
4. aller au fast-food
5. rester à la maison
6. regarder la télé
7. travailler
8. sortir avec des amis

Modèles:

étudier le français
Student A: As-tu étudié le français hier?
Student B: Oui, j'ai étudié le français hier./Non, je n'ai pas étudié le français hier.

aller au cinéma
Student B: Es-tu allé(e) au cinéma hier?
Student A: Oui, je suis allé(e) au cinéma hier./Non, je ne suis pas allé(e) au cinéma hier.

Communication

9 Imagine that you've just returned home after a one-week stay in Paris with some of your classmates. During your trip you were so busy going places and seeing things that you didn't have time to write in your journal. Instead, you just wrote brief notes. Now that you have more time, put your notes from the first two days into sentences so that you will have a more complete account of what you did.

> *1ᵉʳ jour – 12.7*
>
> *banque – chèques de voyage*
> *Louvre – la Joconde*
> *librairie – plan de Paris*
> *jardins des Tuileries – fleurs,*
> *   enfants*
> *restaurant – Le Petit Zinzin,*
> *   poulet, frites, coca*

> *2ᵉ jour – 13.7*
>
> *avenue des Champs-Élysées*
> *magasin – Prisunic, tee-shirt*
> *   arc de triomphe*
> *Drugstore – glace au chocolat*
> *tabac – timbres*
> *cinéma – film américain*

10 *Trouvez une personne qui....* (Find someone who . . . .) Interview your classmates to find out who did various things this past weekend. On a separate sheet of paper, number from 1 to 15. Circulate around the classroom asking your classmates, one at a time, questions based on the phrases that follow. When someone says that he or she did a specific thing, have that person write his or her name next to the number of the appropriate phrase. Continue asking questions, trying to find a different person who did each thing.

1. jouer au basket
2. manger de la pizza
3. rester au lit samedi matin
4. acheter des vêtements
5. travailler
6. sortir avec des amis
7. aller au cinéma
8. regarder la télé
9. étudier le français
10. aller au centre commercial
11. dormir jusqu'à dix heures dimanche
12. perdre quelque chose
13. aller au fast-food
14. finir les devoirs
15. nager

Modèle:

Jean-Paul: Tu as joué au basket?
Clémence: Oui, j'ai joué au basket.
(Writes her name beside number 1.)

Oui, j'ai joué au basket samedi après-midi.

11 Write a paragraph in which you describe what you did this past weekend. For each day, tell where you went, what you did at each place and whether or not you worked. Add any interesting details. Some verbs you may be able to include are **regarder, parler, jouer, manger, étudier, travailler, dormir, voyager, acheter, finir, aller, rentrer, rester** and **sortir.** While writing your paragraph in the **passé composé,** be sure to use the appropriate helping verb to describe each action.

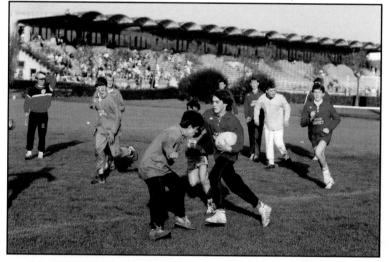

Benoît a joué au foot samedi.

Prononciation

The sound [k]

The sound [k] is written as **c** (before **a, o** or **u**), **k** or **qu.** The sound [k] in French is different from the English sound "k." In producing the French sound, no air escapes from the mouth. To see if you pronounce the French [k] correctly, hold a sheet of paper about two inches in front of your mouth. Then say the following sentences without making the paper move.

De quelle couleur est le costume?

Caroline et Colette prennent du coca et du ketchup.

Les carottes coûtent quatre francs.

Combien de Canadiens ont des coiffeurs américains?

À quelle heure commence le cours?

The paper should move only when you pronounce the English equivalent of each of these words:

café	Canada
cuisine	cassette
camping	cousin

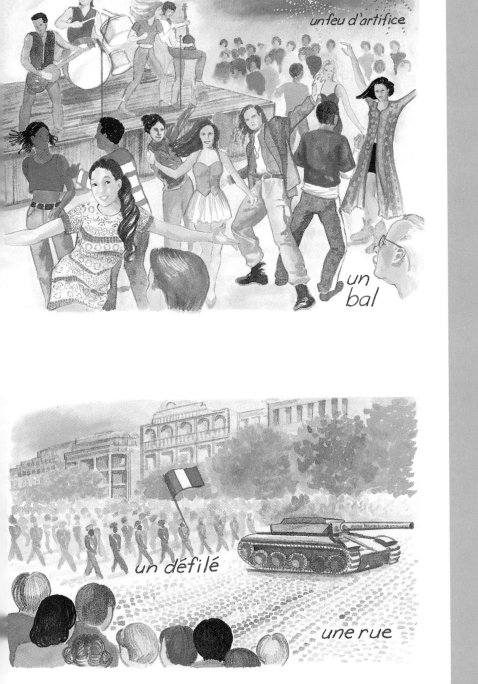

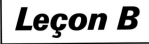

Leçon B

In this lesson you will be able to:

➤ **describe past events**

➤ **sequence events**

➤ **express need and necessity**

Karine continues to write in her journal, describing a busy week in Paris.

le 17 juillet

J'ai passé une bonne semaine. Lundi j'ai vu le Centre Pompidou où je suis montée jusqu'au cinquième étage pour bien voir Paris. Puis, j'ai pris un coca sur la place et j'ai regardé des musiciens. Mardi matin je suis allée à la Défense où j'ai visité l'arche et les magasins modernes. Mardi soir il y a eu un bal dans la rue. J'ai dansé jusqu'à trois heures du matin! Puis, j'ai été obligée de prendre un taxi pour rentrer à l'hôtel, parce qu'on a fermé le métro. Mercredi j'ai regardé le grand défilé du 14 juillet, la fête nationale de la France. On a fait beaucoup de bruit! Puis, le soir j'ai vu un beau feu d'artifice. Jeudi j'ai visité le musée d'Orsay pour voir les tableaux impressionnistes. Vendredi j'ai vu le tombeau de Napoléon aux Invalides et la statue du Penseur au musée Rodin. Une semaine bien chargée, n'est-ce pas?

GRAND FEU D'ARTIFICE DE LA FETE NATIONALE

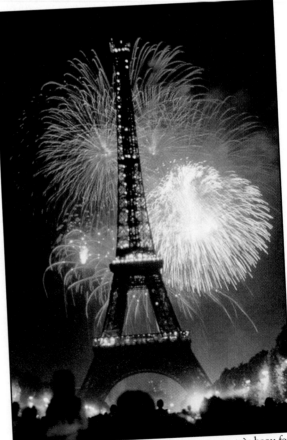

Karine a vu un très beau feu d'artifice mercredi soir. (Paris)

Several modern neighborhoods, such as **la Défense**, have been built on the outskirts of Paris. With its enormous **arche de la Défense**, skyscrapers, apartments, businesses and shops, **la Défense** has changed the skyline of contemporary Paris.

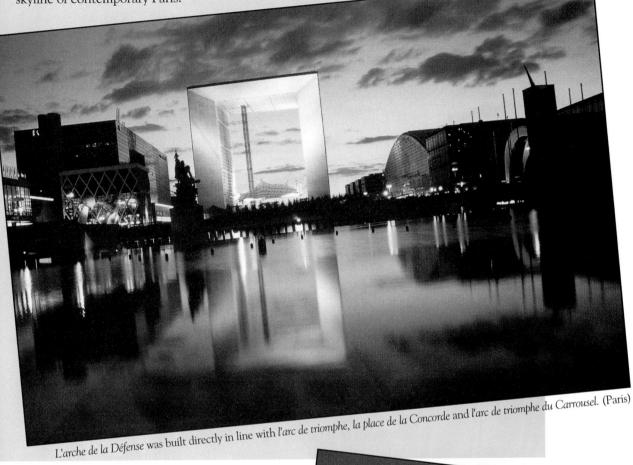

L'arche de la Défense was built directly in line with *l'arc de triomphe, la place de la Concorde* and *l'arc de triomphe du Carrousel*. (Paris)

On July 14 the French celebrate their national holiday. They honor the day in 1789 when the people of Paris captured the **Bastille**, the royal prison. Although only seven non-political prisoners were there at that time, the capture of the old fortress symbolized the beginning of the French Revolution and a spirit of freedom for everyone. The monarchy eventually fell, and the people established a more democratic form of government. Although the **Bastille** itself was demolished shortly after being stormed, a 170-foot column today stands on the **place de la Bastille.**

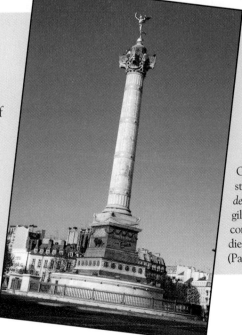

On *la place de la Bastille* stands the bronze *colonne de Juillet*, topped with a gilded spirit of liberty that commemorates those who died there in July, 1830. (Paris)

Students from the École Polytechnique dazzle the crowds during the Bastille Day parade. (Paris)

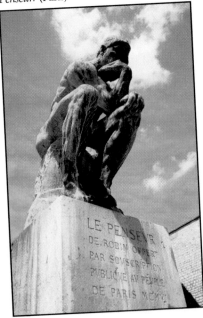

On Bastille Day, Parisians line the parade route hours in advance to have the best possible view of the annual military parade. A flyover with jets trailing blue, white and red smoke starts the parade. Then the French president comes down the parade route, usually **l'avenue des Champs-Élysées**. Both male and female members of the police, the Foreign Legion, **la garde républicaine** and other military units are presented for the inspection of the president and the French people, along with various military hardware. Smaller towns often hold military parades as well. In the evening fireworks explode across the sky. Street dances take place the nights of July 13 and 14. The firefighters of Paris, for example, sponsor dances which last well into the morning hours. People of all ages dance to a variety of music in celebration of their freedom.

1 | *Répondez aux questions avec la lettre de l'expression convenable d'après le journal de Karine.*

1. À quel étage du Centre Pompidou est-ce que Karine est montée?
2. Qui est-ce que Karine a regardé sur la place?
3. Où est-ce qu'il y a une arche moderne?
4. Où est-ce qu'il y a eu un bal?
5. Jusqu'à quelle heure est-ce que Karine a dansé?
6. Comment est-ce que Karine est rentrée?
7. Où sont les tableaux impressionnistes?
8. Où est le tombeau de Napoléon?
9. Où est la statue du *Penseur*?

a. aux Invalides
b. au cinquième
c. au musée d'Orsay
d. des musiciens
e. au musée Rodin
f. en taxi
g. à la Défense
h. dans la rue
i. jusqu'à trois heures du matin

Auguste Rodin a fait la statue du *Penseur*. (Paris)

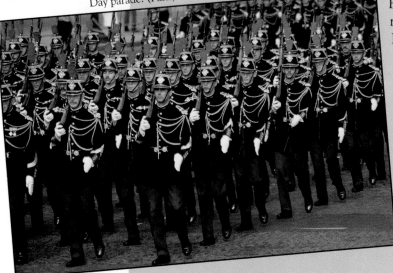

LE PENSEUR
DE RODIN OFFERT
PAR SOUSCRIPTION
PUBLIQUE AU PEUPLE
DE PARIS MCMVI

Invalides

MUSÉE DE L'ARMÉE

L'église du Dôme
Le tombeau de l'Empereur
L'Hôtel national des Invalides

Les armes et armures
14-18 et 39-45
L'artillerie
Les emblèmes
De Louis XIV à
Napoléon III

Identify each of the things or people that Karine saw during her stay in Paris.

Modèle:

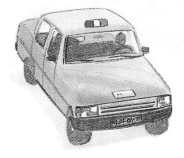

C'est un taxi.

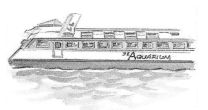

1.

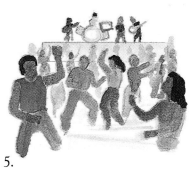

5.

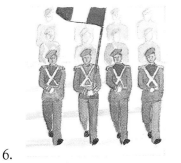

2.

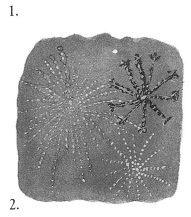

6.

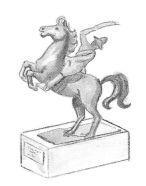

3.

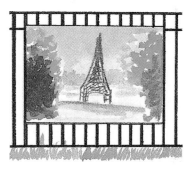

7.

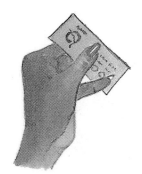

4.

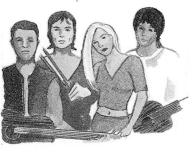

8.

3 *C'est à toi!*

1. Qu'est-ce que tu fais le 4 juillet?
2. Est-ce que tu préfères regarder un défilé ou un feu d'artifice?
3. Est-ce que tu aimes danser?
4. Quel musicien est-ce que tu préfères?
5. Est-ce que tu aimes les tableaux impressionnistes?
6. Dans ta famille, qui fait beaucoup de bruit?
7. Est-ce que tu as passé une bonne semaine? Pourquoi ou pourquoi pas?

Structure

Irregular past participles

Some verbs that form their **passé composé** with **avoir** have irregular past participles.

Verb	Past Participle	Passé Composé	
avoir	**eu**	Il y **a eu** un grand défilé.	*There was a big parade.*
être	**été**	J'**ai été** obligé de prendre le métro.	*I had to (was obliged to) take the subway.*
faire	**fait**	On n'**a** pas **fait** beaucoup de bruit.	*They didn't make a lot of noise.*
prendre	**pris**	Karine **a pris** un café.	*Karine had coffee.*
voir	**vu**	**As**-tu **vu** le feu d'artifice?	*Did you see the fireworks?*

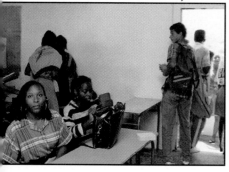

Ces élèves ont eu une interro aujourd'hui.

Pratique

4 Tell what the following people did yesterday.

Modèle:

Karine/du roller

Karine a fait du roller hier.

1. M. Lefebvre/les courses
2. les étudiants/ les devoirs
3. je/du sport
4. ta belle-sœur et toi, vous/ du shopping
5. mes cousins et moi, nous/du vélo
6. tu/un tour en bateau
7. Mme Boucher et son mari/ du footing

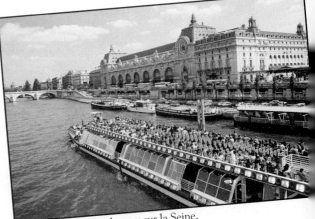

On a fait un tour en bateau sur la Seine.

5 The Troussard family spent a week in Paris. To find out what they did, complete each sentence with the **passé composé** of the appropriate verb from the following list.

avoir	être	faire	prendre	voir

1. M. Troussard... obligé de passer une semaine à Paris. Donc, sa femme et ses fils sont venus à Paris aussi.
2. Ils... le métro pour aller à leur hôtel.
3. La famille Troussard... beaucoup de monuments à Paris.
4. Djamel Troussard... des photos de la tour Eiffel.
5. Le 14 juillet les Troussard sont allés aux Champs-Élysées où il y... un grand défilé.
6. Au défilé, les garçons... beaucoup de bruit!
7. Puis, le soir il y... un feu d'artifice.
8. Le 15 juillet les Troussard... un tour en bateau sur la Seine.

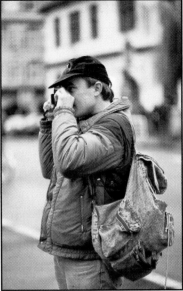

Gérard a pris beaucoup de photos.

6 Marie-Claude made a list of everything she wanted to do yesterday. This morning she checked off those things she was able to get done. Tell whether or not Marie-Claude did the things she wanted to do.

Modèle:

Elle n'a pas dormi jusqu'à dix heures du matin.

    dormir jusqu'à dix heures du matin
✔ *prendre rendez-vous avec le médecin*
    faire les magasins
    voir le nouveau film au Gaumont
✔ *finir les devoirs*
    téléphoner à Cécile
✔ *attendre Daniel à l'aéroport*

Communication

7 Your French-speaking pen pal is curious to know what Americans do to celebrate their national holiday on July 4. Write your pen pal a short letter in which you describe what you, your friends and your family did last Fourth of July. Also tell about some of the special events that took place in your town or city during this holiday, even if you didn't take part in them.

8 With a partner, talk about what you did this past weekend. In preparation, each partner needs to bring to class three props, either real objects or drawings of them, that serve as reminders of some things he or she did. Student A begins by telling Student B about the activity that each of his or her props represents. After each of Student A's sentences, Student B asks Student A a specific follow-up question about that activity, and Student A responds. Then switch roles.

Modèle:

Student A: (shows Student B a movie ad from the newspaper) Je suis allée au cinéma vendredi soir.
Student B: Tu as vu quel film?
Student A: J'ai vu *Pocahontas*.

Mise au point sur... Paris

"If you are lucky enough to have lived in Paris as a young man, then wherever you go for the rest of your life, it stays with you, for Paris is a moveable feast," wrote the American author Ernest Hemingway. Long considered to be the cultural capital of the world, Paris still attracts people interested in the arts. Visitors come from all over the globe to see the famous sights of this cosmopolitan city.

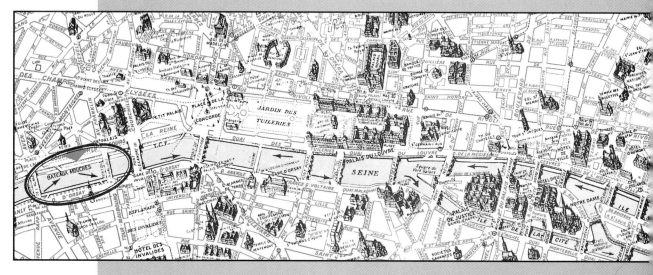

The origins of Paris go back many centuries. The city received its name from the **Parisii,** a Gallic tribe that settled on the **île de la Cité** over 2,000 years ago. The larger of the two islands in the Seine, the **île de la Cité** is called the "cradle" of Paris because the city's history began here. Tourists admire the quaint seventeenth century buildings on the smaller, more residential **île Saint-Louis.** Sightseers needing a break stop at Le Berthillon, a popular establishment known for its delicious ice cream.

Several monuments draw visitors to the **île de la Cité.** The cathedral of **Notre-Dame,** begun in the twelfth century, is a triumph of Gothic architecture with its ribbed vaulting and flying buttresses. These structures support the weight of the cathedral from the outside, allowing for thinner, higher walls filled with richly colored stained glass windows. Gargoyles, waterspouts sculpted in the form of long-necked creatures, and intricately carved statues decorate the church's façade.

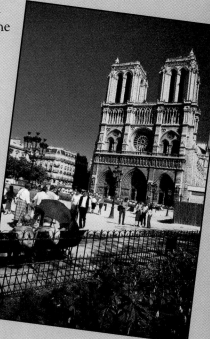

The **Sainte-Chapelle,** a tiny church on the **île de la Cité,** was built in the thirteenth century to house relics from the religious Crusades. Another jewel of Gothic architecture, it contains enough stained glass windows to

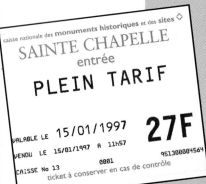

caisse nationale des **monuments historiques** et des **sites** ◊
SAINTE CHAPELLE
entrée
PLEIN TARIF
VALABLE LE 15/01/1997 **27F**
VENDU LE 15/01/1997 A 11h57
951300004564
CAISSE No 13   0001
ticket à conserver en cas de contrôle

The western façade of the cathedral of *Notre-Dame* features three large doors, two tall towers and a central rose window. (Paris)

cover three basketball courts. Since most people couldn't read during the Middle Ages, biblical stories were illustrated through the scenes on these windows, as well as on those of other Gothic churches.

Just a block away lies the **Conciergerie**, which was a state prison during the French Revolution. You can still visit cell number VI where Queen Marie-Antoinette, wife of King Louis XVI, spent her last days before being guillotined in 1793.

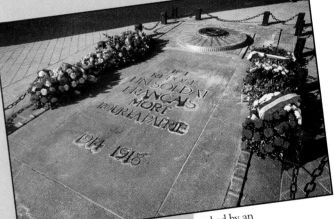

seine rive gauche
3, rue Louise Weiss - 75013 Paris
face 161, rue du Chevaleret - 44.23.80.02
RESTAURANT SALON DE THÉ - Référencé Gault et Millau
ASSIETTES COMPOSÉES RAFFINÉES
PÂTISSERIES MAISON
TERRASSE, OUVERT TOUT L'ÉTÉ

The Seine River divides Paris in half before it continues northwest to the English Channel. The Right Bank (**rive droite**) is north of the Seine; the Left Bank (**rive gauche**) is south of the Seine. More than 30 bridges, such as the **Pont-Neuf** (the oldest) and the **pont Alexandre-III** (the

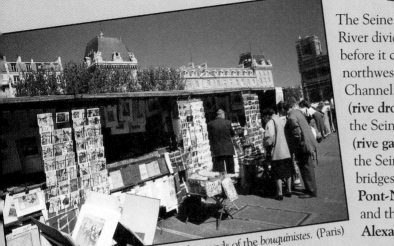

Bargain hunters often like to browse at the stands of the *bouquinistes*. (Paris)

newest and most elaborate), join the two sides of the river. **Les bouquinistes** (*booksellers*) line the banks of the Seine with their stands full of secondhand books, posters, old prints and postcards.

On the Right Bank of the Seine is the **place Charles-de-Gaulle** where Napoléon had the **arc de triomphe** built to commemorate his military victories. Under the arch lies the Tomb of the Unknown Soldier. This square used to be called the **place de l'Étoile** because 12 avenues radiate from its center. The most famous of these streets,

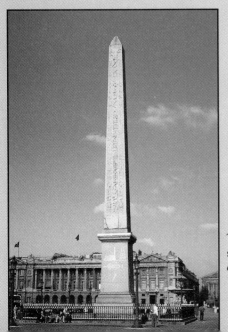

The Tomb of the Unknown Soldier is marked by an eternal flame and a daily bouquet of flowers. (Paris)

the **avenue des Champs-Élysées**, stretches to the **place de la Concorde**, where over one thousand French people were guillotined during the French Revolution. The largest square in western Europe, the **place de la Concorde** has an Egyptian obelisk and beautiful fountains at its center.

The obelisk at the center of *la place de la Concorde* stands 75 feet tall, weighs over 220 tons and is covered with Egyptian hieroglyphics. (Paris)

The **jardins des Tuileries**, the former gardens of French royalty, extend farther east along the river. Next to the gardens is the enormous **musée du Louvre** with its modern steel and glass pyramid designed by the American architect I. M. Pei.

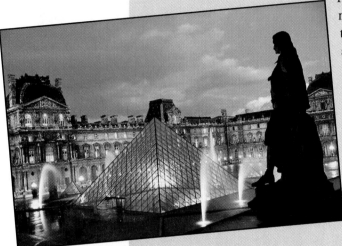

Formerly a royal palace, the **Louvre** houses one of the most extensive art collections in the world. Among its treasures are paintings, such as the *Mona Lisa*, sculptures, such as *Winged Victory*, period furniture, antiquities and the crown jewels of France. If you were to spend three minutes in front of each painting in the museum, it would take you over two and one-half months to view all of them.

On the northern edge of the city, the basilica of **Sacré-Cœur** overlooks Paris from the hill of **Montmartre**, an artistic quarter of the city.

The exterior of the *Louvre* combines classical and modern architecture. (Paris)

The Right Bank has contemporary buildings as well as historical landmarks. The **Centre national d'art et de culture Georges Pompidou**, familiarly called **Beaubourg**, was designed in a bold, functional

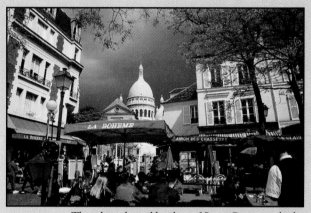

The white-domed basilica of *Sacré-Cœur* overlooks the *place du Tertre*, the artists' quarter. (Paris)

style of architecture.

The pipes, ducts, pillars and stairways of the glass structure are exposed; each is painted a different color according to its function (water, heating, air-conditioning, etc.). A "caterpillar"

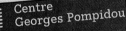

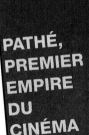

Centre Georges Pompidou

PATHÉ, PREMIER EMPIRE DU CINÉMA

jusqu'au 6 mars

une exposition

et

300 films en Salle Garance

copies rares,
films des premiers temps,
films muets
avec accompagnement musical en direct

escalator brings visitors to the top of the building for a fabulous view of the city. The **Centre Pompidou** contains a computer music center, the city's biggest public library and a modern art museum. The square in front of the building remains a perpetual showcase, with street performers entertaining the public at all hours of the day and night.

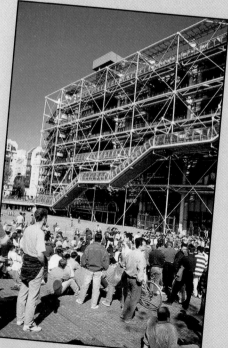

Street performers, such as jugglers, flame throwers, musicians and artists, attract crowds in front of the *Centre Pompidou*. (Paris)

Both the **musée d'Orsay** and the **musée Rodin** are on the Left Bank (**rive gauche**) of the Seine. Built in a former train station, the **musée d'Orsay** features artwork from the years 1848 to 1914. Paintings from such well-known artists as Claude Monet, Vincent Van Gogh, Pierre Auguste Renoir, Édouard Manet, Edgar Degas and Henri de Toulouse-Lautrec hang in this airy museum. The **musée Rodin** and its gardens contain some of the most famous pieces sculpted by Auguste Rodin, such as *The Thinker*, *The Burghers of Calais* and *The Gates of Hell*.

The tomb of Napoléon is located in the **hôtel des Invalides**, a former military hospital and now a military museum. Napoléon's remains are contained within six coffins, one inside the other.

Built by Gustave Eiffel for the World's Fair of 1889, the **tour Eiffel** is the symbol of Paris. Tourists take an elevator to the observation deck on the third level of the tower for a spectacular view of the city, or they may stop at the scenic restaurants on the first and second levels. For many years the tallest structure in the world, the Eiffel Tower was originally scorned by many artists and writers who were offended by its geometric structure. Nevertheless, **la Grande Dame de Paris** has been used for a variety of purposes over the years, serving as a military observation station during World War I, a meteorological post, and a radio and television transmitting station. With new lights illuminating the tower from within, the Eiffel Tower sparkles in the night sky, reminding people that Paris is **la Ville lumière**.

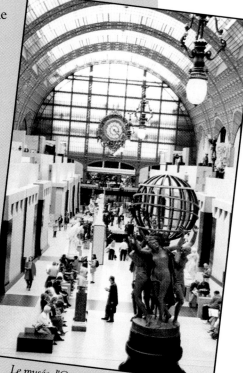

Le musée d'Orsay opened in 1986 and quickly became one of Paris' most popular attractions.

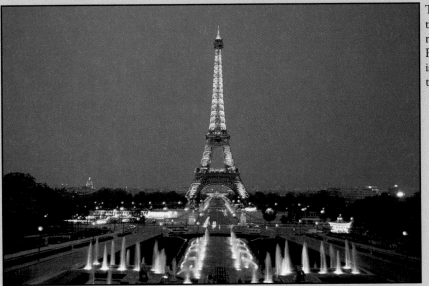

The *tour Eiffel*, the tallest monument in Paris at 985 feet, is the symbol of the city.

An ancient yet beautiful and dynamic city, the Paris of today, including its suburbs, has over 10 million people and is the intellectual, economic, cultural and political center of France. As the German writer Goethe said, **Paris est la capitale du monde**.

Napoléon wanted to be buried near the Seine, and his tomb is in the *hôtel des Invalides* on the Left Bank. (Paris)

9 Answer the following questions.

1. What Gallic tribe settled on the **île de la Cité**?
2. Why is the **île de la Cité** called the "cradle" of Paris?
3. What is the name of the smaller of the two islands in the Seine?
4. What are two characteristics of Gothic architecture?
5. Why were biblical stories told in the stained glass windows of churches?
6. Where was Queen Marie-Antoinette imprisoned?
7. What is the oldest bridge in Paris?
8. Why did Napoléon have the **arc de triomphe** built?
9. Where were many people guillotined during the French Revolution?
10. What are two famous works of art in the **Louvre**?
11. Why do crowds gather outside the contemporary **Centre Pompidou**?
12. What are the names of two artists whose paintings are displayed at the **musée d'Orsay**?
13. Where is Napoléon's tomb?
14. Which monument is considered to be the symbol of Paris?
15. What did Ernest Hemingway mean when he said ". . . Paris is a moveable feast"?

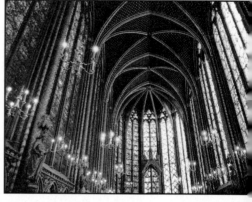

Stained glass windows in the *Sainte-Chapelle* illustrate stories from the Bible in 1,134 scenes. (Paris)

10 Look at the **métro** map of Paris on the next page and answer the following questions.

1. What station is at the opposite end of the line from Porte d'Orléans (on the Left Bank)?
2. How many **métro** lines serve Pasteur (on the Left Bank)?
3. Are there more or less than 15 stations on the line whose end points are Pont de Levallois-Bécon and Gallieni (line 3)?
4. The Voltaire station is on the Right Bank. What are the names of the stations at the end points of the line that passes through this station? What is the number of this line?
5. If you wanted to go from Concorde to Hôtel de Ville (both on the Right Bank), in what direction would you go? (Give the name of the station at the line's end point.)
6. If you were going from Rambuteau to Père-Lachaise (both on the Right Bank), in what direction would you go first? At what station would you transfer? In what direction would you finally go?
7. If you were going from Victor Hugo (on line 2 on the Right Bank) to Jacques Bonsergent (on line 5 on the Right Bank), in what direction would you go first? At what station would you transfer? In what direction would you finally go?

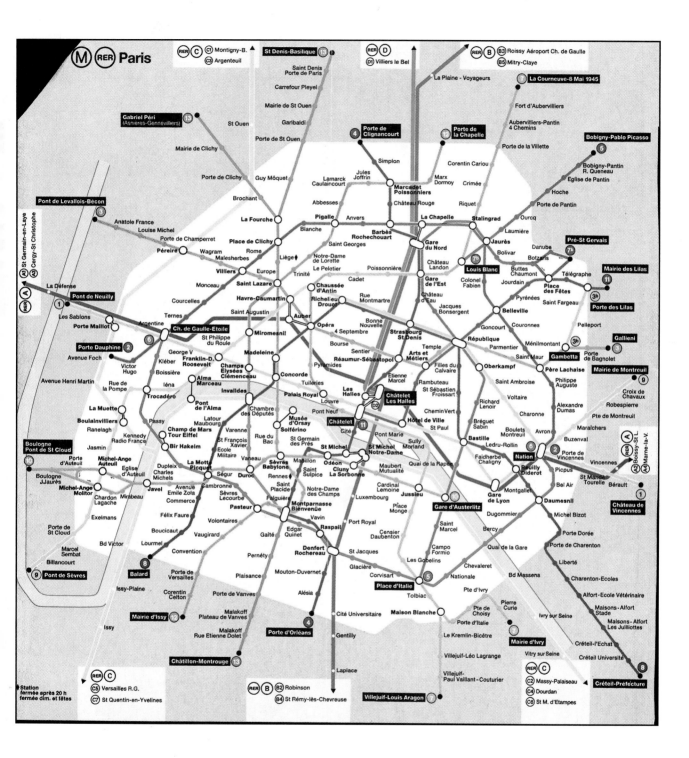

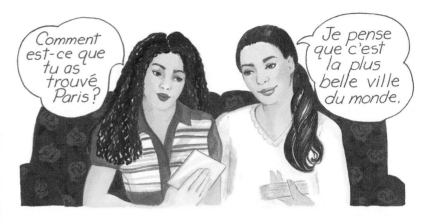

Leçon C

In this lesson you will be able to:

➤ **ask for information**

➤ **give opinions**

➤ **compare things**

➤ **sequence events**

Karine returns to Tahiti and tells her friend Danielle about her trip to Paris.

Danielle: **Comment est-ce que tu as trouvé Paris?**
Karine: **Je pense que c'est la plus belle ville du monde.**
Danielle: **Qu'est-ce que tu as fait?**
Karine: **J'ai vu beaucoup de monuments. La semaine dernière j'ai aussi visité le jardin du Luxembourg. Ce n'est pas le plus grand jardin de Paris, mais il est très joli.**
Danielle: **Quels quartiers sont les plus modernes?**
Karine: **Le Forum des Halles et la Villette.**

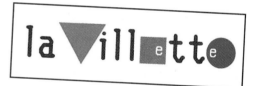

Le Forum des Halles, au centre de Paris, est un quartier très moderne.

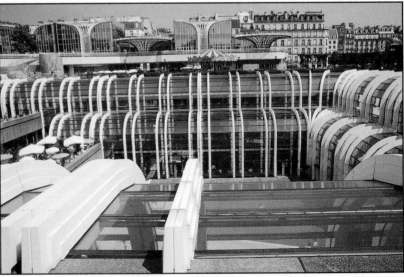

Enquête culturelle

Students from the nearby **Quartier latin** often relax in the **jardin du Luxembourg**. Children push toy boats across the park's large pond with long sticks. In addition to the many public parks in Paris, there are two larger wooded areas, the **bois de Boulogne** on the west side of the city and the **bois de Vincennes** on the east side. Both offer lakes, restaurants, zoos and sporting opportunities for people who want to spend some time away from the busy inner city.

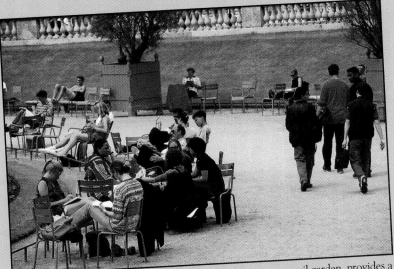

The *jardin du Luxembourg*, a convenient, tranquil garden, provides a perfect place for university students to study or relax. (Paris)

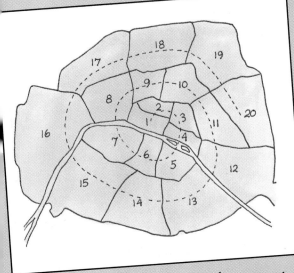

The city of Paris is divided into 20 **arrondissements** (*districts*) for governmental purposes and many **quartiers** (*quarters*) for cultural or artistic reasons. For example, many artists live and work in the **quartier** of **Montmartre**.

Le Forum des Halles is a contemporary, underground shopping mall with restaurants, cafés, snack bars, boutiques and movie theaters on four levels. It also has a branch of Fnac, a large specialty store for those who love music, books, photography and TV. At Fnac you can choose from a wide variety of CDs and also order concert tickets.

La Villette, in the northeastern part of Paris, houses the **Cité des Sciences**, an ultramodern "hands-on" science museum. Here teenagers also enjoy **la Géode**, a movie theater where films are projected 180 degrees above and around the audience.

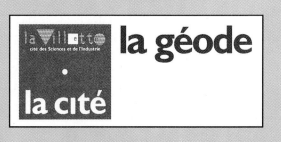

1 Complétez les phrases avec la lettre du mot convenable d'après le dialogue.

1. Qu'est-ce que Karine... de Paris?
2. Quelle est la plus belle ville du...?
3. Qu'est-ce que Karine... fait à Paris?
4. Karine a... beaucoup de monuments.
5. La semaine... elle a visité le... du Luxembourg.
6. La Villette et le... sont des... très modernes.

a. jardin
b. dernière
c. monde
d. vu
e. pense
f. quartiers
g. Forum des Halles
h. a

2 Write a four-sentence paragraph in French that summarizes what Karine tells Danielle about her trip to Paris. Begin by telling what Karine thinks of Paris. Then mention two things that she saw. Next describe the Luxembourg Gardens. Finally, give the name of two modern quarters of Paris.

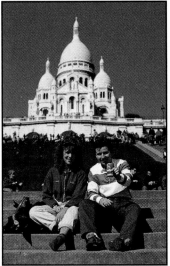

Veux-tu voir le Sacré-Cœur? (Paris)

3 C'est à toi!

1. Quel monument de Paris est-ce que tu veux voir?
2. Quel monument de ta ville ou de ton village est-ce que tu as visité?
3. Comment est-ce que tu trouves ta ville ou ton village?
4. Quel quartier de ta ville ou de ton village est le plus beau?
5. Qu'est-ce que tu as fait hier soir?
6. Est-ce que tu as déjà vu ton professeur d'anglais aujourd'hui?

Structure

Superlative of adjectives

To tell that a person or thing has the most of a certain quality compared to all others, use the superlative construction:

le/la/les	+	**plus**	+	adjective

Je pense que *la Joconde* est le plus beau tableau.

I think that the Mona Lisa is the most beautiful painting.

If an adjective usually precedes a noun, its superlative form also precedes it. If an adjective usually follows a noun, so does its superlative form. Both the definite article and the adjective agree in gender and in number with the noun they describe.

Le Louvre est le plus grand musée.

*The **Louvre** is the largest museum.*

Le Forum des Halles et la Villette sont les quartiers les plus modernes.

*Le **Forum des Halles** and **la Villette** are the most modern neighborhoods.*

Sometimes the superlative is followed by a form of **de** (*in*).

Paris est la plus belle ville du monde.

Paris is the most beautiful city in the world.

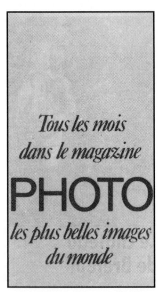

Tous les mois dans le magazine
PHOTO
les plus belles images du monde

Pratique

4 | Describe some of the students and teachers in your school using the superlative construction.

1. M. Poirier (prof généreux)
2. Jérémy et Denise (élèves timides)
3. Anne-Marie et Monique (jolies filles)
4. le professeur de maths et le professeur de dessin (professeurs intelligents)
5. Daniel et Amine (beaux garçons)
6. Mlle Vigier (grande prof)

Modèle:

Caroline (petite fille)
Caroline est la plus petite fille de l'école.

David (garçon bavard)
David est le garçon le plus bavard de l'école.

5 | Comment on some of the sites in Paris. Use a superlative form of one of the adjectives from column A and a noun from column B in stating each of your opinions.

A	B
beau	le cimetière
moderne	l'arche
grand	l'église
joli	le musée
petit	l'avenue
	le monument
	la place
	le quartier
	le jardin

1. la Villette
2. Notre-Dame
3. le cimetière du Père-Lachaise
4. la Cité des Sciences
5. le jardin du Luxembourg
6. la Sainte-Chapelle
7. la tour Eiffel
8. l'arche de la Défense
9. l'avenue des Champs-Élysées
10. la place de la Concorde

Modèle:

le Louvre
Le Louvre est le plus grand musée de Paris.

L'arche de la Défense est l'arche la plus moderne de Paris.

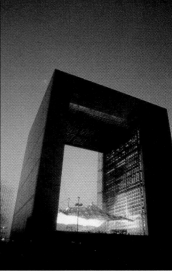

6 | Find out what your partner's opinions are on certain topics. Take turns asking and answering questions using the superlative construction.

1. couleur (moche)
2. repas (grand)
3. élèves (diligent)
4. cours (facile)
5. mois (beau)
6. CD (formidable)
7. légume (mauvais)
8. baskets (cher)

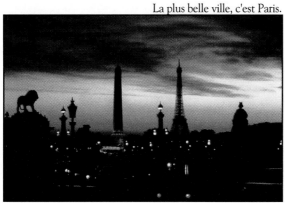

La plus belle ville, c'est Paris.

Modèles:

ville (beau)
Student A: Quelle ville est la plus belle?
Student B: La plus belle ville, c'est Paris.

professeur (sympa)
Student B: Quel professeur est le plus sympa?
Student A: Le professeur le plus sympa, c'est M. Johnson.

Communication

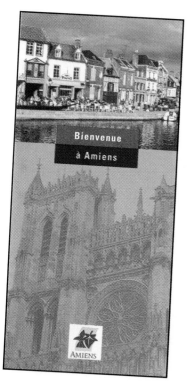

7   Your local tourist bureau has asked your class to help write a French travel brochure about your city, town or area that will be distributed to French-speaking tourists who pass through. Write five sentences in French using the superlative construction. In each sentence describe one of the most important tourist attractions in your area. You might tell which sites are the newest, oldest, most beautiful, largest, smallest, etc.

8   With your classmates, hold an "ultimate" baby contest. Bring to class a picture of you taken when you were either a baby or a toddler. In small groups, come up with five questions using the superlative that students in other groups will be able to answer by looking at your group's baby pictures. (For example, you might ask **Qui a les cheveux les plus blonds?**) Then, select a group member to read these five questions to the entire class. After each group has presented its questions, you and your classmates should choose the ten best questions to use in the contest. In preparation, post your photo on the class bulletin board for your teacher to number and for everyone to see. When the contest begins, one student reads the ten questions, and everyone else votes for the winning baby in each category.

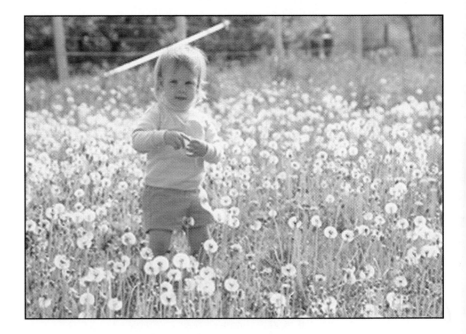

You have already learned several reading strategies that can help you figure out the meaning of French words you don't know, including recognizing cognates and determining the context of the reading. However, there will be times when these strategies won't help you. When all else fails and you need to know the meaning of a word in order to understand the reading as a whole, there is another skill that can help you: using a French-English dictionary.

You may not think you need any special skill to use a dictionary. This is not true! Imagine the different meanings a French speaker will find when looking up the word "kid" in an English dictionary. As a noun, "kid" can mean either "child" or "young goat." As a verb, "kid" means "to joke." Similarly, you know that the French word **glace** means "ice cream." But if you look up **glace** in a French dictionary, you will discover that it can also mean "ice," "glass" or "mirror." The meaning of a word depends entirely on how it is used in a sentence.

The paragraph that follows is the beginning of a historical overview of the **Louvre**. To learn how to use a dictionary effectively, concentrate on the three highlighted examples in this paragraph. After you read it, refer to the dictionary hints that show you how to look up these three words.

XIIIᵉ siècle:

Le château royal du Louvre, fondé par Philippe-Auguste, est situé à Paris sur la rive droite de la Seine et **protège** la ville à l'ouest. La **grosse** tour centrale de cette forteresse **carrée** sert de prison, d'arsenal et de chambre au trésor.

Here are some hints on how to use a French-English dictionary:

1. *Before you look up a word, try to figure out what part of speech it is (noun, verb, adjective, etc.).* As a clue, use the word's position in the sentence. For example, look at the word **carrée**. In the French dictionary there are different meanings for the word as an adjective and as a noun. Looking at its position in the sentence, you'll notice that **carrée** follows **forteresse**, a cognate for the English noun "fortress." You know that most adjectives follow the nouns they describe. Thus, you can figure out that **carrée**, in this sentence, functions as an adjective meaning "square."

2. *Remember that verbs are listed in the dictionary in their infinitive form.* Once you have determined that a word is a verb, try to figure out what its infinitive is before you look it up, keeping in mind that all infinitives end in **-er, -ir** or **-re**. For example, when trying to figure out the infinitive of the verb form **protège**, you should remember that certain forms of **-er** verbs end in **-e**. Thus, you might logically guess that the infinitive of this word is **protéger**, which means "to protect."

3. *Realize that adjectives (and nouns) that have both masculine and feminine forms are listed in the dictionary in their masculine singular form.* For example, once you have determined that **grosse** is a feminine adjective, try to figure out what it's masculine form is before you look it up in the dictionary. You know that some feminine adjectives are formed by doubling the final consonant of a masculine adjective and adding an **e**. So, you might logically guess that the masculine form of **grosse** is **gros**.

Sur la bonne piste

4. *When you look up a word in the dictionary, be sure to check all its possible meanings.* Don't just assume that the first meaning given is the one you need. For example, the adjective **grosse** can mean "big," "large," "thick," "heavy" or "fat." Use the context of the sentence it appears in to figure out which meaning applies. **Grosse** modifies **la tour**, which you know means "tower." This information can help you determine that the correct meaning for **grosse** in this sentence is "big" or "large."

Now read the rest of the historical description of the **Louvre**. Use all the reading strategies you have learned up to this point to figure out the meaning of words you don't know.

XIVe siècle:

Charles V embellit le château et le transforme en demeure habitable.

XVIe siècle:

François Ier démolit la forteresse et commence le palais. Amateur d'art italien, il y installe ses tableaux préférés, *la Joconde* incluse. Pierre Lescot élève la partie sud-ouest de la Cour Carrée.

Fin du XVIe, début du XVIIe siècle:

Pour joindre le Louvre au Palais des Tuileries, la Petite Galerie et la Grande Galerie sont construites le long de la Seine.

XVIIe siècle:

Louis XIII et Louis XIV donnent à la Cour Carrée ses proportions actuelles. Claude Perrault est un des auteurs de la Colonade qui, à l'est, fait face à l'église Saint-Germain-l'Auxerrois.

XVIIIe siècle:

Napoléon Ier achève la Cour Carrée et son décor. Il commence l'aile Richelieu qui longe la rue de Rivoli. Demeure des rois de France, siège des Académies, le Louvre devient musée pendant la Révolution en 1793.

XIXe siècle:

Napoléon III et ses architectes terminent les travaux à l'ouest. Les Tuileries brûlent en 1871 et l'unité de cet immense ensemble de palais est rompue.

XXe siècle:

Ieoh Ming Pei, architecte américain d'origine chinoise, construit une pyramide moderne de verre dans la cour du musée en 1989. Elle fonctionne comme entrée principale et librairie. En 1993 l'aile Richelieu est remise à neuf. Le Carrousel, centre commercial de luxe souterrain, est bâti.

Aujourd'hui:

Le musée devient un des plus riches du monde. Les collections justement célèbres ne font que croître.

9 Now make a list of the words you still don't know that you feel are essential to understanding the reading as a whole. By answering the following questions, the meaning of some of these words may become clear.

1. Realizing that the word **embellit** is a verb form, what do you think its infinitive is?
2. The word **amateur** can mean either "amateur" or "lover (of something)." Which meaning applies here?
3. The word **élève** can function as a noun or as a verb. Which part of speech applies here?
4. The word **actuelles** is an adjective. What is its masculine singular form?
5. The word **ensemble** can function as an adverb or as a noun. Which part of speech applies here?
6. The word **neuf** can mean either "nine" or "new." Which meaning applies here?
7. The word **devient** looks similar to a verb form you have already learned. What is it? What do you think its infinitive is?
8. Choose three of the words you still don't understand from the list you made and answer the following questions about each word.
   a. What part of speech is the word?
   b. If it is a verb form, what is its infinitive?
   c. If it is an adjective, what is its masculine singular form?
   d. When you look it up in a French-English dictionary, how many different meanings does it have?
   e. Which meaning applies here?

Nathalie et Raoul

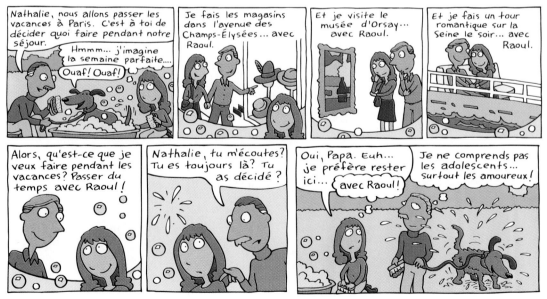

C'est à moi!

Now that you have completed this unit, take a look at what you should be able to do in French. Can you do all of these tasks?

➤ I can write a journal entry.

➤ I can talk about what happened in the past.

➤ I can talk about things sequentially.

➤ I can say what needs to be done.

➤ I can ask for information.

➤ I can give my opinion by saying what I think.

➤ I can make comparisons by saying who or what has the most of a certain quality.

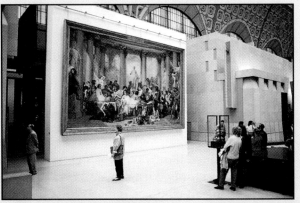

Vous êtes obligé(e) de visiter le musée d'Orsay! (Paris)

Here is a brief checkup to see how much you understand about French culture. Decide if each statement is **vrai** or **faux**.

1. *La Joconde*, the French name for Leonardo da Vinci's masterpiece, can be found in the **musée d'Orsay** in Paris.
2. The **R.E.R.**, an expansion of the Paris **métro** system, serves the suburbs with fewer stops in the center of the city.
3. France and the United States both have their national holiday on July 4.
4. The French celebrate Bastille Day with a military parade, fireworks and street dances.
5. **Notre-Dame,** the **Sainte-Chapelle** and the **Conciergerie** are all located on the **île de la Cité** in the Seine River.

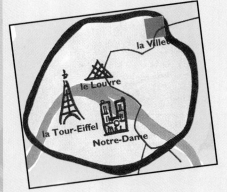

What cathedral is located on the *île de la Cité*? (Paris)

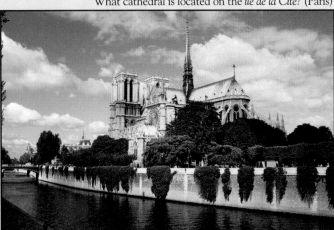

6. Napoléon's **arc de triomphe** is the site where he had over one thousand people guillotined during the French Revolution.

7. The **Centre Pompidou** has a modern, functional style of architecture with its pipes, ducts, pillars and stairways on the outside of the building.

8. To view the paintings by such great French artists as Monet, Renoir and Toulouse-Lautrec, visit the **Louvre**.

9. The **tour Eiffel** is best known because both the Tomb of the Unknown Soldier and the tomb of Jim Morrison lie underneath it.

10. Modern **quartiers** of Paris include **la Défense, la Villette** and **le Forum des Halles.**

Communication orale

Imagine that you and your partner have returned from separate one-week trips to Paris. One partner went there as part of a group of tourists specifically interested in seeing the sites. The other partner went there to visit a former French exchange student and stayed with the student's family. Consequently, both partners have different memories of Paris. The second partner didn't see as many sites as the first partner, but took part in more family-related activities and did things that French teenagers do. Begin your conversation by greeting each other. Then ask and tell each other how you liked Paris. Next ask and tell when you arrived in Paris. Finally, ask and tell where you went and what you saw and did. Finish your conversation by asking and telling each other when you returned home.

Communication écrite

Your teacher is curious to find out what you and your partner did in Paris and how you liked the city. Write a composition in French that describes the similarities and differences between your trip and your partner's trip, based on the information you exchanged in your previous conversation. To help you organize your composition, you may first want to make intersecting circles. In the first circle list only the things that you did and saw; in the second circle list only the things that your partner did and saw; in the section where the circles intersect list the things that both of you did and saw.

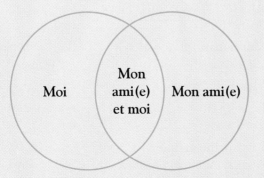

Moi | Mon ami(e) et moi | Mon ami(e)

Communication active

To write journal entries, use:

le 5 juillet   *July 5*

To describe past events, use:

J'ai regardé de beaux tableaux.   *I looked at some beautiful paintings.*

J'ai fini la journée en bateau sur la Seine.   *I finished the day on a boat on the Seine.*

J'ai perdu mon plan de métro.   *I lost my subway map.*

Karine a vu le pont Alexandre-III. (Paris)

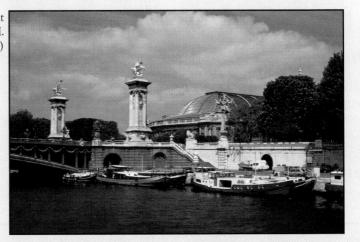

J'ai vu le Centre Pompidou.   *I saw the **Centre Pompidou**.*

J'ai pris un café sur la place.   *I had coffee on the square.*

Il y a eu un bal dans la rue.   *There was a street dance.*

J'ai été obligé(e) de rentrer.   *I had to (was obliged to) come back.*

On a fait beaucoup de bruit.   *People made a lot of noise.*

Je suis monté(e) au cinquième étage.   *I went up to the fifth floor.*

To sequence events, use:

D'abord, j'ai marché sur l'avenue des Champs-Élysées.   *First I walked on the **Champs-Élysées**.*

Puis, j'ai continué mon chemin jusqu'au Louvre.   *Then I continued on my way (up) to the **Louvre**.*

Alors, je suis allée au guichet du métro.   *Then I went to the subway ticket window.*

Mardi matin je suis allé(e) à la Défense.   *Tuesday morning I went to **la Défense**.*

Mercredi j'ai regardé le défilé.   *Wednesday I watched the parade.*

Le soir j'ai vu un beau feu d'artifice.   *In the evening I saw some beautiful fireworks.*

La semaine dernière j'ai aussi visité le jardin du Luxembourg.   *Last week I also visited the Luxembourg Gardens.*

To express need and necessity, use:

> **J'ai été obligé(e) de** prendre un taxi à l'hôtel.

> *I had to (was obliged to) take a taxi to the hotel.*

To ask for information, use:

> **Comment est-ce que tu as trouvé** Paris?

> *How did you like Paris?*

To give opinions, use:

> **Je pense que** c'est la plus belle ville du monde.

> *I think that it's the most beautiful city in the world.*

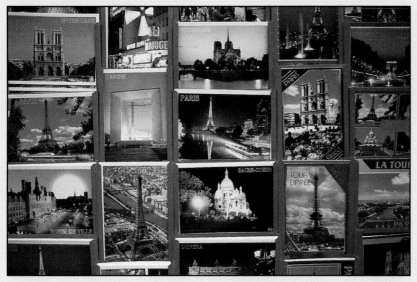

Paris est la plus belle ville du monde, n'est-ce pas?

To compare things, use:

> Le Louvre est **le plus grand** musée de Paris.

> *The **Louvre** is the largest museum in Paris.*

Nathalie et Raoul

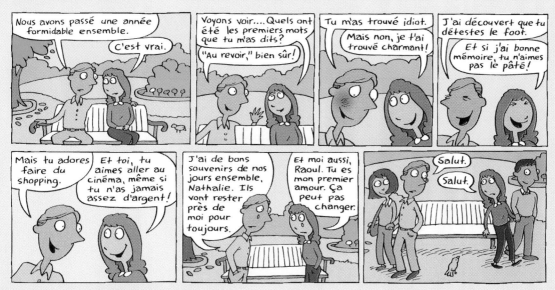

Grammar Summary

Subject Pronouns

Singular	Plural
je	nous
tu	vous
il/elle/on	ils/elles

Indefinite Articles

Singular		Plural
Masculine	Feminine	
un	une	des

Definite Articles

Singular			Plural
Before a Consonant Sound		Before a Vowel Sound	
Masculine	Feminine		
le	la	l'	les

À + Definite Articles

Singular			Plural
Before a Consonant Sound		Before a Vowel Sound	
Masculine	Feminine		
au	à la	à l'	aux

De + Definite Articles

Singular			Plural
Before a Consonant Sound		Before a Vowel Sound	
Masculine	Feminine		
du	de la	de l'	des

Partitive Articles

Before a Consonant Sound		Before a Vowel Sound
Masculine	**Feminine**	
du pain	**de la** glace	**de l'**eau

In negative sentences the partitive article becomes *de (d')*.

Expressions of Quantity

combien	how much, how many
assez	enough
beaucoup	a lot, many
(un) peu	(a) little, few
trop	too much, too many

These expressions are followed by *de (d')* before a noun.

Question Words

combien	how much, how many
comment	what, how
où	where
pourquoi	why
qu'est-ce que	what
quand	when
quel, quelle	what, which
qui	who, whom

Question Formation

1. By a rising tone of voice
   Vous travaillez beaucoup?
2. By beginning with *est-ce que*
   Est-ce que vous travaillez beaucoup?
3. By adding *n'est-ce pas?*
   Vous travaillez beaucoup, n'est-ce pas?
4. By inversion
   Travaillez-vous beaucoup?

Possessive Adjectives

Singular			Plural
Masculine	Feminine before a Consonant Sound	Feminine before a Vowel Sound	
mon	ma	mon	mes
ton	ta	ton	tes
son	sa	son	ses
notre	notre	notre	nos
votre	votre	votre	vos
leur	leur	leur	leurs

Demonstrative Adjectives

	Masculine before a Consonant Sound	Masculine before a Vowel Sound	Feminine
Singular	ce	cet	cette
Plural	ces	ces	ces

Quel

	Masculine	Feminine
Singular	quel	quelle
Plural	quels	quelles

Agreement of Adjectives

	Masculine	Feminine
add **e**	Il est bavard.	Elle est bavarde.
no change	Il est suisse.	Elle est suisse.
change **-er** to **-ère**	Il est cher.	Elle est chère.
change **-eux** to **-euse**	Il est paresseux.	Elle est paresseuse.
double consonant + **e**	Il est gros.	Elle est grosse.

Irregular Feminine Adjectives

Masculine before a Consonant Sound	Masculine before a Vowel Sound	Feminine
blanc		blanche
frais		fraîche
long		longue
beau	bel	belle
nouveau	nouvel	nouvelle
vieux	vieil	vieille

Position of Adjectives

Most adjectives usually follow their nouns. But adjectives expressing beauty, age, goodness and size precede their nouns. Some of these preceding adjectives are:

autre	joli
beau	mauvais
bon	nouveau
grand	petit
gros	vieux
jeune	

Comparative of Adjectives

plus	+	adjective	+	**que**
moins	+	adjective	+	**que**
aussi	+	adjective	+	**que**

Superlative of Adjectives

le/la/les	+	**plus**	+	adjective

Regular Verbs—Present Tense

-er **parler**			
je	parle	nous	parlons
tu	parles	vous	parlez
il/elle/on	parle	ils/elles	parlent

-ir **finir**			
je	finis	nous	finissons
tu	finis	vous	finissez
il/elle/on	finit	ils/elles	finissent

-re **perdre**			
je	perds	nous	perdons
tu	perds	vous	perdez
il/elle/on	perd	ils/elles	perdent

Irregular Verbs

acheter			
j'	achète	nous	achetons
tu	achètes	vous	achetez
il/elle/on	achète	ils/elles	achètent

aller			
je	vais	nous	allons
tu	vas	vous	allez
il/elle/on	va	ils/elles	vont

avoir			
j'	ai	nous	avons
tu	as	vous	avez
il/elle/on	a	ils/elles	ont

devoir			
je	dois	nous	devons
tu	dois	vous	devez
il/elle/on	doit	ils/elles	doivent

être			
je	suis	nous	sommes
tu	es	vous	êtes
il/elle/on	est	ils/elles	sont

faire			
je	fais	nous	faisons
tu	fais	vous	faites
il/elle/on	fait	ils/elles	font

falloir	
il	faut

mettre			
je	mets	nous	mettons
tu	mets	vous	mettez
il/elle/on	met	ils/elles	mettent

pleuvoir	
il	pleut

pouvoir			
je	peux	nous	pouvons
tu	peux	vous	pouvez
il/elle/on	peut	ils/elles	peuvent

préférer			
je	préfère	nous	préférons
tu	préfères	vous	préférez
il/elle/on	préfère	ils/elles	préfèrent

prendre			
je	prends	nous	prenons
tu	prends	vous	prenez
il/elle/on	prend	ils/elles	prennent

venir			
je	viens	nous	venons
tu	viens	vous	venez
il/elle/on	vient	ils/elles	viennent

voir			
je	vois	nous	voyons
tu	vois	vous	voyez
il/elle/on	voit	ils/elles	voient

vouloir			
je	veux	nous	voulons
tu	veux	vous	voulez
il/elle/on	veut	ils/elles	veulent

Regular Imperatives

-er parler	-ir finir	-re perdre
parle	finis	perds
parlez	finissez	perdez
parlons	finissons	perdons

Verbs + Infinitive

adorer	devoir	regarder
aimer	falloir	venir
aller	pouvoir	vouloir
désirer	préférer	

Negation in Present Tense

ne... jamais	Je **ne** vois **jamais** Hélène.
ne... pas	Vous **ne** mangez **pas.**
ne... personne	Il **n'**y a **personne** ici.
ne... plus	Tu **ne** fais **plus** de footing?
ne... rien	Nous **ne** faisons **rien.**

Numbers

0 = zéro	18 = dix-huit	71 = soixante et onze
1 = un	19 = dix-neuf	72 = soixante-douze
2 = deux	20 = vingt	80 = quatre-vingts
3 = trois	21 = vingt et un	81 = quatre-vingt-un
4 = quatre	22 = vingt-deux	82 = quatre-vingt-deux
5 = cinq	30 = trente	90 = quatre-vingt-dix
6 = six	31 = trente et un	91 = quatre-vingt-onze
7 = sept	32 = trente-deux	92 = quatre-vingt-douze
8 = huit	40 = quarante	100 = cent
9 = neuf	41 = quarante et un	101 = cent un
10 = dix	42 = quarante-deux	102 = cent deux
11 = onze	50 = cinquante	200 = deux cents
12 = douze	51 = cinquante et un	201 = deux cent un
13 = treize	52 = cinquante-deux	1.000 = mille
14 = quatorze	60 = soixante	1.001 = mille un
15 = quinze	61 = soixante et un	2.000 = deux mille
16 = seize	62 = soixante-deux	1.000.000 = un million
17 = dix-sept	70 = soixante-dix	2.000.000 = deux millions

Ordinal Numbers

1er	= premier	6e	= sixième
2e	= deuxième	7e	= septième
3e	= troisième	8e	= huitième
4e	= quatrième	9e	= neuvième
5e	= cinquième	10e	= dixième

Passé Composé—Regular Past Participles

jouer			
j'ai	joué	nous avons	joué
tu as	joué	vous avez	joué
il/elle/on a	joué	ils/elles ont	joué

finir			
j'ai	fini	nous avons	fini
tu as	fini	vous avez	fini
il/elle/on a	fini	ils/elles ont	fini

attendre			
j'ai	attendu	nous avons	attendu
tu as	attendu	vous avez	attendu
il/elle/on a	attendu	ils/elles ont	attendu

Passé Composé—Irregular Past Participles

Infinitive	Past Participle
avoir	eu
être	été
faire	fait
prendre	pris
voir	vu

Passé Composé with *Être*

aller		
je	suis	allé
je	suis	allée
tu	es	allé
tu	es	allée
il	est	allé
elle	est	allée
on	est	allé
nous	sommes	allés
nous	sommes	allées
vous	êtes	allé
vous	êtes	allés
vous	êtes	allée
vous	êtes	allées
ils	sont	allés
elles	sont	allées

Some of the verbs that use *être* as the helping verb in the *passé composé* are:

Infinitive	Past Participle
aller	allé
arriver	arrivé
entrer	entré
partir	parti
rentrer	rentré
rester	resté
sortir	sorti
venir	venu

Vocabulary
French/English

All words and expressions introduced as active vocabulary in *C'est à toi!* appear in this end vocabulary. The number following the meaning of each word or expression indicates the unit in which it appears for the first time. If there is more than one meaning for a word or expression and it has appeared in different units, the corresponding unit numbers are listed.

A

à to 2; at 4; in 6; *À bientôt.* See you soon. 1; *À demain.* See you tomorrow. 2; *à droite* to (on) the right 9; *à gauche* to (on) the left 9; *À tes souhaits!* Bless you! 10

acheter to buy 7

adorer to love 7

un **aéroport** airport 11

une **affiche** poster 4

l' **Afrique (f.)** Africa 11

l' **âge (m.)** age 5; *Tu as quel âge?* How old are you? 5

un **agent de police** police officer 6

ah oh 1

aimer to like, to love 2

l' **Algérie (f.)** Algeria 11

algérien, algérienne Algerian 11

l' **Allemagne (f.)** Germany 6

l' **allemand (m.)** German (language) 4

allemand(e) German 6

aller to go 2; *allons-y* let's go (there) 3

allô hello (on telephone) 1

alors (well) then 2

américain(e) American 6

un(e) **ami(e)** friend 6

amoureux, amoureuse in love 12

un **an** year 5; *J'ai... ans.* I'm ... years old. 5

l' **anglais (m.)** English (language) 4

anglais(e) English 6

l' **Angleterre (f.)** England 6

un **anniversaire** birthday 5

un **anorak** ski jacket 7

août August 5

un **appartement** apartment 9

après after 6

l' **après-midi (m.)** afternoon 10

un **arbre** tree 9

un **arc** arch 12

une **arche** arch 12

l' **argent (m.)** money 11

une **armoire** wardrobe 9

arriver to arrive 1

assez rather, quite 7; *assez de* enough 8

une **assiette** plate 9

attendre to wait (for) 8

au to (the), at (the) 2; in (the) 6; *au moins* at least 12; *au revoir* good-bye 1; *Au secours!* Help! 10; *au-dessus de* above 9

aujourd'hui today 6

aussi also, too 2; as 8

aussitôt que as soon as 10

l' **automne (m.)** autumn, fall 6

autre other 6; *un(e) autre* another 6

aux to (the), at (the), in (the) 7

avec with 4

une **avenue** avenue 11

un **avion** airplane 11

un(e) **avocat(e)** lawyer 6

avoir to have 4; *avoir besoin de* to need 4; *avoir bonne/mauvaise mine* to look well/sick 10; *avoir chaud* to be warm, hot 10; *avoir envie de* to want, to feel like 11; *avoir faim* to be hungry 4; *avoir froid* to be cold 10; *avoir mal (à...)* to hurt, to have a/an ... ache, to have a sore ... 10; *avoir mal au cœur* to feel nauseous 10; *avoir peur (de)* to be afraid (of) 10; *avoir quel âge* to be how old 5; *avoir soif* to be thirsty 4; *avoir... ans* to be ... (years old) 5

avril April 5

B

une **baguette** long, thin loaf of bread 8

une **baignoire** bathtub 9

un **bain: une salle de bains** bathroom 9

baisser to lower 10

un **bal** dance 12

un **balcon** balcony 9

une **banane** banana 8

une **banque** bank 11

des **bas (m.)** (panty) hose 7

le **basket (basketball)** basketball 2

des **baskets (f.)** hightops 7

un **bateau** boat 12

un **bâton** ski pole 10

bavard(e) talkative 5

beau, bel, belle beautiful, handsome 5

beaucoup a lot, (very) much 2; *beaucoup de* a lot of, many 8

un **beau-frère** stepbrother, brother-in-law 5

un **beau-père** stepfather, father-in-law 5

beige beige 7

belge Belgian 11

la **Belgique** Belgium 11

une **belle-mère** stepmother, mother-in-law 5

une **belle-sœur** stepsister, sister-in-law 5

ben: bon ben well then 2

le **besoin: avoir besoin de** to need 4

bête stupid, dumb 5

Beurk! Yuk! 7

le **beurre** butter 8

une **bibliothèque** library 11

bien well 1; really 2; *bien sûr* of course 9

Bienvenue! Welcome! 9

un **billet** ticket 12

la **biologie** biology 4

une **bise** kiss 11

blanc, blanche white 7

bleu(e) blue 5

blond(e) blond 5

un **blouson** jacket (outdoor) 7

le **bœuf** beef 8

une **boisson** drink, beverage 3

une **boîte** dance club 2; can 8

un **bol** bowl 9

bon, bonne good 2; *bon ben* well then 2; *bon marché* cheap 7

bonjour hello 1

bonsoir good evening 9

une **botte** boot 7

une **bouche** mouth 10

une **boucherie** butcher shop 8

une **bouillabaisse** fish soup 8

une **boulangerie** bakery 8

une **boum** party 7

une **bouteille** bottle 8

une **boutique** shop, boutique 7

un **bras** arm 10

un **bruit** noise 12

brun(e) dark (hair), brown 5

un **bureau** desk 4

C

c'est this is, it's 1; he is, she is 5; that's 6

ça that, it 3; *Ça fait....* That's/It's . . . . 3; *Ça fait combien?* How much is it/that? 3; *Ça va?* How are things going? 1; *Ça va bien.* Things are going well. 1

un **cabinet** (doctor or dentist's) office 10

un **cadeau** gift, present 5

un **café** café; coffee 3

un **cahier** notebook 4

un **calendrier** calendar 4

une **cassette** cassette 4

le **camembert** Camembert cheese 8

le **camping** camping 2

un **camping** campground 11

le **Canada** Canada 6

canadien, canadienne Canadian 6

un **canapé** couch, sofa 9

une **cantine** cafeteria 4

une **carotte** carrot 8

une **carte** map 4

une **cassette** cassette 4

un **CD** CD 4

ce, cet, cette; ces this, that; these, those 8

ce sont they are, these are, those are 5

cent (one) hundred 3

un **centre** center 12; *un centre commercial* shopping center, mall 7

une **cerise** cherry 8

une **chaise** chair 4

une **chambre** bedroom 9

un **champignon** mushroom 8

la **chance** luck 6

un **chapeau** hat 7

une **charcuterie** delicatessen 8

chargé(e) full 12

un **chat** cat 5

chaud(e) warm, hot 6; *avoir chaud* to be warm, hot 10

une **chaussette** sock 7

une **chaussure** shoe 7

un **chemin** path, way 12

une **chemise** shirt 7

un **chèque de voyage** traveler's check 11

cher, chère expensive 7; dear 11

chercher to look for 7

un **cheval** horse 5

des **cheveux (m.)** hair 5

chez to the house/home of 2; at the house/home of 11; *chez moi* to my house 2

un **chien** dog 5

la **chimie** chemistry 4

la **Chine** China 6

chinois(e) Chinese 6

des **chips (m.)** snacks 9

le **chocolat** chocolate 3

une **chose** thing 7; *quelque chose* something 7

ciao bye 1

un **cimetière** cemetery 12

le **cinéma** movies 2

cinq five 1

cinquante fifty 3

cinquième fifth 11

un **coca** Coke 3

un **cœur** heart 10; *avoir mal au cœur* to feel nauseous 10

un **coiffeur, une coiffeuse** hairdresser 6

combien how much 3; *combien de* how much, how many 8

comme like, for 3; *comme ci, comme ça* so-so 3

commencer to begin 4

comment what 1; how 3; *Comment vas-tu?* How are you? 3

un(e) **comptable** accountant 6

la **confiture** jam 8

continuer to continue 12

une **corbeille** wastebasket 4

un **corps** body 10

un **costume** man's suit 7

la **Côte-d'Ivoire** Ivory Coast 11

un **cou** neck 10

une **couleur** color 7

un **cours** course, class 4

les **courses: faire les courses** to go grocery shopping 8

court(e) short 7

le **couscous** couscous 9

un(e) **cousin(e)** cousin 5

un **couteau** knife 9

coûter to cost 3

un **couvert** table setting 9

un **crabe** crab 8

un **crayon** pencil 4

une **crémerie** dairy store 8

une **crêpe** crêpe 3

une **crevette** shrimp 8

un **croissant** croissant 8

une **cuiller** spoon 9

une **cuisine** kitchen 9

un **cuisinier, une cuisinière** cook 6

une **cuisinière** stove 9

D

d'abord first 8

d'accord OK 1

d'après according to 12

dans in 4

danser to dance 2

une **date** date 5

de (d') of, from 4; a, an, any 6; some 9; in, by 12

décembre December 5

décider (de) to decide 12

un **défilé** parade 12

déjà already 3

le **déjeuner** lunch 9; *le petit déjeuner* breakfast 9

demain tomorrow 2

demander to ask for 12

demi(e) half 4; *et demi(e)* thirty (minutes), half past 4

un **demi-frère** half-brother 5

une **demi-sœur** half-sister 5

une **dent** tooth 10

un(e) **dentiste** dentist 6

dernier, dernière last 12

derrière behind 4

des some 3; from (the), of (the) 6; any 8

désirer to want 3; *Vous désirez?* What would you like? 3

un **dessert** dessert 3

le **dessin** drawing 4

dessus: au-dessus de above 9

deux two 1

deuxième second 11

devant in front of 4

devoir to have to 10

les **devoirs (m.)** homework 2

un **dictionnaire** dictionary 4

diligent(e) hardworking 5

dimanche (m.) Sunday 4

le **dîner** dinner, supper 9

dis say 2

une **disquette** diskette 4

dix ten 1

dix-huit eighteen 1

dixième tenth 11

dix-neuf nineteen 1

dix-sept seventeen 1

un **docteur** doctor 10

un **doigt** finger 10; *un doigt de pied* toe 10

un **dollar** dollar 7

donc so, then 9

donner to give 3; *Donnez-moi....* Give me 3

dormir to sleep 2

un **dos** back 10

une **douche** shower 9

douze twelve 1

la **droite: à droite** to (on) the right 9

du from (the), of (the) 6; some, any 8; in (the) 12

E

l' **eau (f.)** water 3; *l'eau minérale (f.)* mineral water 3

une **école** school 4

écoute listen 1

écouter to listen (to) 2; *écouter de la musique* to listen to music 2

une **église** church 11

égoïste selfish 5

Eh! Hey! 1

un(e) **élève** student 4

elle she, it 2

elles they (f.) 2

un **emploi du temps** schedule 4

en to (the) 2; on 5; in 6; *en solde* on sale 7

enchanté(e) delighted 9

encore still 9

un(e) **enfant** child 5

ensemble together 4

un **ensemble** outfit 7

une **entrée** entrance 9

entrer to enter, to come in 9

l' **envie (f.): avoir envie de** to want, to feel like 11

une **épaule** shoulder 10

un **escalier** stairs, staircase 9

l' **Espagne (f.)** Spain 6

l' **espagnol (m.)** Spanish (language) 4

espagnol(e) Spanish 6

est is 3

l' **est (m.)** east 11

est-ce que? (phrase introducing a question) 6

et and 2

un **étage** floor, story 9

les **États-Unis (m.)** United States 6

l' **été (m.)** summer 6

être to be 5; *Nous sommes le (+ date).* It's the (+ date). 5

un(e) **étudiant(e)** student 4

étudier to study 2; *Étudions....* Let's study 4

euh uhm 8

l' **Europe (f.)** Europe 11

un **évier** sink 9

excusez-moi excuse me 7

F

facile easy 10

la **faim: J'ai faim.** I'm hungry. 3

faire to do, to make 2; *faire du (+ number)* to wear size (+ number) 7; *faire du footing* to go running 2; *faire du roller* to go in-line skating 2; *faire du shopping* to go shopping 2; *faire du sport* to play sports 2; *faire du vélo* to go biking 2; *faire le tour* to take a tour 9; *faire les courses* to go grocery shopping 8; *faire les devoirs* to do homework 2; *faire les magasins* to go shopping 7; *faire un tour* to go for a ride 6

fait: Ça fait.... That's/It's . . . 3; *Quel temps fait-il?* What's the weather like? How's the weather? 6; *Il fait beau.* It's (The weather's) beautiful/ nice. 6; *Il fait chaud.* It's (The weather's) hot/warm. 6; *Il fait du soleil.* It's sunny. 6; *Il fait du vent.* It's windy. 6; *Il fait frais.* It's (The weather's) cool. 6; *Il fait froid.* It's (The weather's) cold. 6; *Il fait mauvais.* It's (The weather's) bad. 6

falloir to be necessary, to have to 10

une **famille** family 5

un **fast-food** fast-food restaurant 3

fatigué(e) tired 10

faut: il faut it is necessary, one has to/must, we/you have to/must 10

un **fauteuil** armchair 9

une **femme** wife; woman 5; *une femme au foyer* housewife 6; *une femme d'affaires* businesswoman 6

une **fenêtre** window 4

fermer to close 12

un **fermier, une fermière** farmer 6

une **fête** holiday, festival 12

un **feu d'artifice** fireworks 12

une **feuille de papier** sheet of paper 4

février February 5

la **fièvre** fever 10

une **figure** face 10

une **fille** girl 4; daughter 5

un **film** movie 2

un **fils** son 5

finir to finish 4

une **fleur** flower 9

une **fois** time 12

le **foot (football)** soccer 2

le **footing** running 2

une **forme: être en bonne/mauvaise forme** to be in good/bad shape 10

formidable great, terrific 11

un **four** oven 9

une **fourchette** fork 9

frais, fraîche cool, fresh 6

une **fraise** strawberry 8

un **franc** franc 3

le **français** French (language) 4

français(e) French 6

la **France** France 6

un **frère** brother 5

un **frigo** refrigerator 9

des **frissons (m.)** chills 10

des **frites (f.)** French fries 3

froid(e) cold 6; *avoir froid* to be cold 10

le **fromage** cheese 3

un **fruit** fruit 8

G

un **garage** garage 9

un **garçon** boy 4

garder to keep 10

une **gare** train station 11

un **gâteau** cake 8

la **gauche: à gauche** to (on) the left 9

généreux, généreuse generous 5

un **genou** knee 10

gentil, gentille nice 9

la **géographie** geography 4

une **glace** ice cream 3; *une glace à la vanille* vanilla ice cream 3; *une glace au chocolat* chocolate ice cream 3

une **gorge** throat 10

le **goûter** afternoon snack 9

grand(e) tall, big, large 7

une **grand-mère** grandmother 5

un **grand-père** grandfather 5

un **grenier** attic 9

la **grippe** flu 10

gris(e) gray 5

gros, grosse big, fat, large 11

la **Guadeloupe** Guadeloupe 5

un **guichet** ticket window 12

H

habiter to live 9

un **hamburger** hamburger 3

des **haricots verts (m.)** green beans 8

l' **heure (f.)** hour, time, o'clock 3; *Quelle heure est-il?* What time is it? 3

hier yesterday 11

l' **histoire (f.)** history 4

l' **hiver (m.)** winter 6

un **homme** man 6; *un homme au foyer* househusband 6; *un homme d'affaires* businessman 6

un **horaire** schedule, timetable 11

un **hot-dog** hot dog 3

un **hôtel** hotel 12

huit eight 1

huitième eighth 11

I

ici here 6

il he, it 2

il y a there is, there are 7

ils they (m.) 2

imaginer to imagine 12

un **immeuble** apartment building 9

impressionniste Impressionist 12

un **infirmier,** une **infirmière** nurse 6

un **informaticien,** une **informaticienne** computer specialist 6

l' **informatique (f.)** computer science 4

un **ingénieur** engineer 6

intelligent(e) intelligent 5

une **interro (interrogation)** quiz, test 2

inviter to invite 2

l' **Italie (f.)** Italy 6

italien, italienne Italian 6

ivoirien, ivoirienne from the Ivory Coast 11

J

j' I 1

jamais: ne (n')... jamais never 10

une **jambe** leg 10

le **jambon** ham 3

janvier January 5

le **Japon** Japan 6

japonais(e) Japanese 6

un **jardin** garden, lawn 9; park 12

jaune yellow 7

le **jazz** jazz 2

je I 1

un **jean** (pair of) jeans 7

jeudi (m.) Thursday 4

jeune young 12

des **jeux vidéo (m.)** video games 2

joli(e) pretty 7

jouer to play 2; *jouer au basket* to play basketball 2; *jouer au foot* to play soccer 2; *jouer au tennis* to play tennis 2; *jouer au volley* to play volleyball 2; *jouer aux jeux vidéo* to play video games 2

un **jour** day 4

un(e) **journaliste** journalist 6

une **journée** day 12

juillet July 5

juin June 5

une **jupe** skirt 7

le **jus d'orange** orange juice 3; *le jus de fruit* fruit juice 9; *le jus de pomme* apple juice 3; *le jus de raisin* grape juice 3

jusqu'à up to, until 12

juste just, only 4

K

le **ketchup** ketchup 8

un **kilogramme (kilo)** kilogram 8

un **kilomètre** kilometer 5

L

là there, here 4

là-bas over there 7

le **lait** milk 8

une **lampe** lamp 9

le **latin** Latin (language) 4

le, la, l' the 2; *le (+ day of the week)* on (+ day of the week) 4; *le (+ number)* on the (+ ordinal number) 1

un **légume** vegetable 8

les the 2

leur their 5

la **liberté** liberty 12

une **librairie** bookstore 11

une **limonade** lemon-lime soda 3

lire to read 2

un **lit** bed 9

un **livre** book 4

loin far 11

long, longue long 7

une **lumière** light 12

lundi (m.) Monday 4

le **Luxembourg** Luxembourg 11

luxembourgeois(e) from Luxembourg 11

M

m'appelle: je m'appelle my name is 1

Madame (Mme) Mrs., Ma'am 1

Mademoiselle (Mlle) Miss 1

un **magasin** store 7; *un grand magasin* department store 7

un **magnétoscope** VCR 4

mai May 5

un **maillot de bain** swimsuit 7

une **main** hand 10

maintenant now 8

une **mairie** town hall 11

mais but 2

une **maison** house 9

mal bad, badly 3; *avoir mal (à...)* to hurt, to have a/an ... ache, to have a sore ... 10

malade sick 10

maman (f.) Mom 8

manger to eat 2; *manger de la pizza* to eat pizza 2; *une salle à manger* dining room 9

un **manteau** coat 7

un(e) **marchand(e)** merchant 8

un **marché** market 8

marcher to walk 12

mardi (m.) Tuesday 4

un **mari** husband 5

le **Maroc** Morocco 11

marocain(e) Moroccan 11

marre: J'en ai marre! I'm sick of it! I've had it! 4

marron brown 7

mars March 5

la **Martinique** Martinique 5

les **maths (f.)** math 4

un **matin** morning 8; *le matin* in the morning 8

mauvais(e) bad 6

la **mayonnaise** mayonnaise 8

me (to) me 11

méchant(e) mean 5

un **médecin** doctor 6

un **melon** melon 8

un **membre** member 5

même even 9

une **mer** sea 11

merci thanks 1

mercredi (m.) Wednesday 4

une **mère** mother 5

Messieurs-Dames ladies and gentlemen 3

un **métro** subway 12

mettre to put (on), to set 9

mexicain(e) Mexican 6

le **Mexique** Mexico 6

un **micro-onde** microwave 9

midi noon 3

mille (one) thousand 4

un **million** million 5

la **mine: avoir bonne/mauvaise mine** to look well/sick 10

minuit midnight 3

une **minute** minute 4

moche ugly 7

moderne modern 12

moi me, I 2

moins minus 4; less 8; *au moins* at least 12; *moins le quart* quarter to 4

un **mois** month 5

mon, ma; mes my 5

le **monde** world 12

Monsieur Mr., Sir 1

monter to go up 12

montrer to show 4; *Montrez-moi....* Show me.... 4

un **monument** monument 12

un **morceau** piece 8

la **moutarde** mustard 8

mûr(e) ripe 8

un **musée** museum 11

un **musicien, une musicienne** musician 12

la **musique** music 2

N

n'est-ce pas? isn't that so? 5

nager to swim 2

une **nappe** tablecloth 9

national(e) national 12

ne (n')... jamais never 10

ne (n')... pas not 2

ne (n')... personne no one, nobody, not anyone 10

ne (n')... plus no longer, not anymore 10

ne (n')... rien nothing, not anything 10

neiger: Il neige. It's snowing. 6

neuf nine 1

neuvième ninth 11

un **nez** nose 10

noir(e) black 5

non no 1

le **nord** north 11

notre; nos our 5

nous we 2; us 5

nouveau, nouvel, nouvelle new 7

novembre November 5

O

obligé(e): être obligé(e) de to be obliged to, to have to 12

octobre October 5

un **œil** eye 10

un **œuf** egg 8

oh oh 4; *Oh là là!* Wow! Oh no! Oh dear! 10

un **oignon** onion 8

un **oiseau** bird 5

OK OK 8

une **omelette** omelette 3

on they, we, one 2; *On y va?* Shall we go (there)? 2

un **oncle** uncle 5

onze eleven 1

orange orange 7

une **orange** orange 3

un **ordinateur** computer 4

une **oreille** ear 10

ou or 3

où where 4

ouais yeah 8

l' **ouest (m.)** west 11

oui yes 1

P

le **pain** bread 8

un **pantalon** (pair of) pants 7

par per 4

le **paradis** paradise 12

parce que because 5

pardon excuse me 1

un **parent** parent; relative 5

paresseux, paresseuse lazy 5

parler to speak, to talk 6

partir to leave 11

pas not 1

un **passeport** passport 11

passer to show (a movie) 2; to spend (time) 12

une **pastèque** watermelon 8

le **pâté** pâté 8

une **pâtisserie** pastry store 8

une **pêche** peach 8

une **pendule** clock 4

penser (à) to think (of) 12

perdre to lose 12

un **père** father 5

une **personne: ne (n')... personne** no one, nobody, not anyone 10

petit(e) short, little, small 7; *le petit déjeuner* breakfast 9

des **petits pois (m.)** peas 8

(un) **peu** (a) little 2; *(un) peu de* (a) little, few 8

la **peur: avoir peur (de)** to be afraid (of) 10

peut-être maybe 7

la **philosophie** philosophy 4

une **photo** photo, picture 5

la **physique** physics 4

une **pièce** room 9

un **pied** foot 10; *un doigt de pied* toe 10

une **piscine** swimming pool 11

une **pizza** pizza 2

un **placard** cupboard 9

la **place** room, space 10; *une place* (public) square 11

une **plage** beach 11

plaît: ... me plaît.
I like 11

un **plan** map 12

pleuvoir: Il pleut. It's
raining. 6

plus more 8; *le/la/les plus* (+
adjective) the most (+
adjective) 12; *ne (n')... plus*
no longer, not anymore 10

une **poire** pear 8

les **pois (m.): des petits pois
(m.)** peas 8

un **poisson** fish 5; *un poisson
rouge* goldfish 5

le **poivre** pepper 9

une **pomme** apple 3; *une pomme
de terre* potato 8

le **porc** pork 8

une **porte** door 4

porter to wear 7

possible possible 2

une **poste** post office 11

un **pot** jar 8

un **poulet** chicken 8

pour for 2; (in order) to 7

pourquoi why 2

pouvoir to be able to 8

préférer to prefer 2

premier, première first 5

prendre to take, to have (food
or drink) 9; *prendre
rendez-vous* to make an
appointment 10

près (de) near 11

présenter to introduce 1

prie: Je vous en prie. You're
welcome. 3

le **printemps** spring 6

un(e) **prof** teacher 4

un **professeur** teacher 4

une **profession** occupation 6

puis then 8

un **pull** sweater 7

Q

qu'est-ce que what 2; *Qu'est-
ce que c'est?* What is it/this? 4;
Qu'est-ce que tu as? What's
the matter with you? 10

quand when 6

quarante forty 3

un **quart** quarter 4; *et quart*
fifteen (minutes after),
quarter after 4; *moins le
quart* quarter to 4

un **quartier** quarter,
neighborhood 12

quatorze fourteen 1

quatre four 1

quatre-vingt-dix ninety 3

quatre-vingts eighty 3

quatrième fourth 11

que how 5; than, as, that 8;
Que je suis bête! How dumb I
am! 5; *Que vous êtes gentils!*
How nice you are! 9

quel, quelle what, which 3

quelqu'un someone,
somebody 10

quelque chose something 7

quelques some 9

qui who, whom 2

une **quiche** quiche 3

quinze fifteen 1

quitter to leave (a person or
place) 12

quoi what 4

R

un **raisin** grape 3

un(e) **réceptionniste** receptionist 10

regarder to watch 2; to look
(at) 10

le **reggae** reggae 2

regretter to be sorry 10

un **rendez-vous** appointment 10;
prendre rendez-vous to make
an appointment 10

rentrer to come home, to
return, to come back 11

un **repas** meal 8

ressembler à to look like, to
resemble 5

un **restaurant** restaurant 11

rester to stay, to remain 10

revenir to come back, to
return 11

le **rez-de-chaussée** ground
floor 9

un **rhume** cold 10

rien: ne (n')... rien nothing,
not anything 10

une **robe** dress 7

le **rock** rock (music) 2

le **roller** in-line skating 2

rose pink 7

rouge red 5

roux, rousse red (hair) 5

une **rue** street 12

S

s'appelle: elle s'appelle her
name is 1; *il s'appelle* his
name is 1

s'il te plaît please 9; *s'il vous
plaît* please 3

un **sac à dos** backpack 4

une **salade** salad 3

une **salle à manger** dining room 9

une **salle de bains** bathroom 9

une **salle de classe** classroom 4

un **salon** living room 9

salut hi; good-bye 1

samedi (m.) Saturday 4

un **sandwich** sandwich 3; *un
sandwich au fromage* cheese
sandwich 3; *un sandwich au
jambon* ham sandwich 3

la **santé** health 10

le **saucisson** salami 8

les **sciences (f.)** science 4

le **secours: Au secours!**
Help! 10

seize sixteen 1

un **séjour** family room 9;
stay 11

le **sel** salt 9

une **semaine** week 4

le **Sénégal** Senegal 11

sénégalais(e) Senegalese 11

sept seven 1

septembre September 5

septième seventh 11

un **serveur, une serveuse**
server 3

une **serviette** napkin 9

seulement only 12

le **shopping** shopping 2

un **short** (pair of) shorts 7

si yes (on the contrary) 4; so 6

six six 1

sixième sixth 11

skier to ski 2

une **sœur** sister 5

la **soif: J'ai soif.** I'm thirsty. 3

un **soir** evening 7; *ce soir* tonight 8

soixante sixty 3

soixante-dix seventy 3

des **soldes (f.)** sale(s) 7

le **soleil** sun 6

solide steady 10

son, sa; ses his, her, one's, its 5

sortir to go out 2

un **souhait: À tes souhaits!** Bless you! 10

la **soupe** soup 8

sous under 4

un **sous-sol** basement 9

souvent often 6

un **sport** sport 2

un **stade** stadium 11

une **station** station 12

une **statue** statue 12

un **steak** steak 3; *un steak-frites* steak with French fries 3

une **stéréo** stereo 4

un **stylo** pen 4

le **sucre** sugar 9

le **sud** south 11

suisse Swiss 11

la **Suisse** Switzerland 11

super super, terrific, great 2

un **supermarché** supermarket 8

sur on 4; in 6

sûr: bien sûr of course 9

un **sweat** sweatshirt 7

sympa (sympathique) nice 5

T

t'appelles: tu t'appelles your name is 1

un **tabac** tobacco shop 11

une **table** table 9

un **tableau** (chalk)board 4; painting 12

une **taille** size 7

un **taille-crayon** pencil sharpener 4

un **tailleur** woman's suit 7

Tant mieux. That's great. 4

une **tante** aunt 5

un **tapis** rug 9

une **tarte (aux fraises)** (strawberry) pie 8

une **tasse** cup 9

un **taxi** taxi 12

te to you 1

un **tee-shirt** T-shirt 7

la **télé (télévision)** TV, television 2

téléphoner to phone (someone), to make a call 2

une **température** temperature 10

le **temps** weather 6; *Quel temps fait-il?* What's the weather like? How's the weather? 6

des **tennis (m.)** tennis shoes 7

le **tennis** tennis 2

la **terre: une pomme de terre** potato 8

une **tête** head 10

Tiens! Hey! 1

un **timbre** stamp 11

timide timid, shy 5

toi you 3

les **toilettes (f.)** toilet 9

une **tomate** tomato 8

un **tombeau** tomb 12

ton, ta; tes your 5

toucher to cash 11

toujours always 8; still 9

un **tour** trip 6; *le tour* tour 9

une **tour** tower 12

tourner to turn 11

tous les deux both 5

la **Toussaint** All Saints' Day 11

tout all, everything 11; *tout droit* straight ahead 11; *tout le monde* everybody 2

un **train** train 11

une **tranche** slice 8

travailler to work 6

treize thirteen 1

trente thirty 3

très very 3

un **triomphe** triumph 12

trois three 1

troisième third 11

trop too 8; too much 10; *trop de* too much, too many 8

une **trousse** pencil case 4

trouver to find 7

tu you 2

la **Tunisie** Tunisia 11

tunisien, tunisienne Tunisian 11

U

un one 1; a, an 2

une a, an, one 3

V

les **vacances (f.)** vacation 5

un **vase** vase 9

la **veille** night before 11

un **vélo** bicycle, bike 2

un **vendeur, une vendeuse** salesperson 7

vendre to sell 7

vendredi (m.) Friday 4

venir to come 6

le **vent** wind 6

un **ventre** stomach 10

un **verre** glass 9

vert(e) green 5

une **veste** (sport) jacket 7

des **vêtements (m.)** clothes 7

une **vidéocassette** videocassette 4

le **Vietnam** Vietnam 6

vietnamien, vietnamienne Vietnamese 6

vieux, vieil, vieille old 7

un **village** village 11

une **ville** city 11

vingt twenty 1

violet, violette purple 7

visiter to visit (a place) 12

vivre to live 12

voici here is/are 7

voilà here is/are, there is/are 3

voir to see 11

une **voiture** car 9

le **volley (volleyball)** volleyball 2

votre; vos your 5

voudrais would like 3

vouloir to want 8; *vouloir bien* to be willing 9

vous you 2; to you 9

un **voyage** trip 9

voyager to travel 6

voyons let's see 3

vrai(e) true 7

vraiment really 12

W

les **W.-C. (m.)** toilet 9

Y

le **yaourt** yogurt 8

des **yeux (m.)** eyes 5

Z

le **Zaïre** Zaire 11

zaïrois(e) Zairian 11

zéro zero 1

Zut! Darn! 4

Vocabulary

English/French

All words and expressions introduced as active vocabulary in *C'est à toi!* appear in this end vocabulary. The number following the meaning of each word or expression indicates the unit in which it appears for the first time. Verbs are listed in their infinitive forms even though a specific form may appear in an earlier unit. If there is more than one meaning for a word or expression and it has appeared in different units, the corresponding unit numbers are listed.

A

a un 2; une 3; de (d') 6; *a lot* beaucoup 2; *a lot of* beaucoup de 2

to be **able to** pouvoir 8

above au-dessus de 9

according to d'après 12

accountant un(e) comptable 6

ache: to have a/an . . . ache avoir mal (à...) 10

to be **afraid (of)** avoir peur (de) 10

Africa l'Afrique (f.) 11

after après 6

afternoon l'après-midi (m.) 10

age l'âge (m.) 5

ahead: straight ahead tout droit 11

airplane un avion 11

airport un aéroport 11

Algeria l'Algérie (f.) 11

Algerian algérien, algérienne 11

all tout 11; *All Saints' Day* la Toussaint 11

already déjà 3

also aussi 2

always toujours 8

American américain(e) 6

an un 2; une 3; de (d') 6

and et 2

another un(e) autre 6

any de (d') 6; des, du 8

anymore: not anymore ne (n')... plus 10

anyone: not anyone ne (n')... personne 10

anything: not anything ne (n')... rien 10

apartment un appartement 9; *apartment building* un immeuble 9

apple une pomme 3; *apple juice* le jus de pomme 3

appointment un rendez-vous 10; *to make an appointment* prendre rendez-vous 10

April avril 5

arch un arc, une arche 12

arm un bras 10

armchair un fauteuil 9

to **arrive** arriver 1

as aussi, que 8; *as soon as* aussitôt que 10

to **ask for** demander 12

at à 4; *at (the)* au 2, aux 7; *at least* au moins 12

attic un grenier 9

August août 5

aunt une tante 5

autumn l'automne (m.) 6

avenue une avenue 11

B

back un dos 10; *to come back* rentrer, revenir 11

backpack un sac à dos 4

bad mal 3; mauvais(e) 6; *It's bad.* Il fait mauvais. 6

badly mal 3

bakery une boulangerie 8

balcony un balcon 9

banana une banane 8

bank une banque 11

basement un sous-sol 9

basketball le basket (basketball) 2; *to play basketball* jouer au basket 2

bathroom une salle de bains 9

bathtub une baignoire 9

to **be** être 5; *to be . . . (years old)* avoir... ans 5; *to be able to* pouvoir 8; *to be afraid (of)* avoir peur (de) 10; *to be cold* avoir froid 10; *to be how old* avoir quel âge 5; *to be hungry* avoir faim 4; *to be in good/ bad shape* être en bonne/ mauvaise forme 10; *to be necessary* falloir 10; *to be obliged to* être obligé(e) de 12; *to be sorry* regretter 10; *to be thirsty* avoir soif 4; *to be warm/hot* avoir chaud 10; *to be willing* vouloir bien 9

beach une plage 11

beans: green beans des haricots verts (m.) 8

beautiful beau, bel, belle 5; *It's beautiful.* Il fait beau. 6

because parce que 5

bed un lit 9

bedroom une chambre 9

beef le bœuf 8

to **begin** commencer 4

behind derrière 4

beige beige 7

Belgian belge 11

Belgium la Belgique 11

beverage une boisson 3

bicycle un vélo 2

big grand(e) 7; gros, grosse 11

bike un vélo 2

biking: to go biking faire du vélo 2

biology la biologie 4

bird un oiseau 5

birthday un anniversaire 5

black noir(e) 5

Bless you! À tes souhaits! 10

blond blond(e) 5

blue bleu(e) 5

board un tableau 4

boat un bateau 12

body un corps 10

book un livre 4

bookstore une librairie 11

boot une botte 7

both tous les deux 5

bottle une bouteille 8

boutique une boutique 7

bowl un bol 9

boy un garçon 4

bread le pain 8; *long, thin loaf of bread* une baguette 8

breakfast le petit déjeuner 9

brother un frère 5

brother-in-law un beau-frère 5

brown brun(e) 5; marron 7

building: apartment building un immeuble 9

businessman un homme d'affaires 6

businesswoman une femme d'affaires 6

but mais 2

butcher shop une boucherie 8

butter le beurre 8

to **buy** acheter 7

by de (d') 12

bye ciao 1

C

café un café 3

cafeteria une cantine 4

cake un gâteau 8

calendar un calendrier 4

call: to make a call téléphoner 2

Camembert cheese le camembert 8

campground un camping 11

camping le camping 2

can une boîte 8

Canada le Canada 6

Canadian canadien, canadienne 6

car une voiture 9

carrot une carotte 8

to **cash** toucher 11

cassette une cassette 4

cat un chat 5

CD un CD 4

cemetery un cimetière 12

center un centre 12; *shopping center* un centre commercial 7

chair une chaise 4

chalkboard un tableau 4

cheap bon marché 7

check: traveler's check un chèque de voyage 11

cheese le fromage 3; *Camembert cheese* le camembert 8; *cheese sandwich* un sandwich au fromage 3

chemistry la chimie 4

cherry une cerise 8

chicken un poulet 8

child un(e) enfant 5

chills des frissons (m.) 10

China la Chine 6

Chinese chinois(e) 6

chocolate le chocolat 3; *chocolate ice cream* une glace au chocolat 3

church une église 11

city une ville 11

class un cours 4

classroom une salle de classe 4

clock une pendule 4

to **close** fermer 12

clothes des vêtements (m.) 7

club: dance club une boîte 2

coat un manteau 7

coffee un café 3

Coke un coca 3

cold froid(e) 6; *It's cold.* Il fait froid. 6; *to be cold* avoir froid 10

cold un rhume 10

color une couleur 7

to **come** venir 6; *to come back* rentrer, revenir 11; *to come home* rentrer 11; *to come in* entrer 9

computer un ordinateur 4; *computer science* l'informatique (f.) 4; *computer specialist* un informaticien, une informaticienne 6

to **continue** continuer 12

cook un cuisinier, une cuisinière 6

cool frais, fraîche 6; *It's cool.* Il fait frais. 6

to **cost** coûter 3

couch un canapé 9

course un cours 4

couscous le couscous 9

cousin un(e) cousin(e) 5

crab un crabe 8

crêpe une crêpe 3

croissant un croissant 8

cup une tasse 9

cupboard un placard 9

D

dairy store une crémerie 8

dance un bal 12; *dance club* une boîte 2

to **dance** danser 2

dark (hair) brun(e) 5

Darn! Zut! 4

date une date 5

daughter une fille 5

day un jour 4; une journée 12

dear cher, chère 11

December décembre 5

to **decide** décider (de) 12

delicatessen une charcuterie 8

delighted enchanté(e) 9

dentist un(e) dentiste 6

department store un grand magasin 7

desk un bureau 4

dessert un dessert 3

dictionary un dictionnaire 4

dining room une salle à manger 9

dinner le dîner 9

diskette une disquette 4

to **do** faire 2; *to do homework* faire les devoirs 2

doctor un médecin 6; un docteur 10

dog un chien 5

dollar un dollar 7

door une porte 4

drawing le dessin 4

dress une robe 7

drink une boisson 3

dumb bête 5; *How dumb I am!* Que je suis bête! 5

E

ear une oreille 10

east l'est (m.) 11

easy facile 10

to **eat** manger 2; *to eat pizza* manger de la pizza 2

egg un œuf 8

eight huit 1

eighteen dix-huit 1

eighth huitième 11

eighty quatre-vingts 3

eleven onze 1

engineer un ingénieur 6

England l'Angleterre (f.) 6

English anglais(e) 6; *English (language)* l'anglais (m.) 4

enough assez de 8

to **enter** entrer 9

entrance une entrée 9

Europe l'Europe (f.) 11

even même 9

evening un soir 7

everybody tout le monde 2

everything tout 11

excuse me pardon 1; excusez-moi 7

expensive cher, chère 7

eye un œil 10; *eyes* des yeux (m.) 5

F

face une figure 10

fall l'automne (m.) 6

family une famille 5; *family room* un séjour 9

far loin 11

farmer un fermier, une fermière 6

fast-food restaurant un fast-food 3

fat gros, grosse 11

father un père 5

father-in-law un beau-père 5

February février 5

to **feel: to feel like** avoir envie de 11; *to feel nauseous* avoir mal au cœur 10

festival une fête 12

fever la fièvre 10

few (un) peu de 8

fifteen quinze 1; *fifteen (minutes after)* et quart 4

fifth cinquième 11

fifty cinquante 3

to **find** trouver 7

finger un doigt 10

to **finish** finir 4

fireworks un feu d'artifice 12

first premier, première 5; d'abord 8

fish un poisson 5; *fish soup* une bouillabaisse 8

five cinq 1

floor un étage 9; *ground floor* le rez-de-chaussée 9

flower une fleur 9

flu la grippe 10

foot un pied 10

for pour 2; comme 3

fork une fourchette 9

forty quarante 3

four quatre 1

fourteen quatorze 1

fourth quatrième 11

franc un franc 3

France la France 6

French français(e) 6; *French (language)* le français 4; *French fries* des frites (f.) 3

fresh frais, fraîche 6

Friday vendredi (m.) 4

friend un(e) ami(e) 6

fries: French fries des frites (f.) 3; *steak with French fries* un steak-frites 3

from de (d') 4; *from (the)* des 3, du 6

front: in front of devant 4

fruit un fruit 8; *fruit juice* le jus de fruit 9

full chargé(e) 12

G

games: to play video games jouer aux jeux vidéo 2; *video games* des jeux vidéo (m.) 2

garage un garage 9

garden un jardin 9

generous généreux, généreuse 5

geography la géographie 4

German allemand(e) 6; *German (language)* l'allemand (m.) 4

Germany l'Allemagne (f.) 6

gift un cadeau 5

girl une fille 4

to **give** donner 3; *Give me . . . .* Donnez-moi.... 3

glass un verre 9

to **go** aller 2; *let's go (there)* allons-y 3; *Shall we go (there)?* On y va? 2; *to go biking* faire du vélo 2; *to go for a ride* faire un tour 6; *to go grocery shopping* faire les courses 8; *to go in-line skating* faire du roller 2; *to go out* sortir 2; *to go running* faire du footing 2; *to go shopping* faire du shopping 2, faire les magasins 7; *to go up* monter 12

goldfish un poisson rouge 5

good bon, bonne 2; *good evening* bonsoir 9; *good-bye* au revoir, salut 1

grandfather un grand-père 5

grandmother une grand-mère 5

grape un raisin 3; *grape juice* le jus de raisin 3

gray gris(e) 5

great super 2; formidable 11; *That's great.* Tant mieux. 4

green vert(e) 5; *green beans* des haricots verts (m.) 8

ground floor le rez-de-chaussée 9

Guadeloupe la Guadeloupe 5

H

hair des cheveux (m.) 5

hairdresser un coiffeur, une coiffeuse 6

half demi(e) 4; *half past* et demi(e) 4

half-brother un demi-frère 5

half-sister une demi-sœur 5

ham le jambon 3; *ham sandwich* un sandwich au jambon 3

hamburger un hamburger 3

hand une main 10

handsome beau, bel, belle 5

hardworking diligent(e) 5

hat un chapeau 7

to **have** avoir 4; *I've had it!* J'en ai marre! 4; *one has to, we/you have to* il faut 10; *to have (food or drink)* prendre 9; *to have a/an . . . ache, to have a sore . . .* avoir mal 10; *to have to* devoir, falloir 10; être obligé(e) de 12

he il 2; *he is* c'est 5

head une tête 10

health la santé 10

heart un cœur 10

hello bonjour 1; *hello (on telephone)* allô 1

Help! Au secours! 10

her son, sa; ses 5; *her name is* elle s'appelle 1

here là 4; ici 6; *here are* voilà 3, voici 7; *here is* voilà 3, voici 7

Hey! Eh!, Tiens! 1

hi salut 1

hightops des baskets (f.) 7

his son, sa; ses 5; *his name is* il s'appelle 1

history l'histoire (f.) 4

holiday une fête 12

home: at the home of chez 11; *to come home* rentrer 11; *to the home of* chez 2

homework les devoirs (m.) 2; *to do homework* faire les devoirs 2

horse un cheval 5

hot chaud(e) 6; *It's hot.* Il fait chaud. 6; *to be hot* avoir chaud 10

hot dog un hot-dog 3

hotel un hôtel 12

hour l'heure (f.) 3

house une maison 9; *at the house of* chez 11; *to my house* chez moi 2; *to the house of* chez 2

househusband un homme au foyer 6

housewife une femme au foyer 6

how comment 3; que 5; *How are things going?* Ça va? 1; *How are you?* Comment vas-tu? 3; *How dumb I am!* Que je suis bête! 5; *how many* combien de 8; *how much* combien 3, combien de 8; *How much is it/that?* Ça fait combien? 3; *How nice you are!* Que vous êtes gentils! 9;

How old are you? Tu as quel âge? 5; *How's the weather?* Quel temps fait-il? 6

hundred: (one) hundred cent 3

hungry: I'm hungry. J'ai faim. 3; *to be hungry* avoir faim 4

to **hurt** avoir mal (à...) 10

husband un mari 5

I

I j', je 1; moi 2

ice cream une glace 3; *chocolate ice cream* une glace au chocolat 3; *vanilla ice cream* une glace à la vanille 3

to **imagine** imaginer 12

Impressionist impressionniste 12

in dans 4; à, en, sur 6; de (d') 12; *in (the)* au 6, aux 7, du 12; *in front of* devant 4; *in order to* pour 7; *in the morning* le matin 8

in-line skating le roller 2; *to go in-line skating* faire du roller 2

intelligent intelligent(e) 5

to **introduce** présenter 1

to **invite** inviter 2

is est 3; *isn't that so?* n'est-ce pas? 5

it elle, il 2; ça 3; *it is necessary* il faut 10; *it's* c'est 1; *It's . . . .* Ça fait.... 3; *It's bad.* Il fait mauvais. 6; *It's beautiful.* Il fait beau. 6; *It's cold.* Il fait froid. 6; *It's cool.* Il fait frais. 6; *It's hot.* Il fait chaud. 6; *It's nice.* Il fait beau. 6; *It's raining.* Il pleut. 6; *It's snowing.* Il neige. 6; *It's sunny.* Il fait du soleil. 6; *It's the (+ date).* Nous sommes le (+ date). 5; *It's warm.* Il fait chaud. 6; *It's windy.* Il fait du vent. 6

Italian italien, italienne 6

Italy l'Italie (f.) 6

its son, sa; ses 5

Ivory Coast la Côte-d'Ivoire 11; *from the Ivory Coast* ivoirien, ivoirienne 11

J

jacket (outdoor) un blouson 7; *ski jacket* un anorak 7; *sport jacket* une veste 7

jam la confiture 8

January janvier 5

Japan le Japon 6

Japanese japonais(e) 6

jar un pot 8

jazz le jazz 2

jeans: (pair of) jeans un jean 7

journalist un(e) journaliste 6

juice: apple juice le jus de pomme 3; *fruit juice* le jus de fruit 9; *grape juice* le jus de raisin 3; *orange juice* le jus d'orange 3

July juillet 5

June juin 5

just juste 4

K

to **keep** garder 10

ketchup le ketchup 8

kilogram un kilogramme (kilo) 8

kilometer un kilomètre 5

kiss une bise 11

kitchen une cuisine 9

knee un genou 10

knife un couteau 9

L

ladies and gentlemen Messieurs-Dames 3

lamp une lampe 9

large grand(e) 7; gros, grosse 11

last dernier, dernière 12

Latin (language) le latin 4

lawn un jardin 9

lawyer un(e) avocat(e) 6

lazy paresseux, paresseuse 5

least: at least au moins 12

to **leave** partir 11; *to leave (a person or place)* quitter 12

left: to (on) the left à gauche 9

leg une jambe 10

lemon-lime soda une limonade 3

less moins 8

liberty la liberté 12

library une bibliothèque 11

light une lumière 12

like comme 3

to **like** aimer 2; *I like . . . .* ... me plaît. 11; *What would you like?* Vous désirez? 3; *would like* voudrais 3

to **listen (to)** écouter 2; *listen* écoute 1; *to listen to music* écouter de la musique 2

little petit(e) 7; *a little* (un) peu 2, (un) peu de 8

to **live** habiter 9; vivre 12

living room un salon 9

long long, longue 7

longer: no longer ne (n')... plus 10

to **look (at)** regarder 10; *to look for* chercher 7; *to look like* ressembler à 5; *to look well/sick* avoir bonne/ mauvaise mine 10

to **lose** perdre 12

lot: a lot beaucoup 2; *a lot of* beaucoup de 2

love: in love amoureux, amoureuse 12

to **love** aimer 2; adorer 7

to **lower** baisser 10

luck la chance 6

lunch le déjeuner 9

Luxembourg le Luxembourg 11; *from Luxembourg* luxembourgeois(e) 11

M

Ma'am Madame (Mme) 1

to **make** faire 2; *to make a call* téléphoner 2; *to make an appointment* prendre rendez-vous 10

mall un centre commercial 7

man un homme 6

many beaucoup 8; *how many* combien de 8; *too many* trop de 8

map une carte 4; un plan 12

March mars 5

market un marché 8

Martinique la Martinique 5

math les maths (f.) 4

matter: What's the matter with you? Qu'est-ce que tu as? 10

May mai 5

maybe peut-être 7

mayonnaise la mayonnaise 8

me moi 2; me 11; *to me* me 11

meal un repas 8

mean méchant(e) 5

melon un melon 8

member un membre 5

merchant un(e) marchand(e) 8

Mexican mexicain(e) 6

Mexico le Mexique 6

microwave un micro-onde 9

midnight minuit 3

milk le lait 8

million un million 5

mineral water l'eau minérale (f.) 3

minus moins 4

minute une minute 4

Miss Mademoiselle (Mlle) 1

modern moderne 12

Mom maman (f.) 8

Monday lundi (m.) 4

money l'argent (m.) 11

month un mois 5

monument un monument 12

more plus 8

morning un matin 8; *in the morning* le matin 8

Moroccan marocain(e) 11

Morocco le Maroc 11

most: the most (+ adjective) le/la/les plus (+ *adjective*) 12

mother une mère 5

mother-in-law une belle-mère 5

mouth une bouche 10

movie un film 2; *movies* le cinéma 2

Mr. Monsieur 1

Mrs. Madame (Mme) 1

much: how much combien 3; combien de 8; *How much is it/that?* Ça fait combien? 3; *too much* trop de 8, trop 10; *very much* beaucoup 2

museum un musée 11

mushroom un champignon 8

music la musique 2

musician un musicien, une musicienne 12

must: one/we/you must il faut 10

mustard la moutarde 8

my mon, ma; mes 5; *my name is* je m'appelle 1

N

name: her name is elle s'appelle 1; *his name is* il s'appelle 1; *my name is* je m'appelle 1; *your name is* tu t'appelles 1

napkin une serviette 9

national national(e) 12

nauseous: to feel nauseous avoir mal au cœur 10

near près (de) 11

to be **necessary** falloir 10; *it is necessary* il faut 10

neck un cou 10

to **need** avoir besoin de 4

neighborhood un quartier 12

never ne (n')... jamais 10

new nouveau, nouvel, nouvelle 7

nice sympa (sympathique) 5; gentil, gentille 9; *How nice*

you are! Que vous êtes gentils! 9; *It's nice.* Il fait beau. 6

night before la veille 11

nine neuf 1

nineteen dix-neuf 1

ninety quatre-vingt-dix 3

ninth neuvième 11

no non 1; *no longer* ne (n')... plus 10; *no one* ne (n')... personne 10

nobody ne (n')... personne 10

noise un bruit 12

noon midi 3

north le nord 11

nose un nez 10

not pas 1; ne (n')... pas 2; *not anymore* ne (n')... plus 10; *not anyone* ne (n')... personne 10; *not anything* ne (n')... rien 10

notebook un cahier 4

nothing ne (n')... rien 10

November novembre 5

now maintenant 8

nurse un infirmier, une infirmière 6

O

o'clock l'heure (f.) 3

to be **obliged to** être obligé(e) de 12

occupation une profession 6

October octobre 5

of de (d') 4; *of (the)* des, du 6; *of course* bien sûr 9

office (doctor or dentist's) un cabinet 10

often souvent 6

oh ah 1; oh 4; *Oh no! Oh dear!* Oh là là! 10

OK d'accord 1; OK 8

old vieux, vieil, vieille 7; *How old are you?* Tu as quel âge? 5; *I'm ...years old.* J'ai... ans. 5; *to be . . . (years old)* avoir... ans 5; *to be how old* avoir quel âge 5

omelette une omelette 3

on sur 4; en 5; *on (+ day of the week)* le (+ *day of the week*) 4; *on sale* en solde 7; *on the (+ ordinal number)* le (+ *number*) 1

one un 1; on 2; une 3; *no one* ne (n')... personne 10

one's son, sa; ses 5

onion un oignon 8

only juste 4; seulement 12

or ou 3

orange une orange 3; orange 7; *orange juice* le jus d'orange 3

other autre 6

our notre; nos 5

outfit un ensemble 7

oven un four 9

over there là-bas 7

P

painting un tableau 12

pants: (pair of) pants un pantalon 7

panty hose des bas (m.) 7

paper: sheet of paper une feuille de papier 4

parade un défilé 12

paradise le paradis 12

parent un parent 5

park un jardin 12

party une boum 7

passport un passeport 11

pastry store une pâtisserie 8

pâté le pâté 8

path un chemin 12

peach une pêche 8

pear une poire 8

peas des petits pois (m.) 8

pen un stylo 4

pencil un crayon 4; *pencil case* une trousse 4; *pencil sharpener* un taille-crayon 4

pepper le poivre 9

per par 4

philosophy la philosophie 4

to **phone (someone)** téléphoner 2

photo une photo 5

physics la physique 4

picture une photo 5

pie une tarte 8; *strawberry pie* une tarte aux fraises 8

piece un morceau 8

pink rose 7

pizza une pizza 2; *to eat pizza* manger de la pizza 2

plate une assiette 9

to **play** jouer 2; *to play basketball* jouer au basket 2; *to play soccer* jouer au foot 2; *to play sports* faire du sport 2; *to play tennis* jouer au tennis 2; *to play video games* jouer aux jeux vidéo 2; *to play volleyball* jouer au volley 2

please s'il vous plaît 3; s'il te plaît 9

pole: ski pole un bâton 10

police officer un agent de police 6

pool: swimming pool une piscine 11

pork le porc 8

possible possible 2

post office une poste 11

poster une affiche 4

potato une pomme de terre 8

to **prefer** préférer 2

present un cadeau 5

pretty joli(e) 7

purple violet, violette 7

to **put (on)** mettre 9

Q

quarter un quart 4; un quartier 12; *quarter after* et quart 4; *quarter to* moins le quart 4

quiche une quiche 3

quite assez 7

quiz une interro (interrogation) 2

R

to **rain: It's raining.** Il pleut. 6

rather assez 7

to **read** lire 2

really bien 2; vraiment 12

receptionist un(e) réceptionniste 10

red rouge 5; *red (hair)* roux, rousse 5

refrigerator un frigo 9

reggae le reggae 2

relative un parent 5

to **remain** rester 10

to **resemble** ressembler à 5

restaurant un restaurant 11; *fast-food restaurant* un fast-food 3

to **return** rentrer, revenir 11

ride: to go for a ride faire un tour 6

right: to (on) the right à droite 9

ripe mûr(e) 8

rock (music) le rock 2

room une pièce 9; la place 10; *dining room* une salle à manger 9; *family room* un séjour 9; *living room* un salon 9

rug un tapis 9

running le footing 2; *to go running* faire du footing 2

S

saint: All Saints' Day la Toussaint 11

salad une salade 3

salami le saucisson 8

sale(s) des soldes (f.) 7; *on sale* en solde 7

salesperson un vendeur, une vendeuse 7

salt le sel 9

sandwich un sandwich 3; *cheese sandwich* un sandwich au fromage 3; *ham sandwich* un sandwich au jambon 3

Saturday samedi (m.) 4

say dis 2

schedule un emploi du temps 4; un horaire 11

school une école 4

science les sciences (f.) 4

sea une mer 11

second deuxième 11

to **see** voir 11; *let's see* voyons 3; *See you soon.* À bientôt. 1; *See you tomorrow.* À demain. 2

selfish égoïste 5

to **sell** vendre 7

Senegal le Sénégal 11

Senegalese sénégalais(e) 11

September septembre 5

server un serveur, une serveuse 3

to **set** mettre 9

setting: table setting un couvert 9

seven sept 1

seventeen dix-sept 1

seventh septième 11

seventy soixante-dix 3

shape: to be in good/bad shape être en bonne/mauvaise forme 10

sharpener: pencil sharpener un taille-crayon 4

she elle 2; *she is* c'est 5

shirt une chemise 7

shoe une chaussure 7; *tennis shoes* des tennis (m.) 7

shop une boutique 7

shopping le shopping 2; *shopping center* un centre commercial 7; *to go grocery shopping* faire les courses 8; *to go shopping* faire du shopping 2, faire les magasins 7

short court(e), petit(e) 7

shorts: (pair of) shorts un short 7

shoulder une épaule 10

to **show** montrer 4; *Show me ....* Montrez-moi.... 4; *to show (a movie)* passer 2

shower une douche 9

shrimp une crevette 8

shy timide 5

sick malade 10; *I'm sick of it!* J'en ai marre! 4

sink un évier 9

Sir Monsieur 1

sister une sœur 5

sister-in-law une belle-sœur 5

six six 1

sixteen seize 1

sixth sixième 11

sixty soixante 3

size une taille 7

skating: in-line skating le roller 2; *to go in-line skating* faire du roller 2

ski: ski jacket un anorak 7; *ski pole* un bâton 10

to **ski** skier 2

skirt une jupe 7

to **sleep** dormir 2

slice une tranche 8

small petit(e) 7

snacks des chips (m.) 9; *afternoon snack* le goûter 9

snow: It's snowing. Il neige. 6

so si 6; donc 9; *so-so* comme ci, comme ça 3

soccer le foot (football) 2; *to play soccer* jouer au foot 2

sock une chaussette 7

soda: lemon-lime soda une limonade 3

sofa un canapé 9

some des 3; du 8; de (d'), quelques 9

somebody quelqu'un 10

someone quelqu'un 10

something quelque chose 7

son un fils 5

soon: as soon as aussitôt que 10

sore: to have a sore . . . avoir mal (à...) 10

to be **sorry** regretter 10

soup la soupe 8; *fish soup* une bouillabaisse 8

south le sud 11

space la place 10

Spain l'Espagne (f.) 6

Spanish espagnol(e) 6; *Spanish (language)* l'espagnol (m.) 4

to **speak** parler 6

to **spend (time)** passer 12

spoon une cuiller 9

sport un sport 2; *sport jacket* une veste 7; *to play sports* faire du sport 2

spring le printemps 6

square: public square une place 11

stadium un stade 11

staircase, stairs un escalier 9

stamp un timbre 11

station une station 12; *train station* une gare 11

statue une statue 12

stay un séjour 11

to **stay** rester 10

steady solide 10

steak un steak 3; *steak with French fries* un steak-frites 3

stepbrother un beau-frère 5

stepfather un beau-père 5

stepmother une belle-mère 5

stepsister une belle-sœur 5

stereo une stéréo 4

still encore, toujours 9

stomach un ventre 10

store un magasin 7; *department store* un grand magasin 7

story un étage 9

stove une cuisinière 9

straight ahead tout droit 11

strawberry une fraise 8; *strawberry pie* une tarte aux fraises 8

street une rue 12

student un(e) élève, un(e) étudiant(e) 4

to **study** étudier 2; *Let's study . . . .* Étudions.... 4

stupid bête 5

subway un métro 12

sugar le sucre 9

suit: man's suit un costume 7; *woman's suit* un tailleur 7

summer l'été (m.) 6

sun le soleil 6

Sunday dimanche (m.) 4

sunny: It's sunny. Il fait du soleil. 6

super super 2

supermarket un supermarché 8

supper le dîner 9

sweater un pull 7

sweatshirt un sweat 7

to **swim** nager 2

swimming pool une piscine 11

swimsuit un maillot de bain 7

Swiss suisse 11

Switzerland la Suisse 11

T

table une table 9; *table setting* un couvert 9

tablecloth une nappe 9

to **take** prendre 9; *to take a tour* faire le tour 9

to **talk** parler 6

talkative bavard(e) 5

tall grand(e) 7

taxi un taxi 12

teacher un(e) prof, un professeur 4

television la télé (télévision) 2

temperature une température 10

ten dix 1

tennis le tennis 2; *tennis shoes* des tennis (m.) 7; *to play tennis* jouer au tennis 2

tenth dixième 11

terrific super 2; formidable 11

test une interro (interrogation) 2

than que 8

thanks merci 1

that ça 3; ce, cet, cette, que 8; *that's* c'est 6; *That's . . . .* Ça fait.... 3; *That's great.* Tant mieux. 4

the le, la, l', les 2

their leur 5

then puis 8; donc 9; *(well) then* alors 2

there là 4; *there are* voilà 3, il y a 7; *there is* voilà 3, il y a 7; *over there* là-bas 7

these ces 8; *these are* ce sont 5

they on 2; *they (f.)* elles 2; *they (m.)* ils 2; *they are* ce sont 5

thing une chose 7; *How are things going?* Ça va? 1; *Things are going well.* Ça va bien. 1

to **think (of)** penser (à) 12

third troisième 11

thirsty: I'm thirsty. J'ai soif. 3; *to be thirsty* avoir soif 4

thirteen treize 1

thirty trente 3; *thirty (minutes)* et demi(e) 4

this ce, cet, cette 8; *this is* c'est 1

those ces 8; *those are* ce sont 5

thousand: one thousand mille 4

three trois 1

throat une gorge 10

Thursday jeudi (m.) 4

ticket un billet 12; *ticket window* un guichet 12

time l'heure (f.) 3; une fois 12; *What time is it?* Quelle heure est-il? 3

timetable un horaire 11

timid timide 5

tired fatigué(e) 10

to à 2; *in order to* pour 7; *to (the)* au, en 2, aux 7

tobacco shop un tabac 11

today aujourd'hui 6

toe un doigt de pied 10

together ensemble 4

toilet les toilettes (f.), les W.-C. (m.) 9

tomato une tomate 8

tomb un tombeau 12

tomorrow demain 2

tonight ce soir 8

too aussi 2; trop 8; *too many* trop de 8; *too much* trop de 8, trop 10

tooth une dent 10

tour le tour 9; *to take a tour* faire le tour 9

tower une tour 12

town hall une mairie 11

train un train 11; *train station* une gare 11

to **travel** voyager 6

traveler's check un chèque de voyage 11

tree un arbre 9

trip un tour 6; un voyage 9

triumph un triomphe 12

true vrai(e) 7

T-shirt un tee-shirt 7

Tuesday mardi (m.) 4

Tunisia la Tunisie 11

Tunisian tunisien, tunisienne 11

to **turn** tourner 11

TV la télé (télévision) 2

twelve douze 1

twenty vingt 1

two deux 1

U

ugly moche 7

uhm euh 8

uncle un oncle 5

under sous 4

United States les États-Unis (m.) 6

until jusqu'à 12

up to jusqu'à 12

us nous 5

V

vacation les vacances (f.) 5

vanilla ice cream une glace à la vanille 3

vase un vase 9

VCR un magnétoscope 4

vegetable un légume 8

very très 3; *very much* beaucoup 2

video games des jeux vidéo (m.) 2; *to play video games* jouer aux jeux vidéo 2

videocassette une vidéocassette 4

Vietnam le Vietnam 6

Vietnamese vietnamien, vietnamienne 6

village un village 11

to **visit (a place)** visiter 12

volleyball le volley (volleyball) 2; *to play volleyball* jouer au volley 2

W

to **wait (for)** attendre 8

to **walk** marcher 12

to **want** désirer 3; vouloir 8; avoir envie de 11

wardrobe une armoire 9

warm chaud(e) 6; *It's warm.* Il fait chaud. 6; *to be warm* avoir chaud 10

wastebasket une corbeille 4

to **watch** regarder 2

water l'eau (f.) 3; *mineral water* l'eau minérale (f.) 3

watermelon une pastèque 8

way un chemin 12

we nous, on 2

to **wear** porter 7; *to wear size (+ number)* faire du (+ number) 7

weather le temps 6; *The weather's bad.* Il fait mauvais. 6; *The weather's beautiful/nice.* Il fait beau. 6; *The weather's cold.* Il fait froid. 6; *The weather's cool.* Il fait frais. 6; *The weather's hot/warm.* Il fait chaud. 6; *What's the weather like? How's the weather?* Quel temps fait-il? 6

Wednesday mercredi (m.) 4

week une semaine 4

Welcome! Bienvenue! 9; *You're welcome.* Je vous en prie. 3

well bien 1; *well then* alors, bon ben 2

west l'ouest (m.) 11

what comment 1; qu'est-ce que 2; quel, quelle 3; quoi 4; *What is it/this?* Qu'est-ce que c'est? 4; *What time is it?* Quelle heure est-il? 3; *What would you like?* Vous désirez? 3; *What's the matter with you?* Qu'est-ce que tu as? 10; *What's the weather like?* Quel temps fait-il? 6

when quand 6

where où 4

which quel, quelle 3

white blanc, blanche 7

who, whom qui 2

why pourquoi 2

wife une femme 5

to be willing vouloir bien 9

wind le vent 6

window une fenêtre 4; *ticket window* un guichet 12

windy: It's windy. It fait du vent. 6

winter l'hiver (m.) 6

with avec 4

woman une femme 5

to work travailler 6

world le monde 12

would like voudrais 3

Wow! Oh là là! 10

Y

yeah ouais 8

year un an 5; *I'm . . . years old.* J'ai... ans. 5; *to be . . . (years old)* avoir... ans 5

yellow jaune 7

yes oui 1; *yes (on the contrary)* si 4

yesterday hier 11

yogurt le yaourt 8

you tu, vous 2; toi 3; *to you* te 1, vous 9; *You're welcome.* Je vous en prie. 3

young jeune 12

your ton, ta, tes, votre, vos 5; *your name is* tu t'appelles 1

Yuk! Beurk! 7

Z

Zaire le Zaïre 11

Zairian zaïrois(e) 11

zero zéro 1

Grammar Index

Acknowledgments

The following teachers responded to our surveys by offering valuable comments and suggestions in the development of the C'est à toi! series:

Sally Ahrens, Camp Hill High School, Camp Hill, PA

Sonia Alcé, Hyde Park High School, Hyde Park, MA

Missie Babb, Isle of Wight Academy, Isle of Wight, VA

Gerald W. Beauchesne, West Springfield High School, West Springfield, MA

Daniel Beniero, Port Sulphur High School, Port Sulphur, LA

Helen H. Bickell, Hilliard High School, Hilliard, OH

Jacqueline Bodi, Exeter Area High School, Exeter, NH

Coy Boé, Glade Junior High School, LaPlace, LA

Joan Bowers, Tamarend Middle School, Warrington, PA

Susan Boyle, Indian Hills Junior High, Clive, IA

Denise H. Brown, Lima Senior High School, Lima, OH

Kristen Carley, St. Joseph's Episcopal School, Boynton Beach, FL

Amber Challifour, Brebeuf Preparatory School, Indianapolis, IN

Augusta D. Clark, Saint Mary's Hall, San Antonio, TX

Colleen Contrada, St. Augustine's, Andover, MA

Elaine Danford, Sidney High School, Sidney, NY

Kelley DeGraaf, Ionia High School, Ionia, MI

Virginia Delaney, Osceola High School, Osceola, WI

Pauline P. Demetri, Cambridge Rindge and Latin, Cambridge, MA

Margaret Schmidt Dess, St. Joseph Middle School, Waukesha, WI

Elizabeth K. Douglas, Ambridge Area High School, Ambridge, PA

Alma A. Dumareille, First International Language Private School, McAllen, TX

Cathy Dunbar, Chino Valley High School, Chino Valley, AZ

Karen Dymit, Hadley Junior High School, Glen Ellyn, IL

Bob Dzama, Parma High School, Parma, OH

Roy Ellefson, North Sanpete High School, Mt. Pleasant, UT

Nancy Farley, Doddridge County High School, West Union, WV

Candyce Fike, Dallas Senior High School, Dallas, TX

Wilma Franko, Brownsville Area High, Brownsville, PA

Kathy A. Ghiata, Alpena High School, Alpena, MI

William B. Gunn, John S. Burke Catholic High School, Goshen, NY

Jane R. Hill, Alton High School, Alton, IL

Lionel Hogu, Hyde Park High School, Hyde Park, MA

Joseph Holland, Rancocas Valley Regional High School, Mt. Holly, NJ

Danette Hopkin, St. Joseph Regional, Port Vue, PA

Darrylin Keenan, Fort Fairfield High School, Fort Fairfield, ME

James Kolmansberger, Pittston Area High School, Yatesville, PA

Jude-Marie LaFrancis, Grayslake High School, Grayslake, IL

Mark C. Lander, Bacon Academy, Colchester, CT

George Lerrigo, Mt. Anthony Union High School, Bennington, VT

Joy Macy, Stilwell Junior High, West Des Moines, IA

William E. Mann, Clay High School, Clay, WV

Phyllis McCauley, Chopticon High School, Morganza, MD

Theresa Michaud, St. Augustine School, Augusta, ME

Muriel Mikulewicz, Trinity High School, Manchester, NH

Shari Miller, Valley High School, West Des Moines, IA

J. Vincent H. Morrissette, Santa Catalina School, Monterey, CA

Jane Much, East Hills Middle School, Bethlehem, PA

Dale Muegenburg, Santa Clara High School, Ventura, CA

Laura A. Peel, Unami Middle School, Chalfont, PA

Nancy Pond, Bement School, Deerfield, MA

Cherry S. Raley, St. Michael's Academy, Austin, TX

Karen S. Rich, St. Philip Catholic Central High School, Battle Creek, MI

Pamela G. Rogers, Tidewater Academy, Wakefield, VA

Lynn Rouse, Brandywine Junior/Senior High School, Granger, IN

John B. Rudder, St. Margaret's School, Tappahannock, VA

Helene Scarcia, Trexler Middle School, Allentown, PA

George P. Shannon, Littlefield Public Schools, Alanson, MI

Russell J. Sloun, Xavier High School, New York, NY

Marcia Smith, Great Mills High School, Great Mills, MD

Stephanie Snook, Crestwood High School, Mantua, OH

Teri S. Summers, Colonial Heights High School, Colonial Heights, VA

Kim Swanson, Swanson School of Languages, Cincinnati, OH

Magdi S. Tadros, Wallace State College, Hanceville, Alabama

Mignon Taylor, White Oak Middle School, Cincinnati, OH

Sandy Thiernau, Rich South High School, Richton Park, IL

Gabrielle Thomas, Judge Memorial Catholic High School, Salt Lake City, UT

Berthe M. Vandenberg, West Ottawa Senior High School, Holland, MI

Rita Cholet White, Visitation Academy, St. Louis, MO

Patricia Young, Greenville High School, Greenville, IL

Jerauld Zahner, Seymour High School, Payson, IL

Gretchen Zick, Thunder Bay Junior High, Alpena, MI

Photo Credits

Cover: Kelly Stribling Sutherland, *Woman with Jazz Musicians*, original acrylic.

Abbreviations: top (t), bottom (b), left (l), right (r), center (c)

Air France: 379

Antin, Angel: 366 (t)

Armstrong, Rick: 79, 140 (b), 313 (t), 389 (t)

Barbey: xx (b)

Barde, Jean-Luc/French Government Tourist Office: 325 (t)

Barnes, David/The Stock Market: 320 (b)

Berndt, Eric R./Unicorn Stock Photos: 80 (t)

Bordis, E./Leo de Wys Inc.: 41 (tl)

Bourgeois, Steve: xxi (c)

Brown, Steve/Leo de Wys Inc.: xxii(t), 16-17, 32

Burgess, Michele: xxiv (t, c, b), 359, 366 (c), 388 (tr), 398 (b), 400 (b), 402, 404 (c), 406 (r), 418

Camille/French Government Tourist Office: 411 (t)

Chirol/French Government Tourist Office: 396

Comnet/Leo de Wys Inc.: 6 (bc), 343

Damm, Fridmar/Leo de Wys Inc.: 291

Dratch, Howard/Leo de Wys Inc.: v (b)

Flipper, Florent/Unicorn Stock Photos: 398 (t)

Fly, James L./Unicorn Stock Photos: 341 (c)

French Government Tourist Office: xvi, xxi (b), 358, 388 (b), 389 (b)

Fried, Robert: viii (b), ix, x (b), xi, 2 (t), 4, 10 (b), 14 (t), 20 (t), 23 (b), 26, 33 (t), 41 (tr), 45, 51, 52-53, 56 (tl, tr, b), 57 (t), 58, 66, 70, 71, 72, 74, 80 (b), 81 (t), 82 (b), 83 (t), 86, 90 (t), 119, 122-23, 127, 132 (tl, bl), 138 (t), 146 (t), 147 (t), 153, 164 (l), 166 (t), 178 (t, b), 185 (b), 186 (t, b), 187 (b), 198 (c, b), 205 (t), 206 (t, b), 215 (t), 226 (b), 228, 229, 238, 240-41, 243, 244 (b), 245 (t, c, b), 246 (t), 249, 254 (b), 256, 257 (b), 259, 260, 262 (t), 263 (t, b), 267, 269, 276, 286, 295 (b), 306 (c), 320 (t), 327, 335, 347 (t), 349, 350, 361, 371 (b), 381 (t), 388 (tl), 397 (b), 403 (t), 404 (b), 405 (t, b), 406 (l), 408, 409, 416 (t), 419

Garnett, R./Visual Contact: 386 (b)

Garry, Jean-Marc: 147 (b)

Geppert, Rollin/Frozen Images: xxv (b)

Gerda, Paul/Leo de Wys Inc.: 341 (t)

Gratien/French Government Tourist Office: 330 (t)

Greater Montreal Convention and Tourism Bureau: xiv

Greenberg, Jeff/Unicorn Stock Photos: 348 (c)

Higgins, Jean/Unicorn Stock Photos: xxii (b)

Hill, Justine: 21, 23 (tl), 264 (t), 268, 305 (tr), 306 (t)

Hille, W./Leo de Wys Inc.: 136 (cr)

Johnson, Everett/Frozen Images: 385

Larson, June: vi, 2 (cl, b), 19 (b), 22 (tc), 90 (cl), 98, 130, 137, 146 (b), 157, 158, 170 (t), 237 (b), 255 (tr), 257 (c), 262 (b), 264 (bl), 283 (t), 301 (t), 331, 378

Last, Victor: v (t), 34, 184 (l), 185 (c), 208 (b), 212, 232, 255 (tl), 284 (tr, b), 304, 347 (b), 373 (t), 386 (t), 388 (c), 391 (b)

Lyons, Dave/Unicorn Stock Photos: 187 (t)

Magnuson, Mike/Frozen Images: 42 (b)

Matheson, Rob/The Stock Market: 382-83

Messerschmidt, J./Leo de Wys Inc.: 202-3, 292 (t)

Meszaros, Gary/Dembinsky Photo Associates: 318 (t)

Moss, Margo/Unicorn Stock Photos: 185 (t)

Nacivet, Jean-Paul/Leo de Wys Inc.: xii (t), xv, 164 (r), 319 (t)

Nelson, Tom/Frozen Images: 272

Pinson/Sipa/Leo de Wys Inc.: xxiii (b)

Rameu, H./Unicorn Stock Photos: xxiii (t)

Robl, Ernest H.: 411 (b), 416 (b)

Rondel, Benjamin/The Stock Market: 344-45

Simmons, Ben/The Stock Market: 387

Simson, David: vii, viii (t), x (t), xii (b), xiv (t), xx (t), 2 (cr), 5 (t, b), 6 (tl, tr, c, bl, br), 7, 8, 10 (t), 12, 14 (c), 19 (t), 20 (c), 22 (tl, tr, bl, bc, br), 23 (tr), 28, 31, 33 (c, b), 35, 41 (bl, br), 42 (t), 43, 50, 56 (c), 57 (b), 65, 68 (t), 81 (b), 82 (t), 83 (b), 90 (ctr, cbr, b), 92, 93, 95, 97, 101, 102 (t, b), 104 (t, b), 105, 106 (t, b), 107 (b), 108 (t, b), 112, 114 (t, b), 118, 121 (t, b), 128, 131 (t, b), 132 (tc, tr, bcl, bcr, br), 136 (t, cl), 138 (b), 139, 140 (tl), 142, 150, 151, 152, 154, 159, 165 (t, b), 166 (b), 167 (t, b), 168 (t, bl, bc, br), 169 (tl, tc, tr, bc, br), 170 (b), 176, 179, 180, 181, 190, 192 (t, b), 194 (t, b), 198 (t), 200, 201, 205 (b), 208 (t), 210, 215 (b), 216, 220 (t), 221, 224 (t), 226 (t), 230, 231 (t, b), 234 (l, r), 237 (t), 239, 242 (tr), 246 (b), 248, 257 (t), 264 (br), 265, 275, 282, 283 (b), 284 (tl), 285, 292 (b), 294, 296 (t), 297 (t), 299, 300 (b), 301 (b), 305 (b), 306 (b), 307, 308, 311, 317, 318 (b), 319 (b), 324 (l, r), 326 (t, b), 328, 330 (c, b), 336 (t, b), 337 (t, b), 342, 348 (b), 351, 352, 360 (t, b), 363 (t, b), 371 (t), 372, 373 (b), 380, 381 (b), 391 (t), 393, 394, 400 (t), 401, 403 (c, b), 410

Sipa, Benoît/Leo de Wys Inc.: 404 (t)

Skubic, Ned: xxvi-1, 211, 224 (b), 293 (t), 366 (b)

Sternberg, Will: iv, xiii, 110, 160-61, 254 (t), 293 (b), 295 (t), 296 (b), 297 (b), 305 (tl), 312, 313 (b), 325 (b), 354

Swiss National Tourist Office: 314-15, 323 (l, r), 341 (b)

Taylor, Randy G./Leo de Wys Inc.: 15

Teubner, Christian: 47, 68 (b), 73 (t, b), 244 (t), 255 (b), 277, 278-79, 300 (t), 348 (t)

Uemura, Masa/Leo de Wys Inc.: xxi (t), xxv (t)

Unicorn Stock Photos: 214

Vaillancourt, Sarah: 37, 88-89, 107 (t), 120

Vidler, Steve/Leo de Wys Inc.: xxii (c), 184 (r)

Wassman, Bill/The Stock Market: 397 (t)

Additional Credits

Bravo Girl!, August 16, 1993 (advertisements): 235

Femme Actuelle, N° 424 (article): 339

Office de Tourisme (map of Les Saintes-Maries-de-la-Mer): 368-69, 375

RATP, Petit Plan de Paris (subway map): 407

La Redoute, AH. 94/95 (photos): 288-89

Yondo, Elalongué Epanya, *Kamerun! Kamerun!*, Présence Africaine, 1960 (poem): 376